BILLY, ME & YOU

Nicola Streeten

BILLY, ME

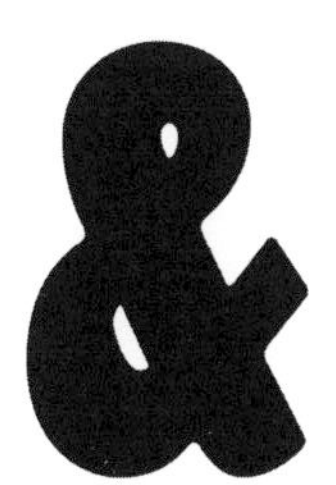

A MEMOIR OF GRIEF AND RECOVERY

YOU

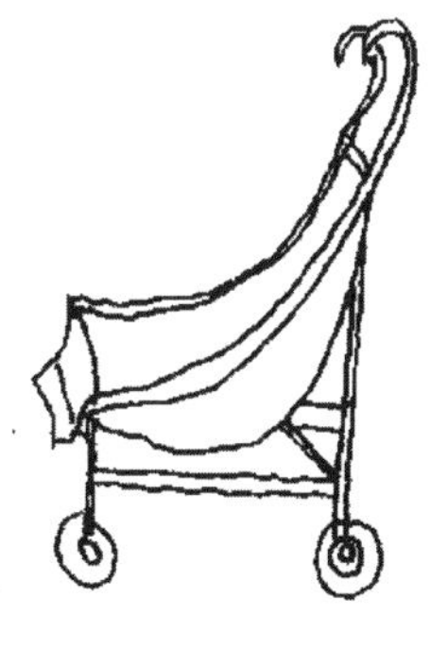

First published in 2011 by

Myriad Editions
59 Lansdowne Place
Brighton BN3 1FL, UK

www.MyriadEditions.com

1 3 5 7 9 10 8 6 4 2

A CIP catalogue record for this book is available from the British Library.

ISBN: 978-0-9565599-4-4

Printed in China on paper sourced from sustainable forests.

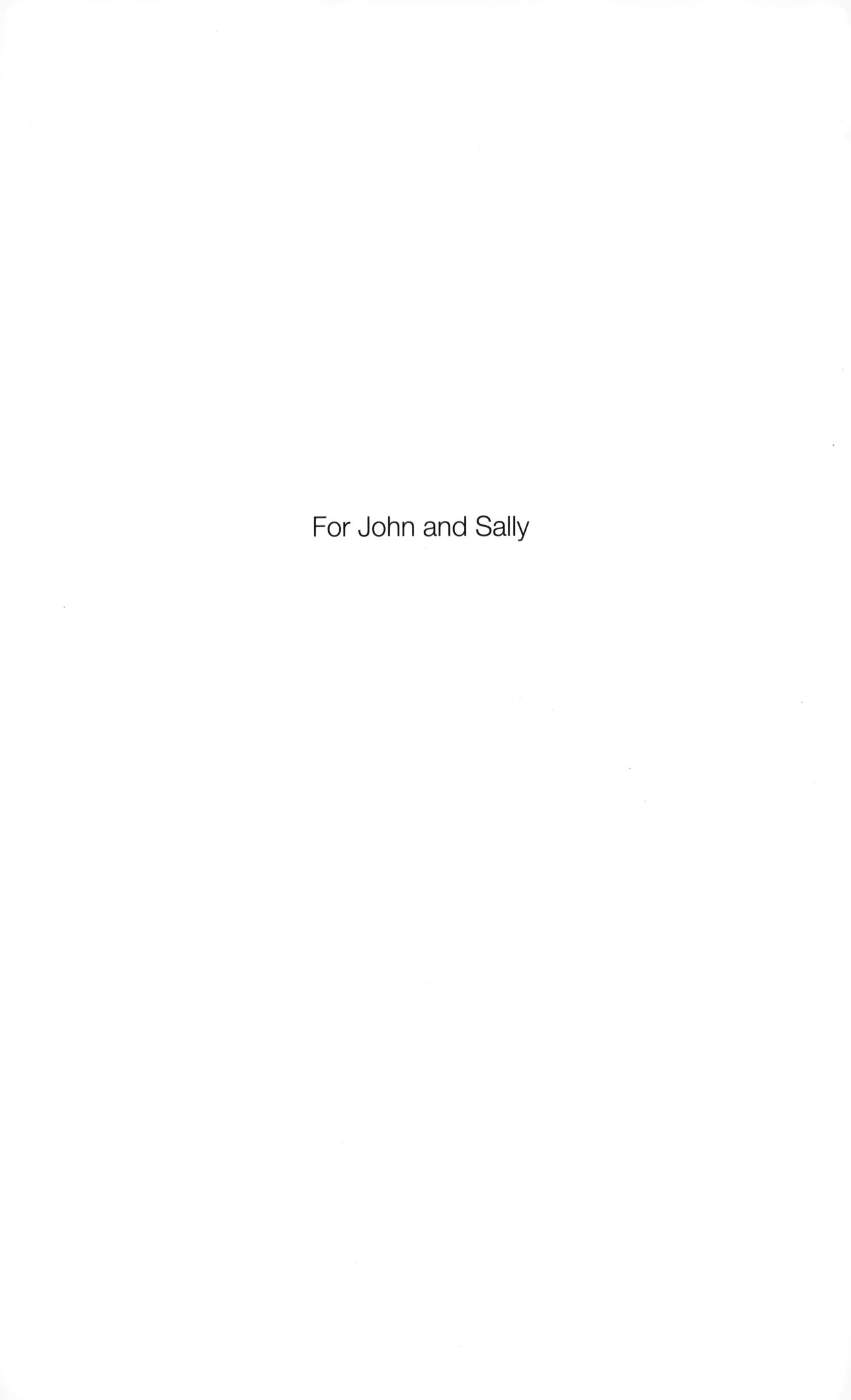

For John and Sally

PART ONE

Wed	Thu	Fri	Sat	Sun	Mon	Tue	Wed	Thu	Fri	Sat	Sun	Mon	Tue	Wed	Thu	Fri	Sat	Sun	Mon	Tue	Wed	Thu	Fri	Sat	Sun	Mon	Tue	Wed	Th
2	3	4	5	6	7	8	9	10	11	12	13	14	15	16	17	18	19	20	21	22	23	24	25	26	27	28	29	30	31

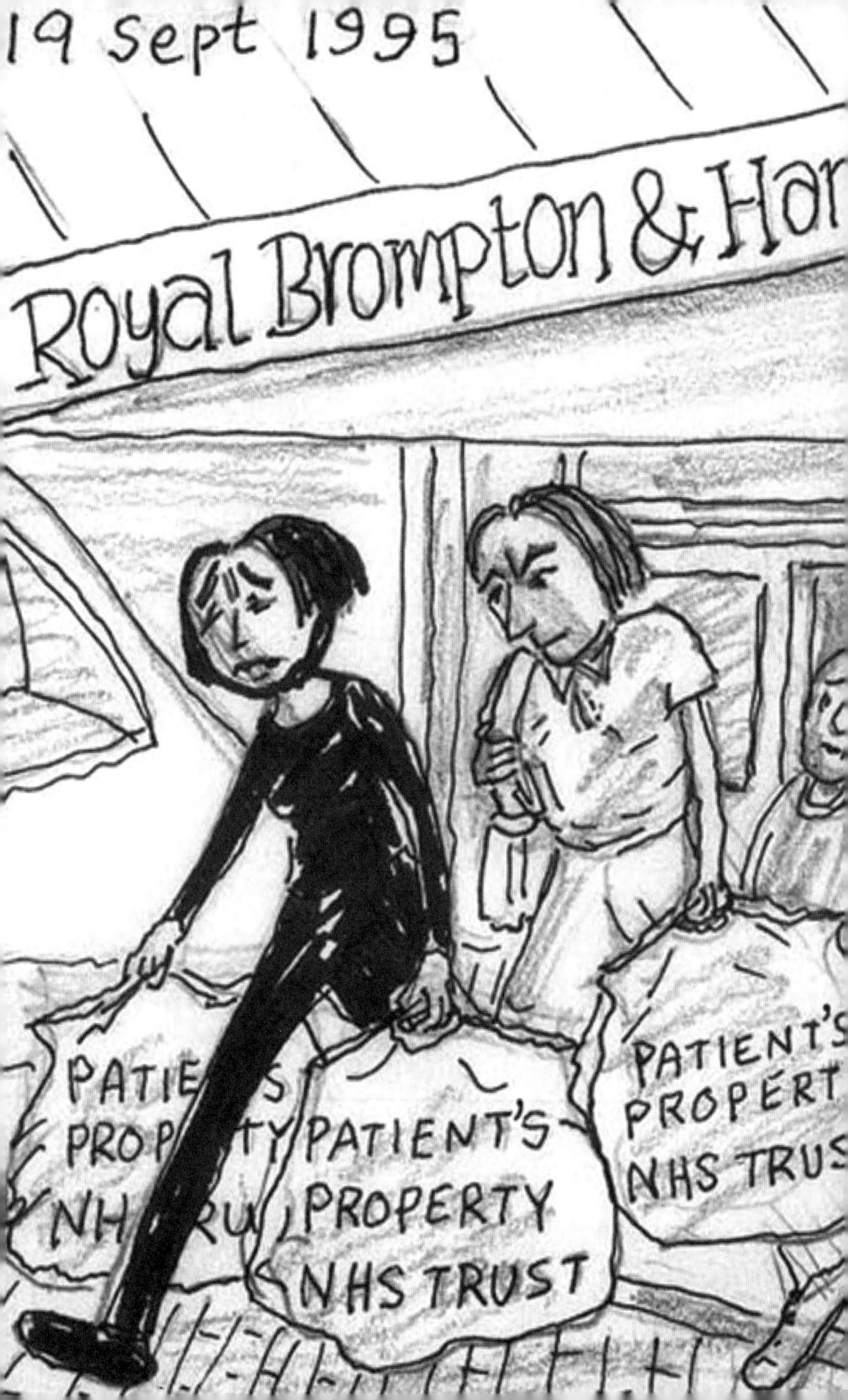

19 Sept 1995

Royal Brompton & Har
PATIENT'S PROPERTY NHS TRUST
PATIENT'S PROPERT NHS TRUS

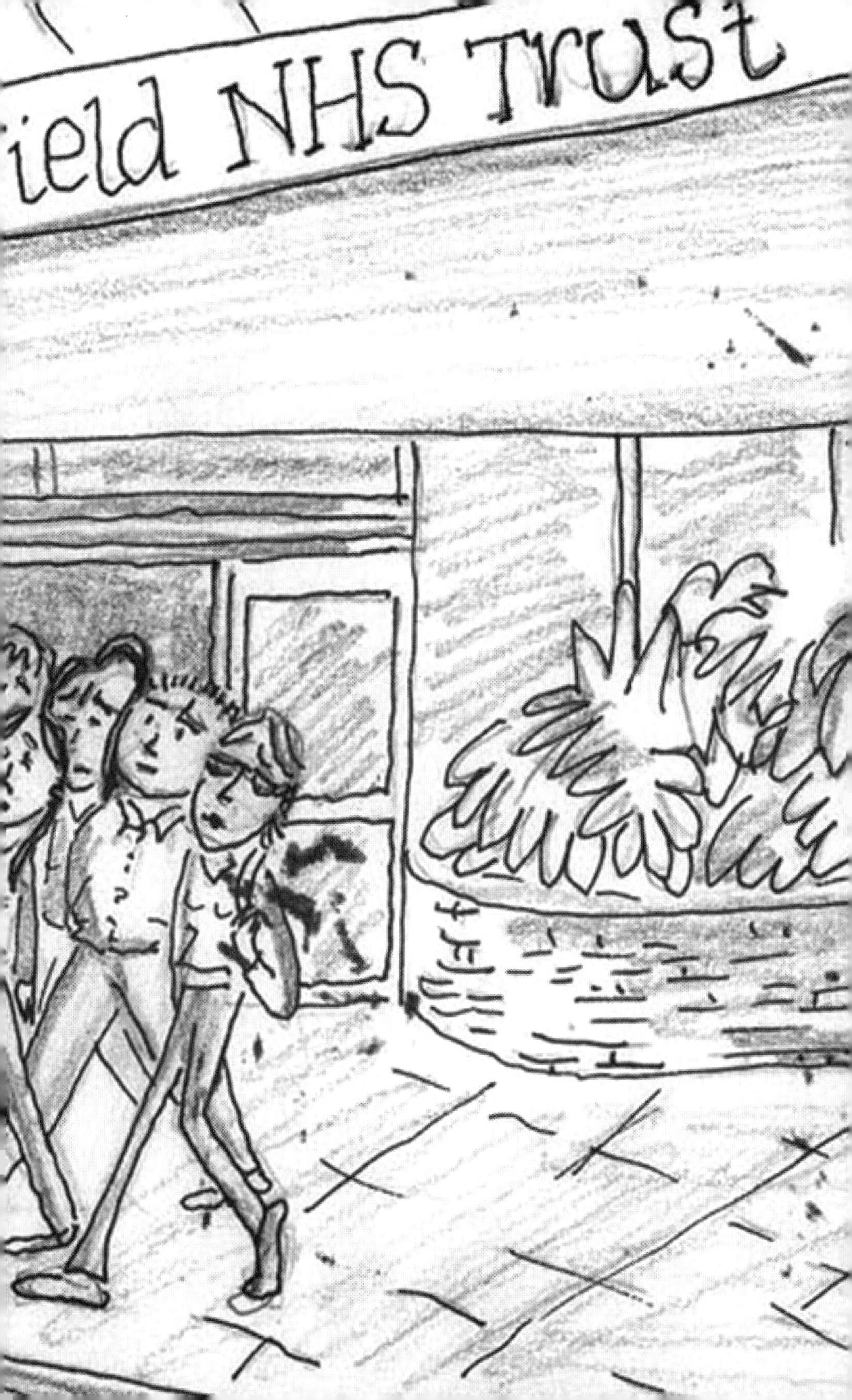
ield NHS Trust

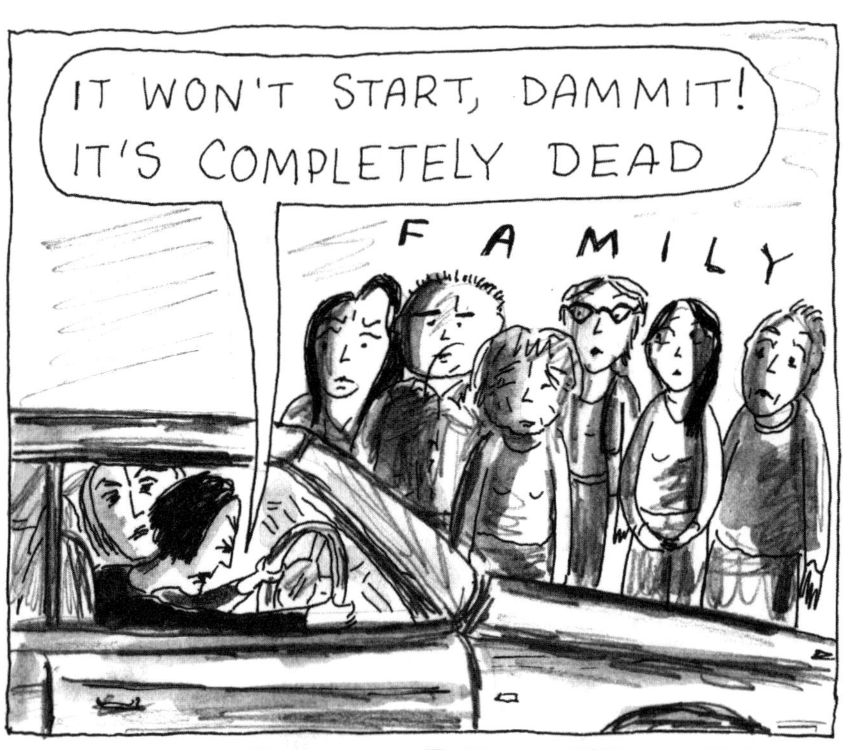
IT WON'T START, DAMMIT! IT'S COMPLETELY DEAD
FAMILY

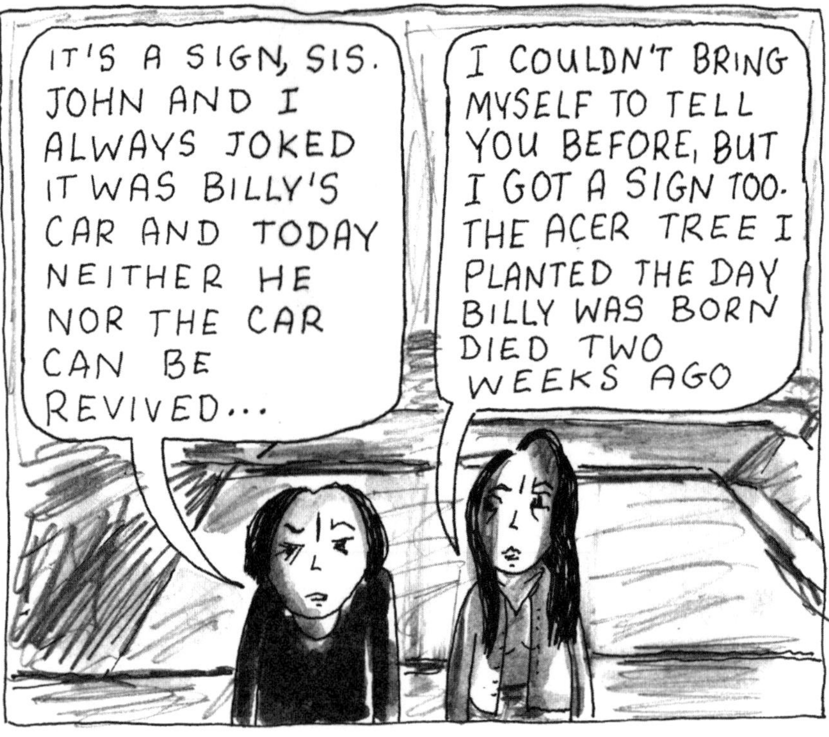
IT'S A SIGN, SIS. JOHN AND I ALWAYS JOKED IT WAS BILLY'S CAR AND TODAY NEITHER HE NOR THE CAR CAN BE REVIVED...
I COULDN'T BRING MYSELF TO TELL YOU BEFORE, BUT I GOT A SIGN TOO. THE ACER TREE I PLANTED THE DAY BILLY WAS BORN DIED TWO WEEKS AGO

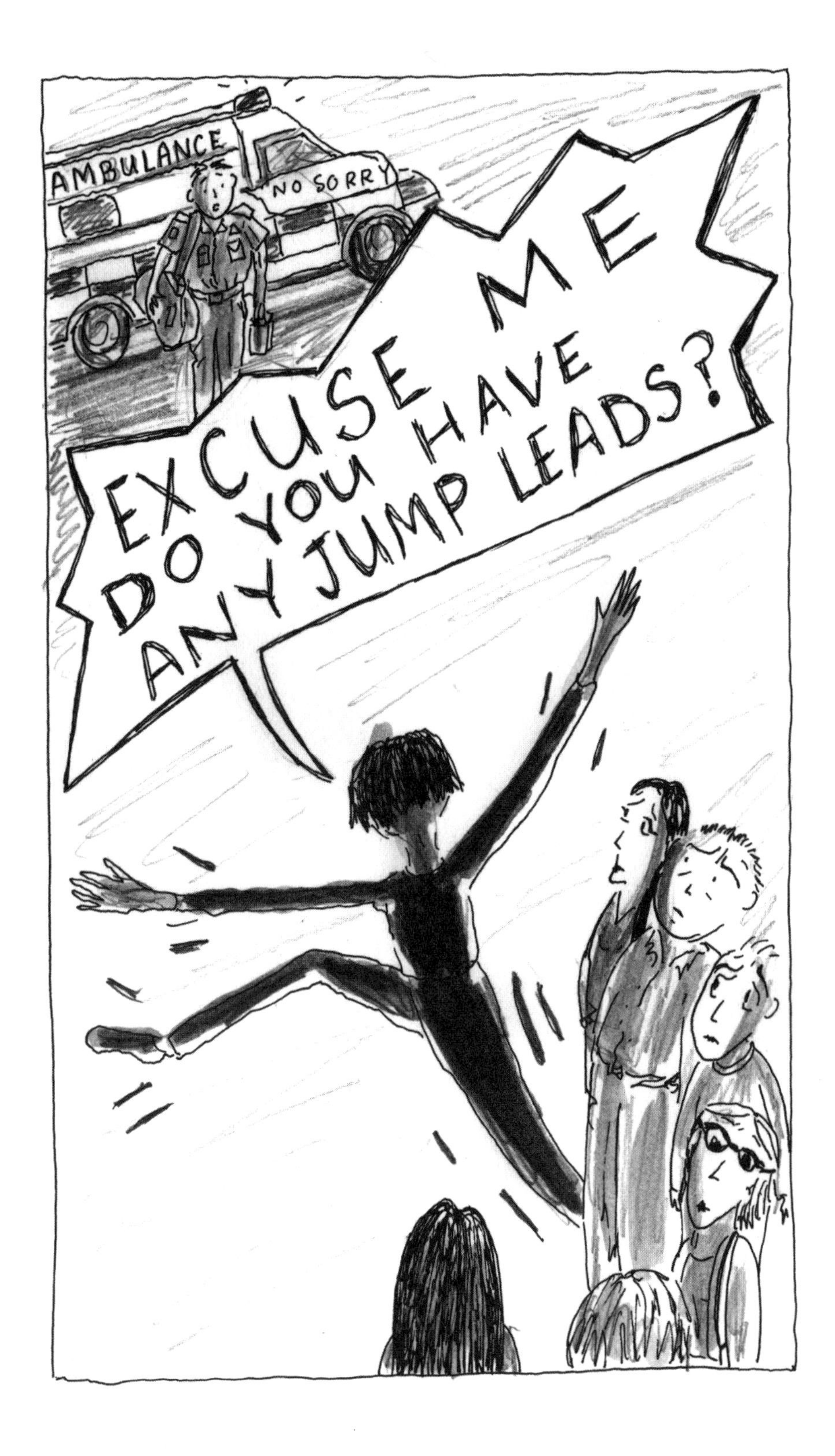
AMBULANCE
NO SORRY
EXCUSE ME
DO YOU HAVE
ANY JUMP LEADS?

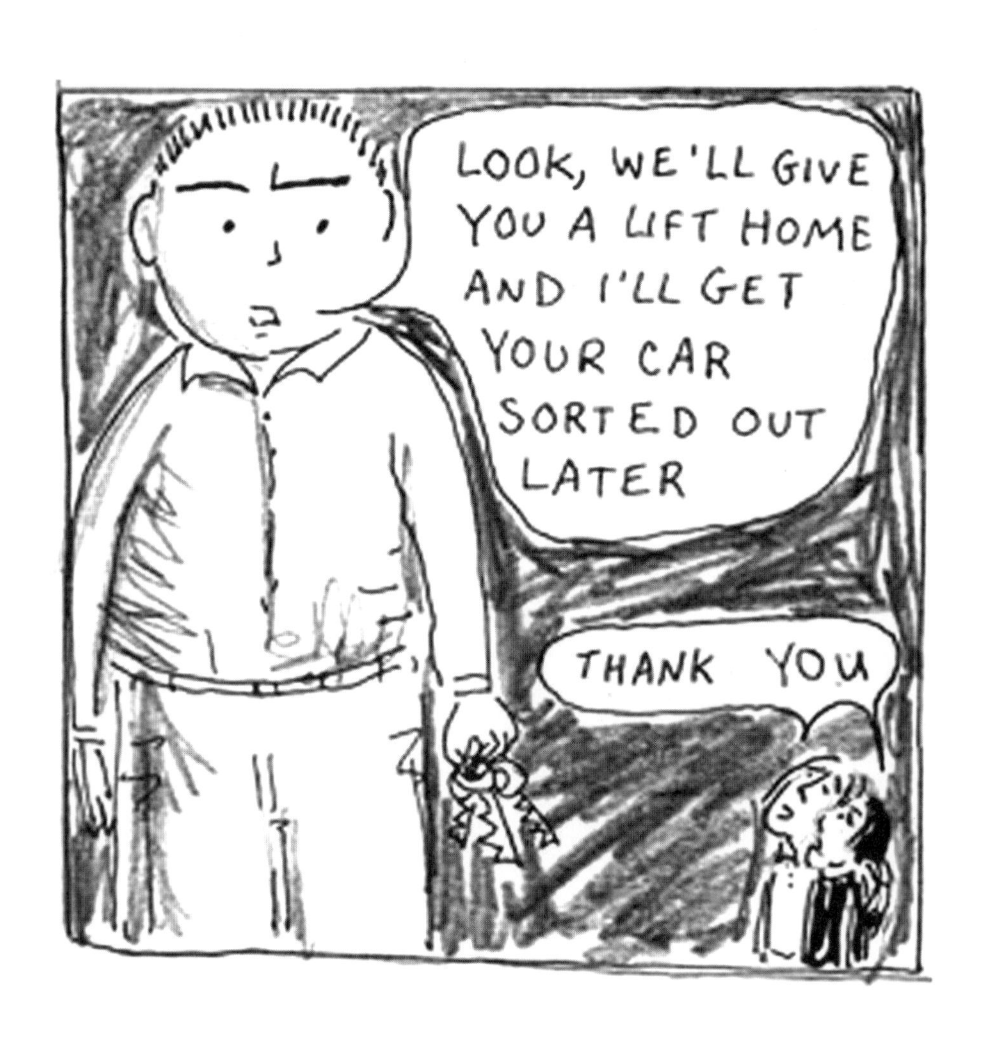
LOOK, WE'LL GIVE YOU A LIFT HOME AND I'LL GET YOUR CAR SORTED OUT LATER
THANK YOU

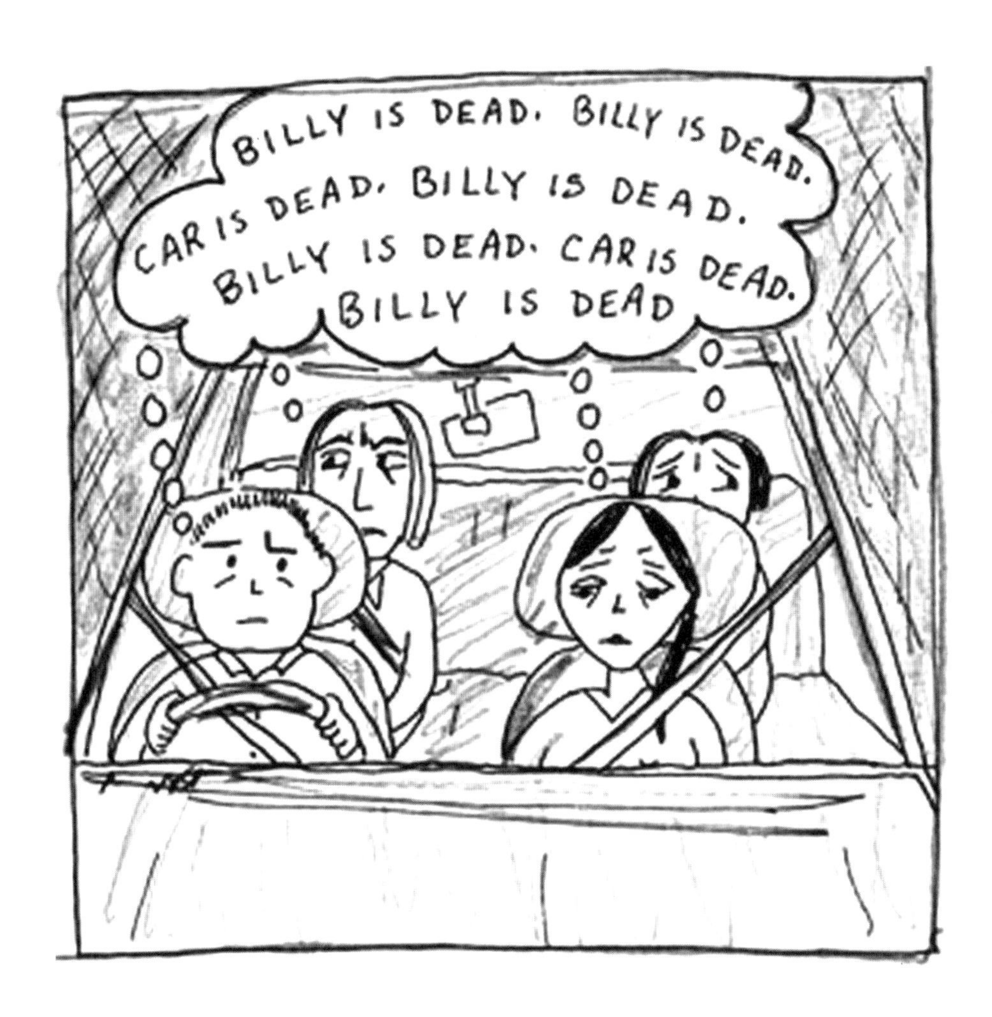
BILLY IS DEAD. BILLY IS DEAD.
CAR IS DEAD. BILLY IS DEAD.
BILLY IS DEAD. CAR IS DEAD.
BILLY IS DEAD

I HAD HELD BACK MY TEARS AT THE HOSPITAL. RIDICULOUS, BUT I HADN'T WANTED TO FURTHER UPSET OUR FAMILIES. BACK HOME, IT FELT SAFE TO RELEASE MY EMOTIONS.

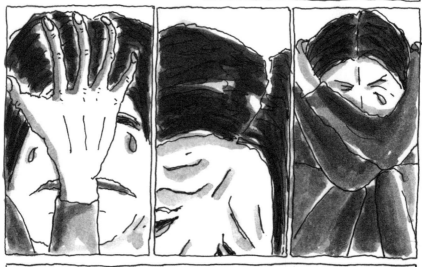

THE CRYING THING WAS SO STRANGE. I CRIED EVERY DAY FOR A YEAR AFTER BILLY DIED, BUT ONLY EVER IN FRONT OF JOHN OR THE PSYCHOLOGIST. ...NOT EVEN IN FRONT OF MY MOTHER... NOT EVEN AT THE FUNERAL.

THIS DAILY CRYING WAS A PSYCHOLOGICAL NECESSITY, LIKE A BOWEL MOVEMENT.

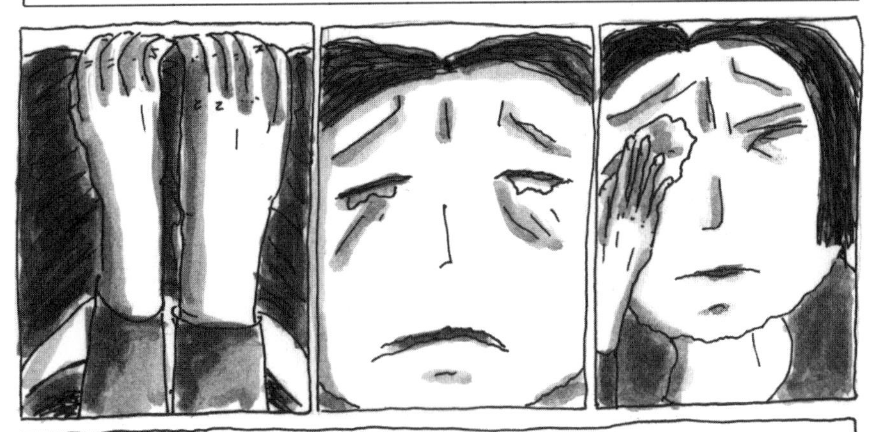

BUT I WAS TERRIFIED BY THE SURROUNDING TABOO —THE SOCIAL LIMITS TO THE DISPLAY OF GRIEF AND THE INVOLUNTARY JUDGEMENTS OF OTHERS.

AT THE SAME TIME I KNEW I WOULD LOSE MY MIND IF I BOTTLED UP SUCH INTENSE PAIN.

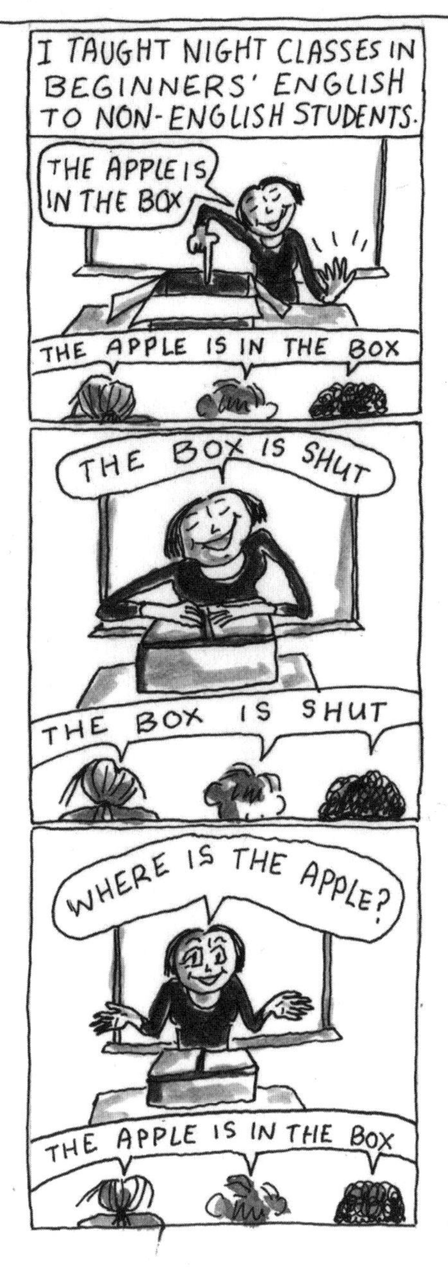

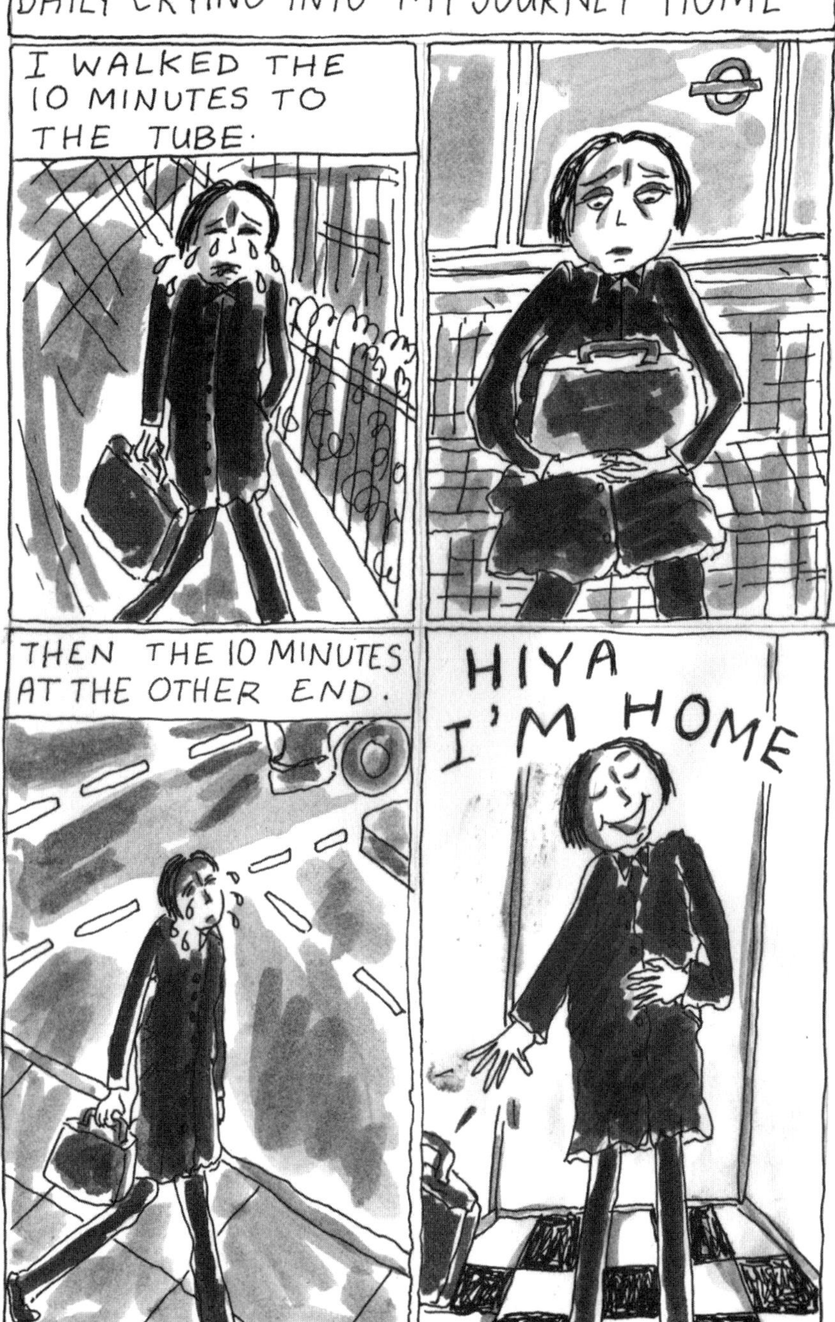
AFTER CLASSES I INCORPORATED THE DAILY CRYING INTO MY JOURNEY HOME.
I WALKED THE 10 MINUTES TO THE TUBE.
THEN THE 10 MINUTES AT THE OTHER END.
HIYA I'M HOME

I KNEW THAT TALKING ABOUT IT WAS ALLOWED – POSITIVELY ENCOURAGED, WITHIN THE LIBERAL CIRCLES IN WHICH I MIXED.

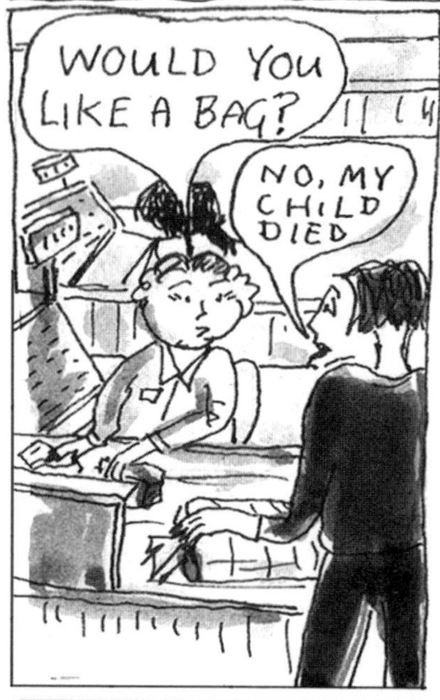
WOULD YOU LIKE A BAG?
NO, MY CHILD DIED

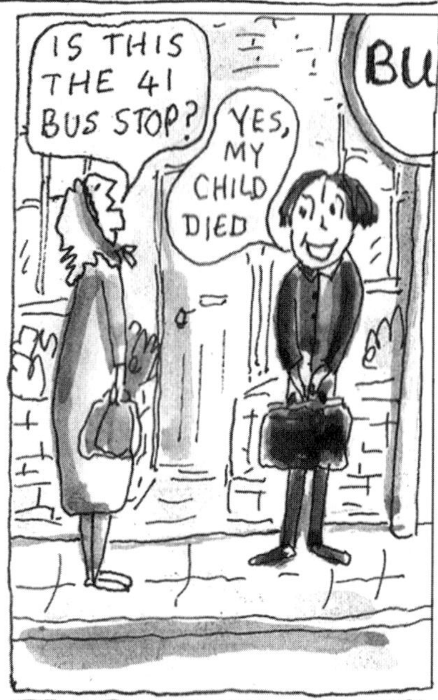
IS THIS THE 41 BUS STOP?
YES, MY CHILD DIED
BU

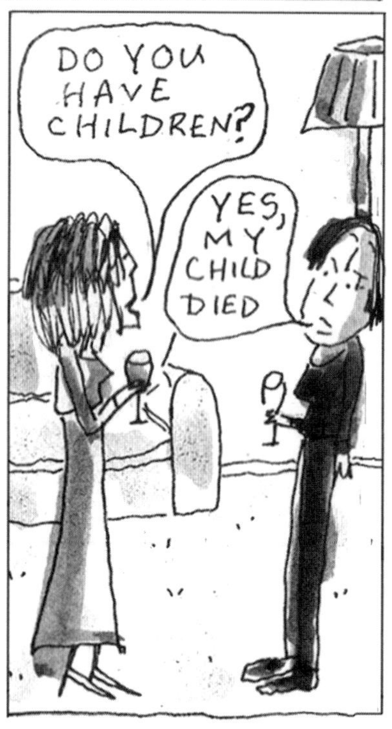
DO YOU HAVE CHILDREN?
YES, MY CHILD DIED

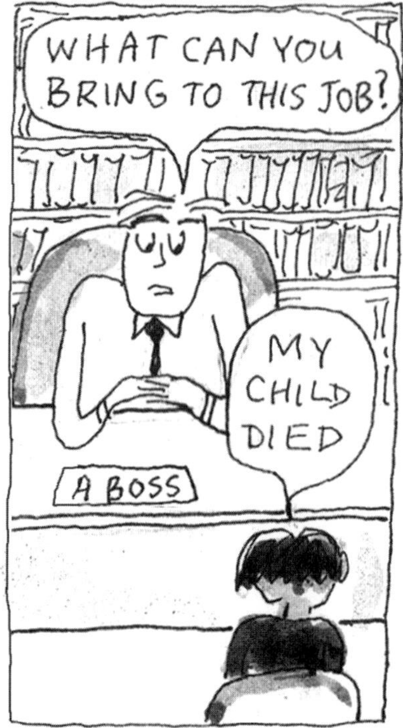
WHAT CAN YOU BRING TO THIS JOB?
MY CHILD DIED
A BOSS

THE MORE I TOLD PEOPLE, THE MORE INTRIGUED I BECAME AT THEIR RESPONSES... I FOUND MYSELF JUDGING PEOPLE BY THEIR REACTIONS.

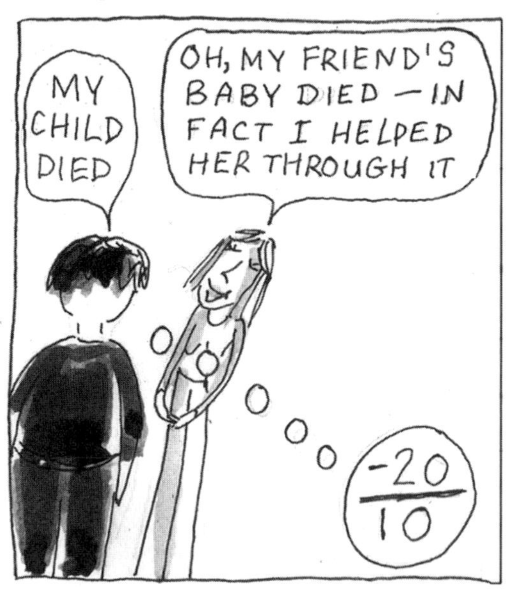
MY CHILD DIED
OH, MY FRIEND'S BABY DIED — IN FACT I HELPED HER THROUGH IT
-20/10

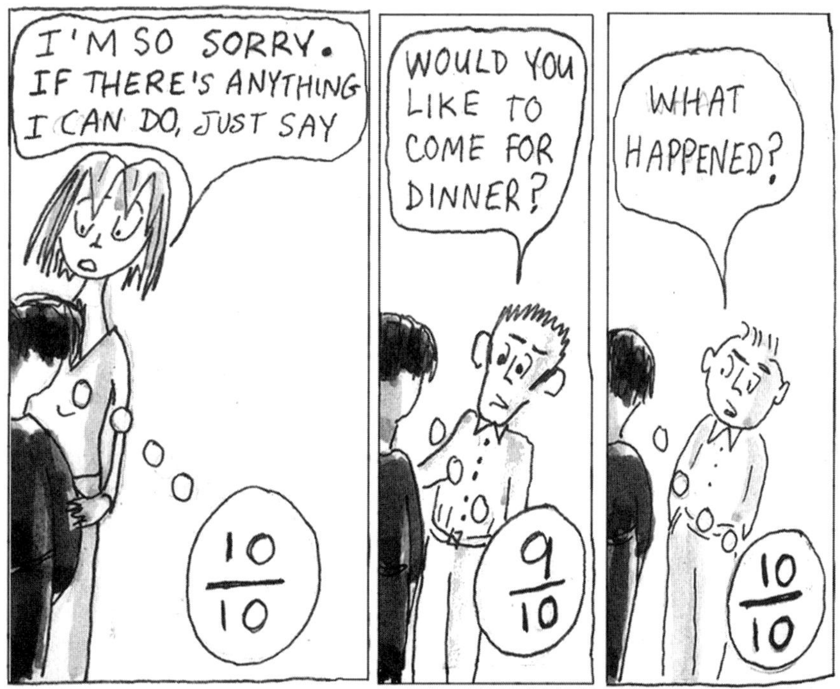
I'M SO SORRY. IF THERE'S ANYTHING I CAN DO, JUST SAY
10/10
WOULD YOU LIKE TO COME FOR DINNER?
9/10
WHAT HAPPENED?
10/10

THE MOST COMMON RESPONSE WAS FOR PEOPLE, EVEN STRANGERS, TO GET WATERY-EYED. THIS FASCINATED ME THE MOST... DID THEY GET THAT EVERY TIME THEY WATCHED STORIES OF DEAD CHILDREN ON THE NEWS?

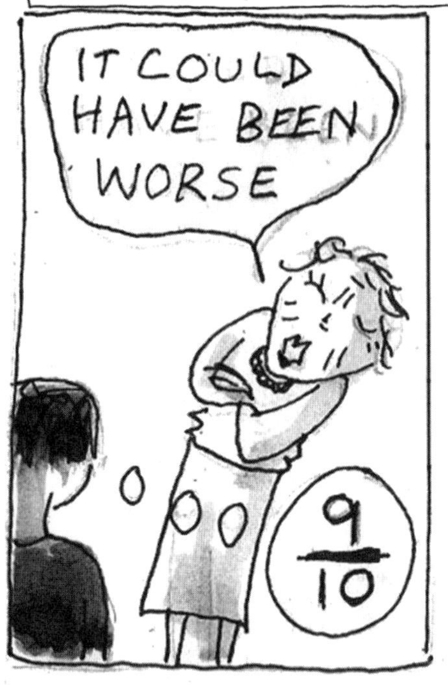
IT COULD HAVE BEEN WORSE
9/10

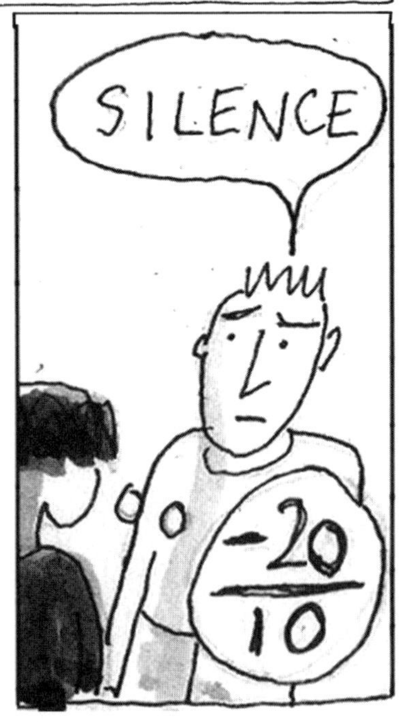
SILENCE
-20/10

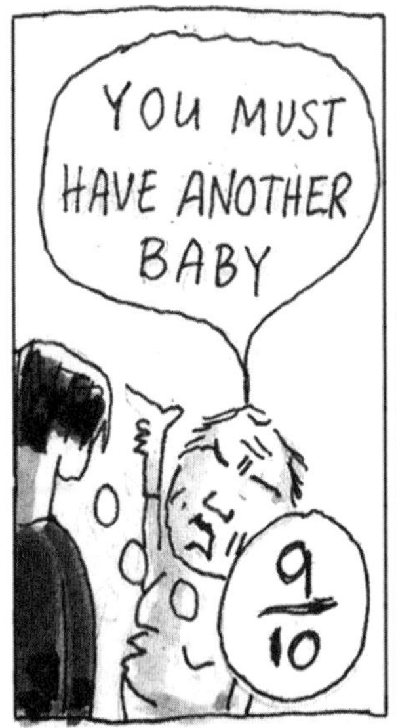
YOU MUST HAVE ANOTHER BABY
9/10

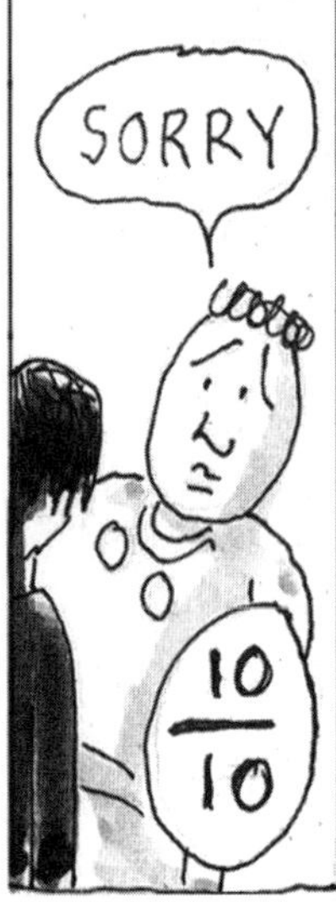
SORRY
10/10

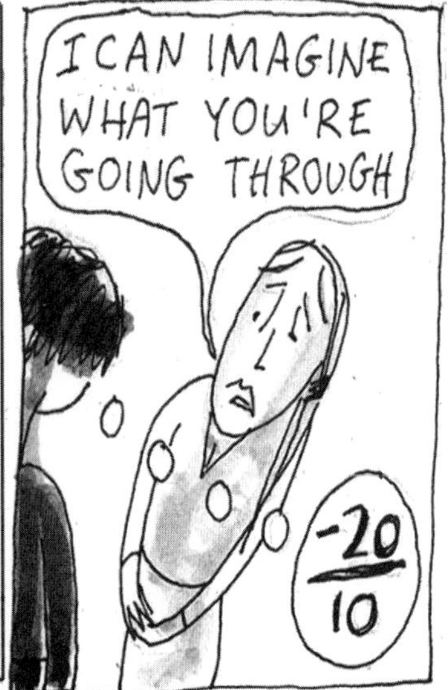
I CAN IMAGINE WHAT YOU'RE GOING THROUGH
-20/10

THE WINNING REPLIES WERE FROM TWO OF MY STUDENTS, HAKIMA AND KARIM, IN SPITE OF THEIR LIMITED ENGLISH.

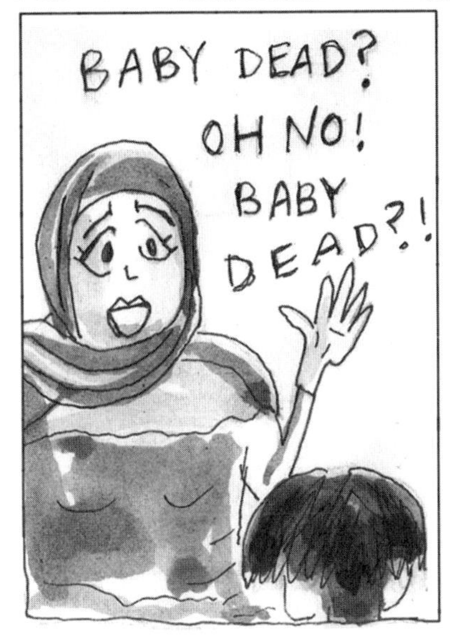
BABY DEAD?
OH NO! BABY DEAD?!

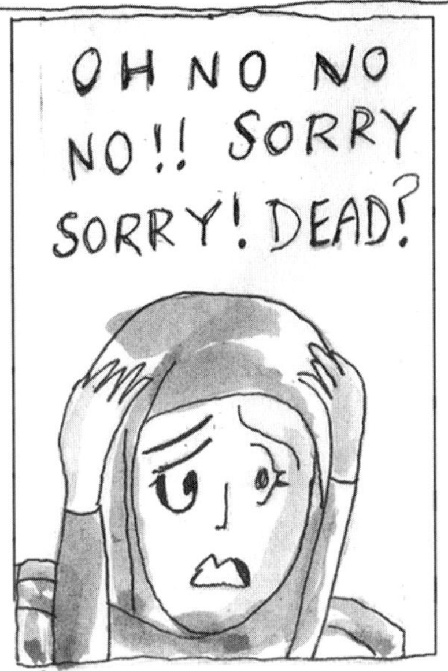
OH NO NO NO!! SORRY SORRY! DEAD?

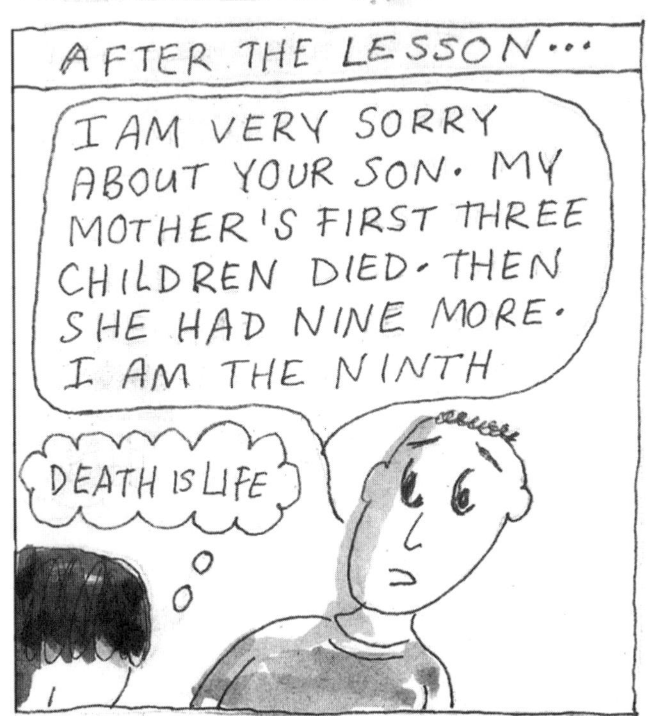
AFTER THE LESSON...
I AM VERY SORRY ABOUT YOUR SON. MY MOTHER'S FIRST THREE CHILDREN DIED. THEN SHE HAD NINE MORE. I AM THE NINTH
DEATH IS LIFE

BUT ON THE DAY BILLY DIED, I STILL HAD A LONG JOURNEY AHEAD.

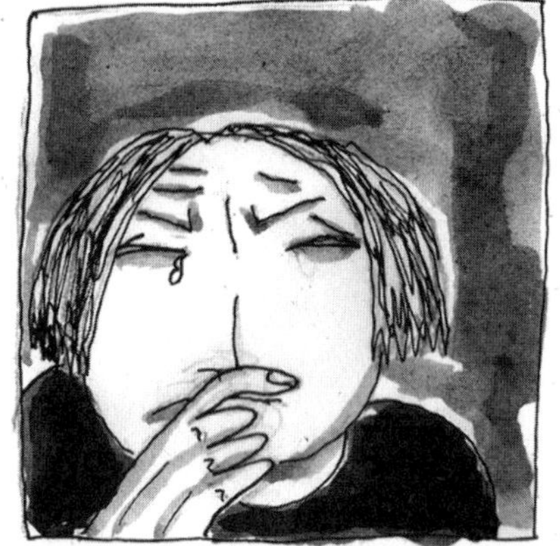

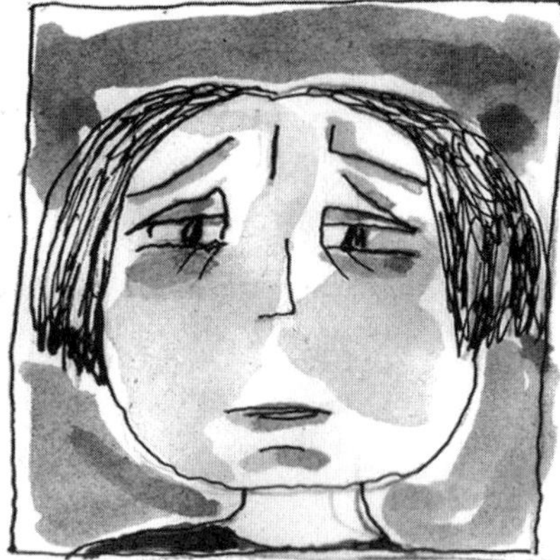

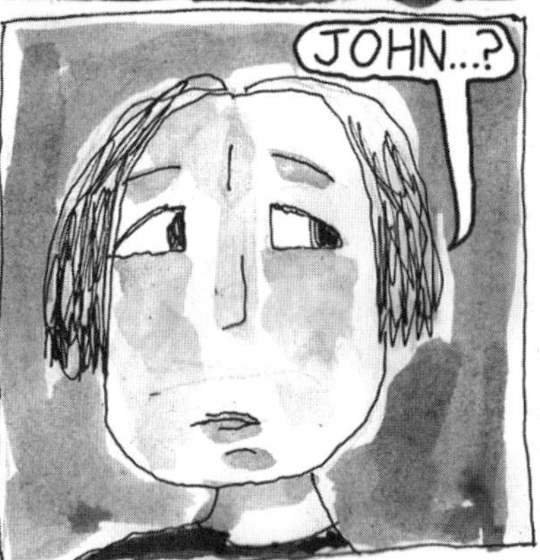

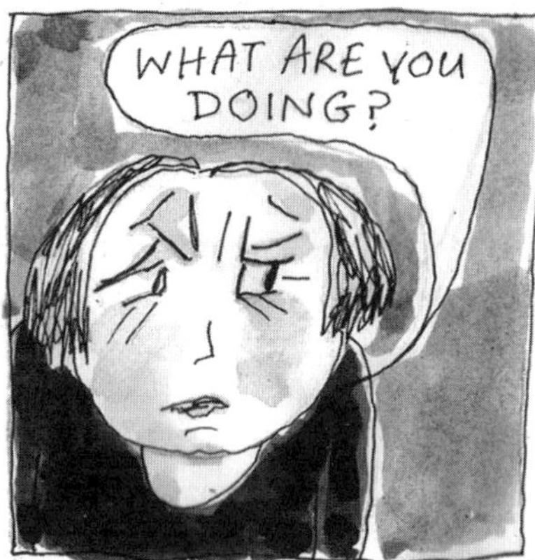

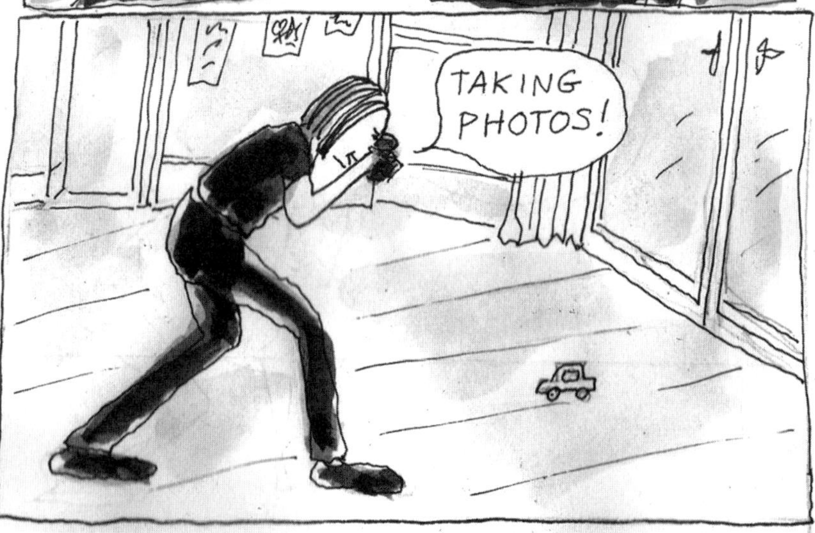

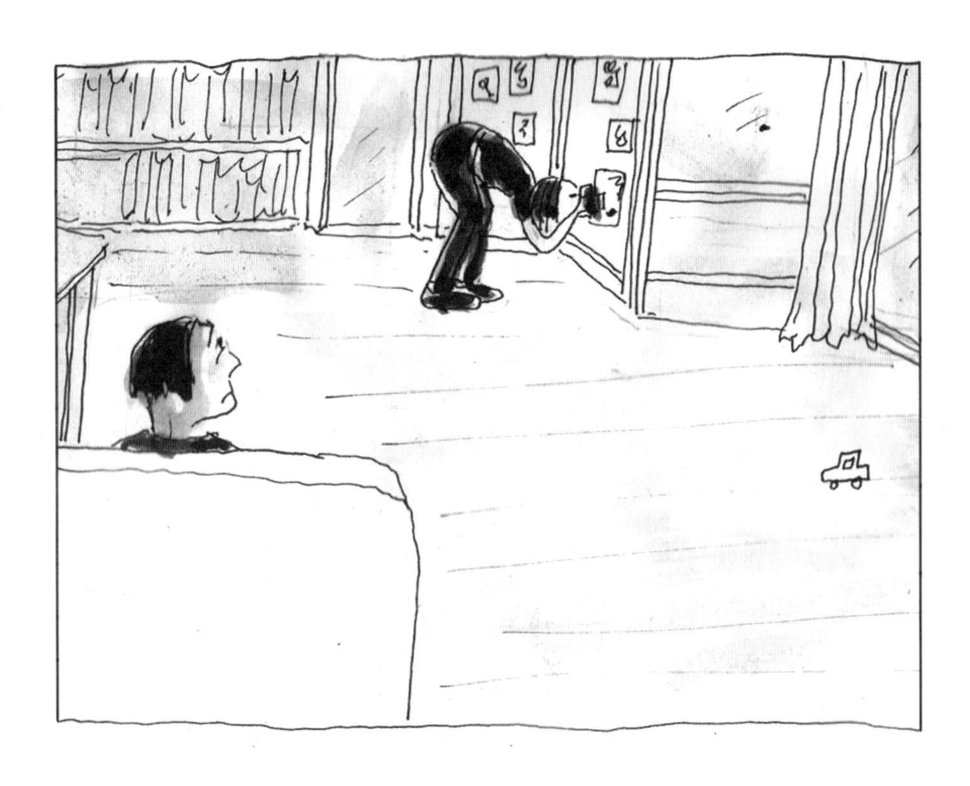

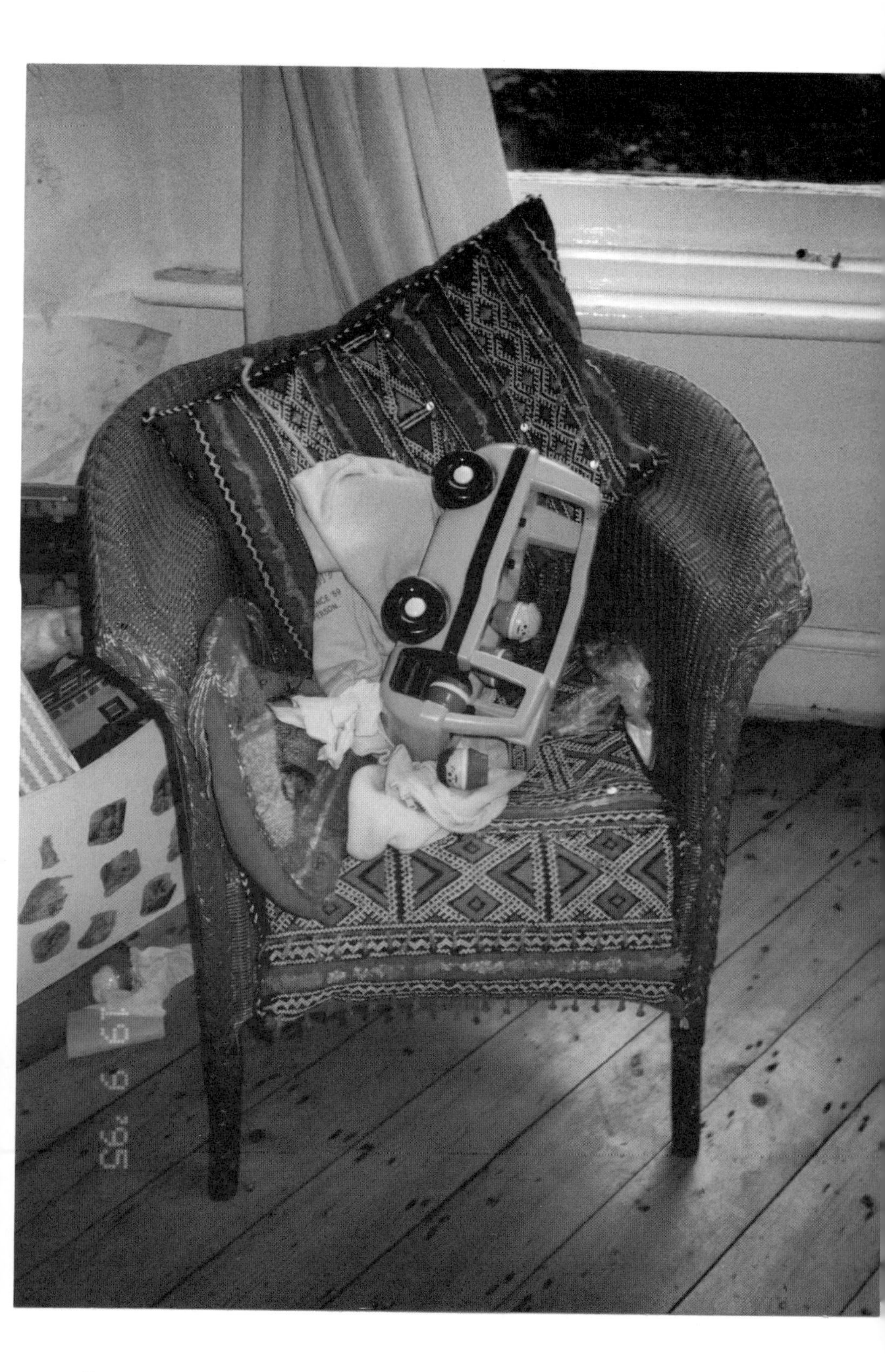
'95 6 19

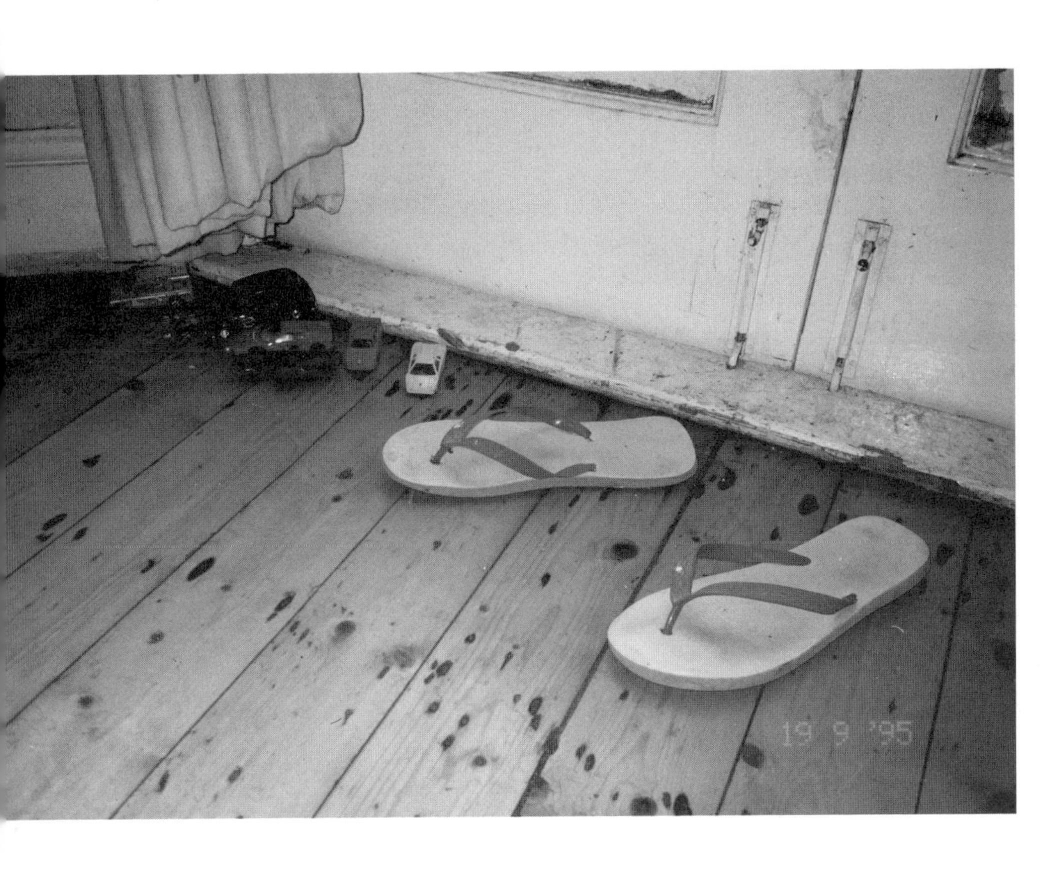
19 9 '95

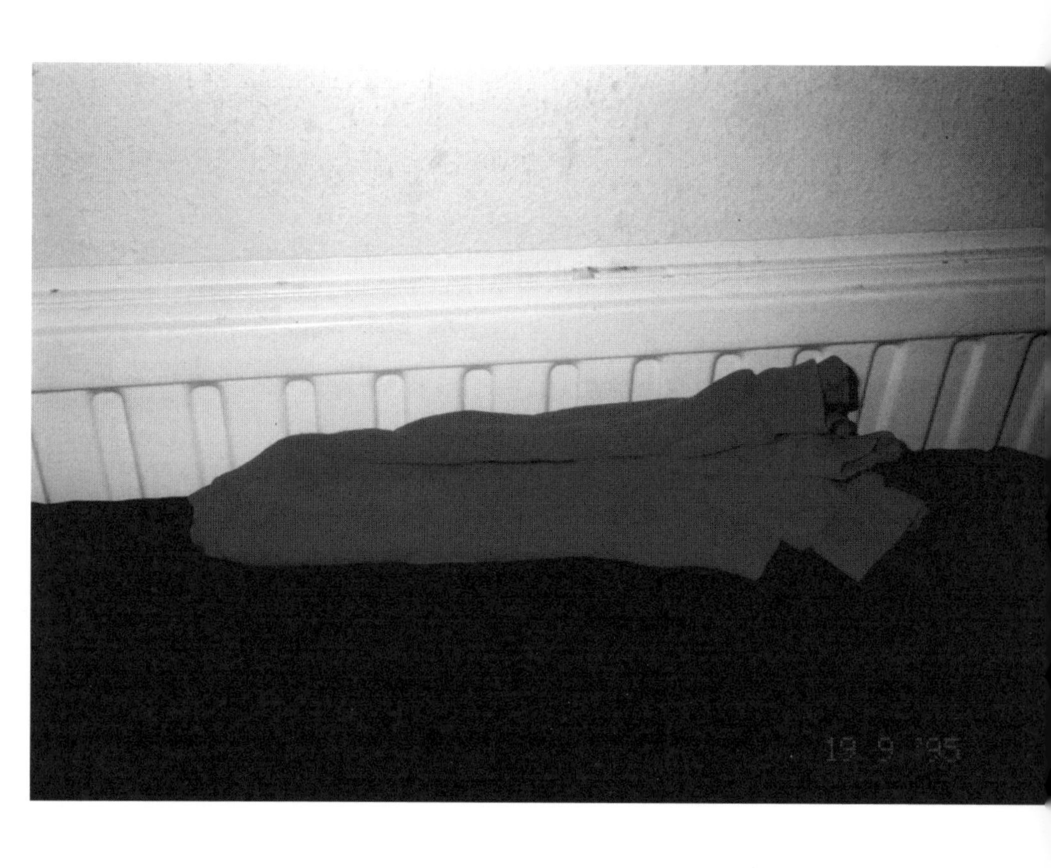
19 9 '95

LATER, DON AND MEL BROUGHT THE CAR BACK AND STAYED FOR A CUP OF TEA. MEL MOVED BILLY'S TOP OUT OF THE WAY AS SHE SAT DOWN.

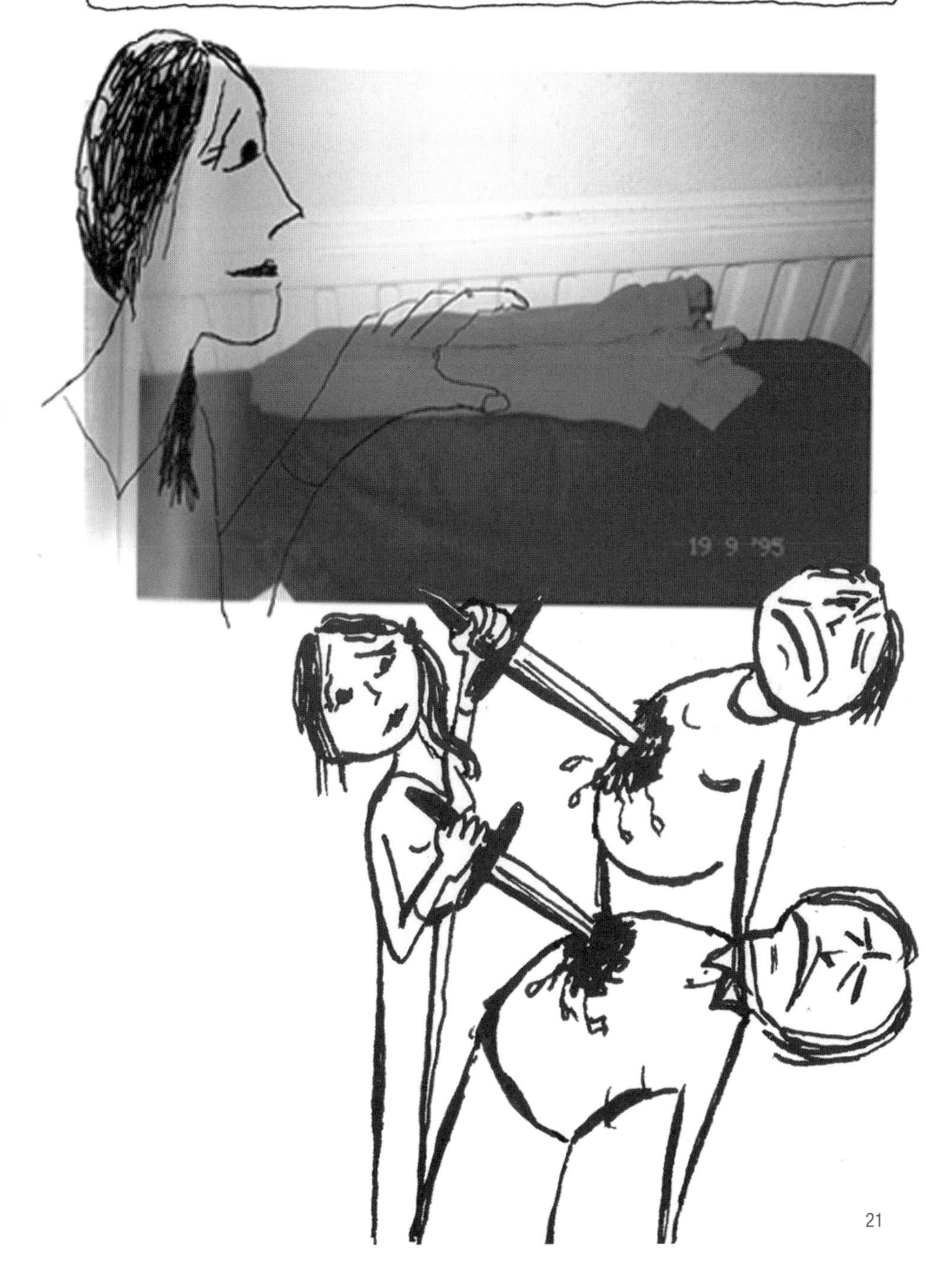

SO THIS WAS GRIEF. A THING WITH A LIFE OF ITS OWN – CONTROLLING AND DISTORTING OUR UNDERSTANDING OF THE WORLD – TURNING THE INNOCENT GESTURES OF KIND PEOPLE WHO LOVED US INTO MALICIOUS ACTS OF SPITE.

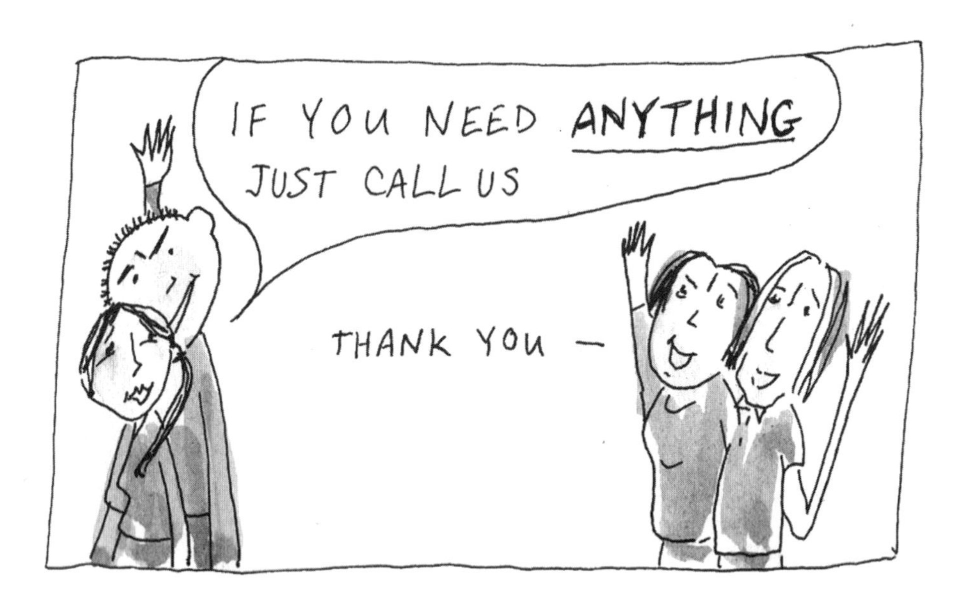

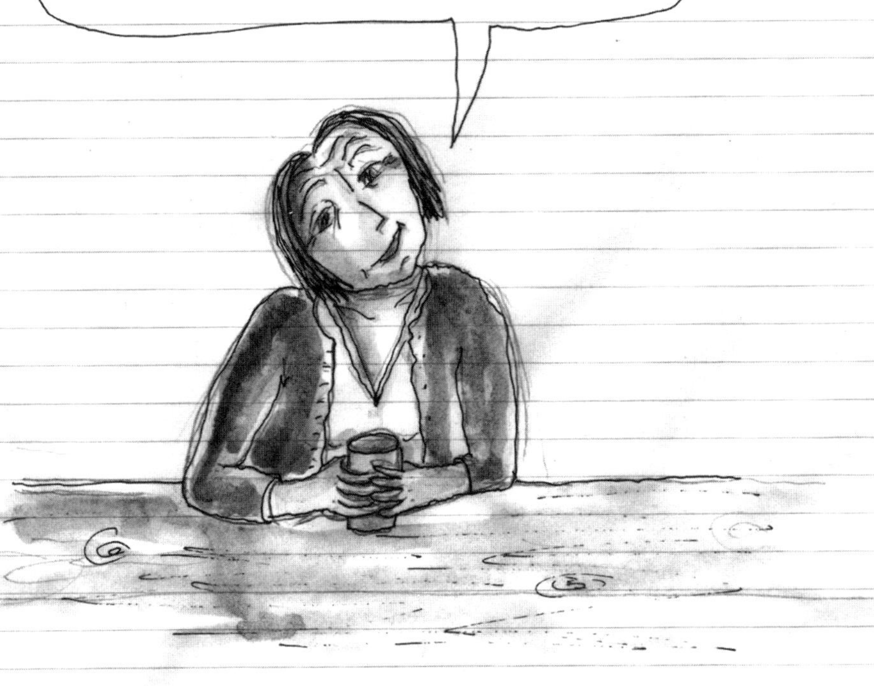
PEOPLE ASK IF THIS BOOK IS CATHARTIC... FOR JOHN AND ME THE CATHARSIS TOOK PLACE AT THE TIME

	Sat	Sun	Mon	Tue	Wed	Thu	Fri	Sat	Sun	Mon	Tue	Wed	Thu	Fri	Sat	Sun	Mon	Tue	Wed	Thu	Fri	Sat	Sun	Mon	Tue	Wed	Thu	Fr
ber	1	2	3	4	5	6	7	8	9	10	11	12	13	14	15	16	17	18	19	20	21	22	23	24	25	26	27	2

AT FIRST WE ATTENDED A "DEAD BABY CLUB" IN SOMEONE'S HOME.

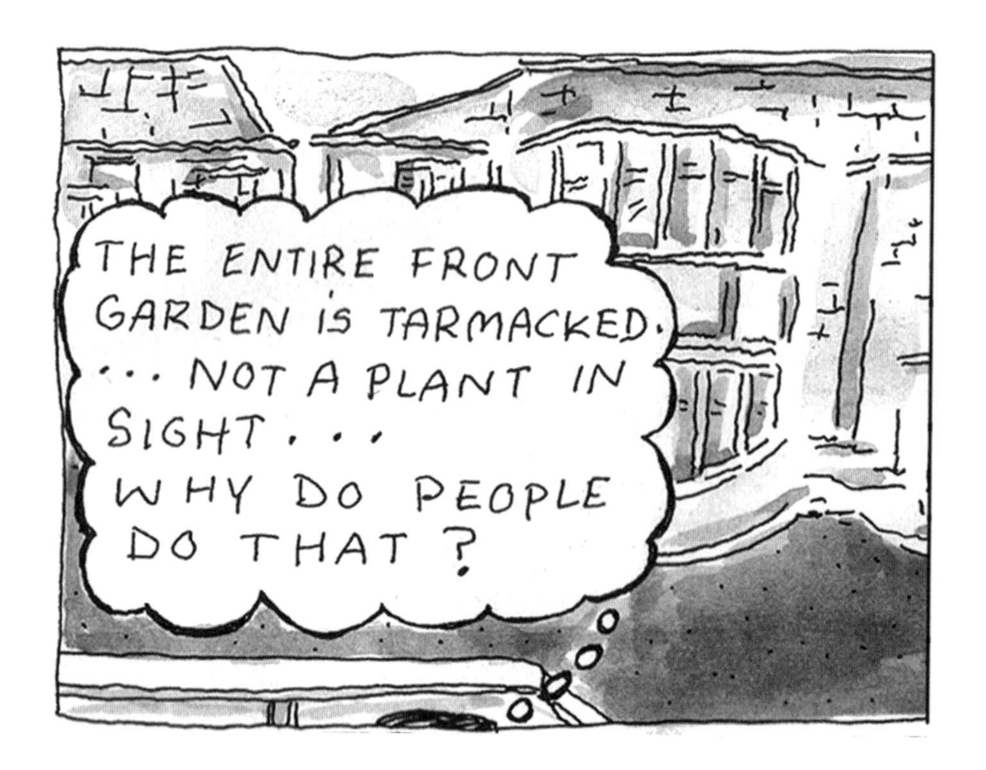
THE ENTIRE FRONT GARDEN IS TARMACKED. ... NOT A PLANT IN SIGHT... WHY DO PEOPLE DO THAT?

WE WERE WARMLY WELCOMED IN BY A HUSBAND AND WIFE.

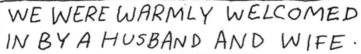

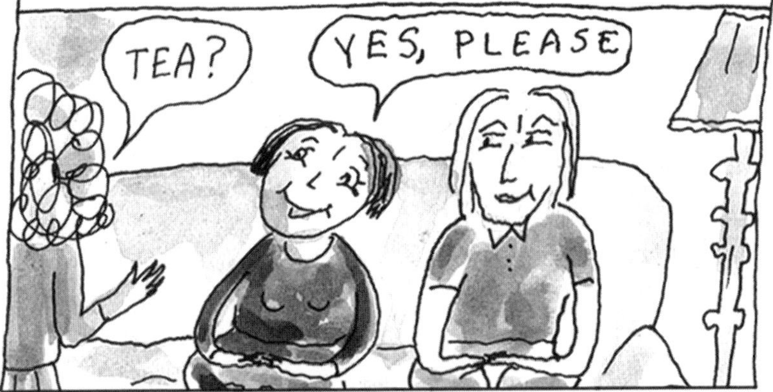
TEA?
YES, PLEASE

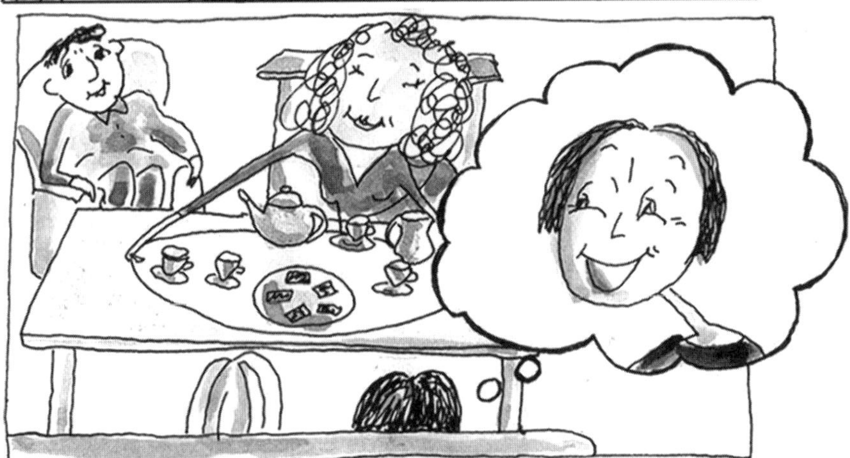

IT WAS AN UTTERLY PERFECT CUP OF TEA ... WITH THE CORRECT BISCUITS.

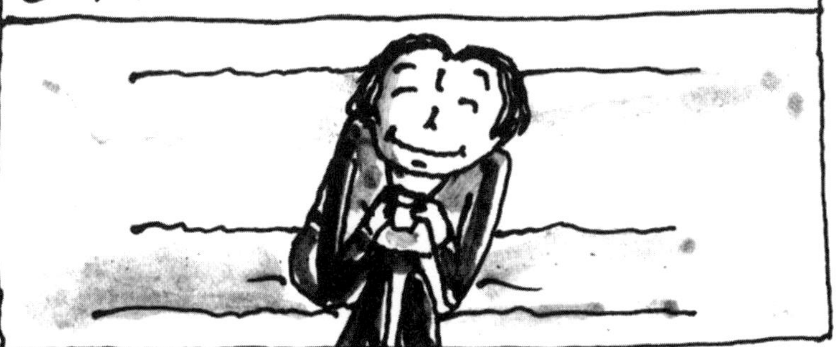

SINCE BILLY DIED I'D BEEN OBSESSING ABOUT TOP-SHELF BISCUITS (BISCUIT PORN?) YOU KNOW THE KIND... OVERPRICED, CONTINENTAL, QUALITY CHOCOLATE, HARDLY ANY IN A PACKET, SERVED WITH GOOD TEA.

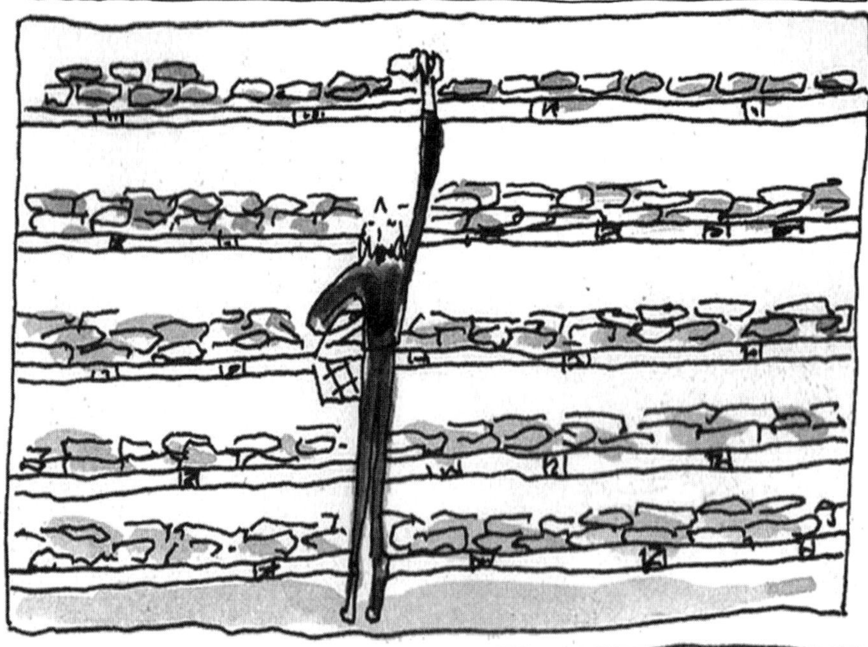

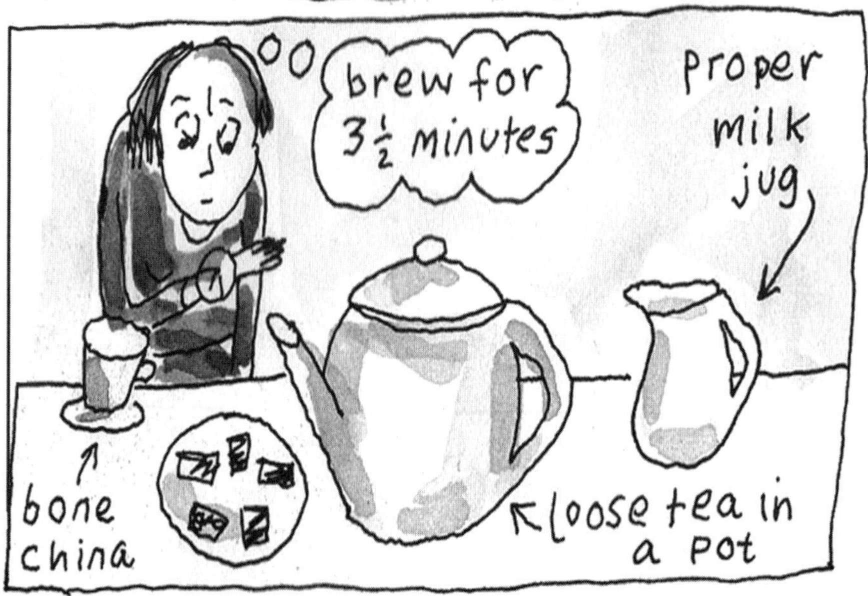

SO THE MAIN THINGS IN MY LIFE HAD SPIRALLED OUT OF CONTROL BUT A COMFORTING ORDER COULD BE CREATED THROUGH THE DETAIL. SHE KNEW THAT—THIS WOMAN WHO LOST HER BABY SIX YEARS AGO.

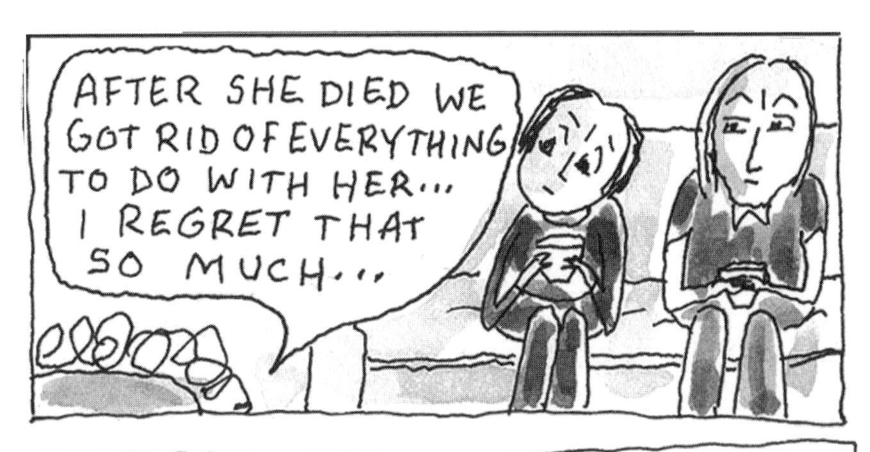

AFTER SHE DIED WE GOT RID OF EVERYTHING TO DO WITH HER... I REGRET THAT SO MUCH...

THE FORMAT WAS SIMILAR TO A MOTHER AND BABY GROUP WHERE YOU SWAP BIRTH STORIES AND EXCHANGE TIPS FOR COPING WITH YOUR NEW STATUS.

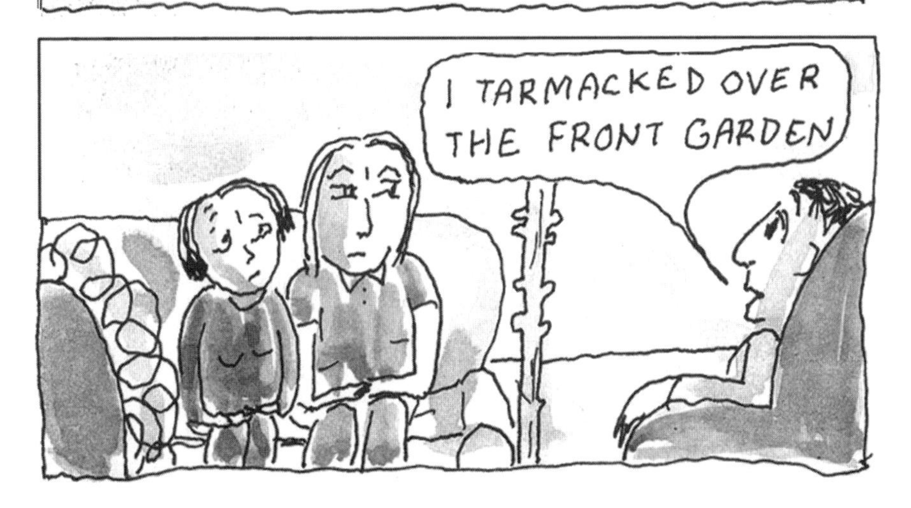

I TARMACKED OVER THE FRONT GARDEN

SOME WEEKS LATER WE ATTENDED A GROUP AT THE HOSPITAL RUN BY A FRIENDLY NURSE. IT WAS OUR FIRST VISIT BACK TO THE HOSPITAL.

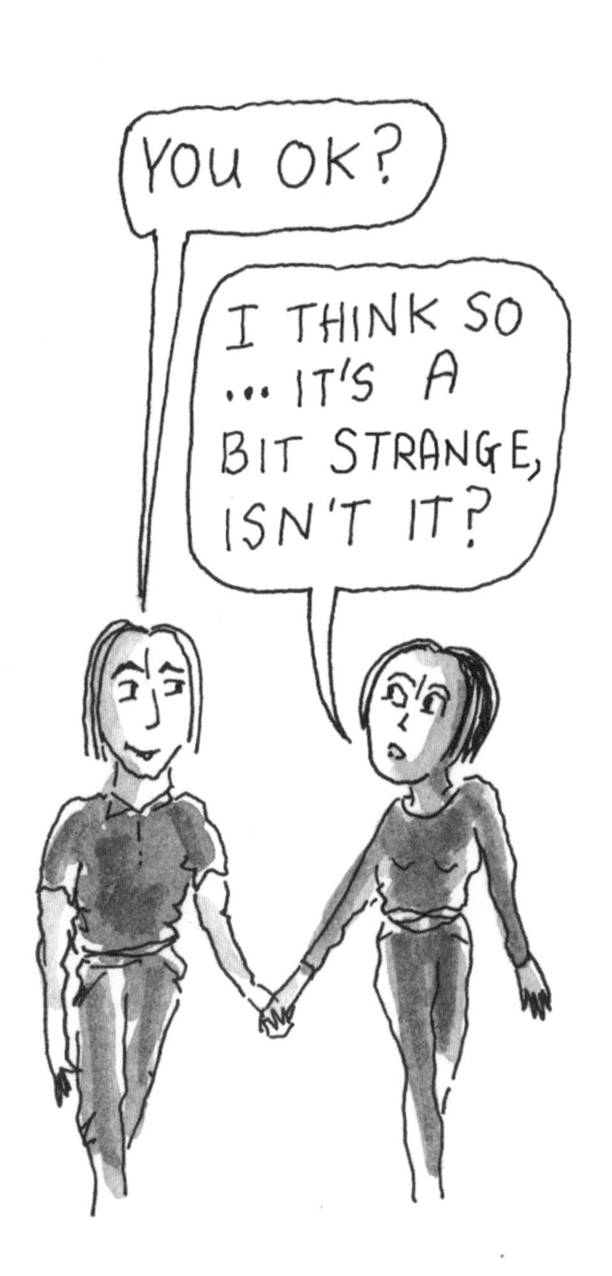
YOU OK?
I THINK SO ... IT'S A BIT STRANGE, ISN'T IT?

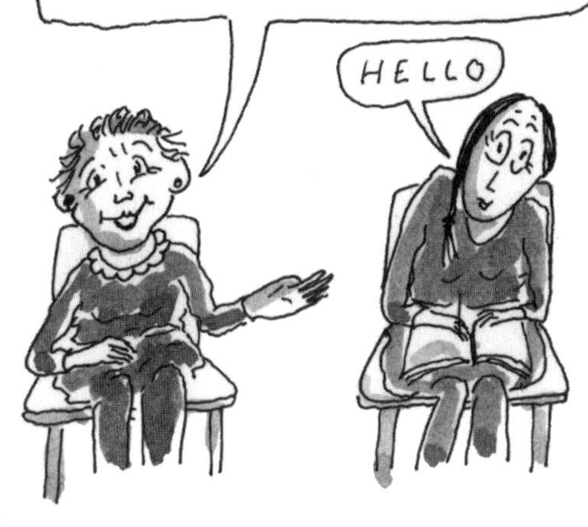
WE'LL GO ROUND THE CIRCLE. BUT FIRST, I'D LIKE TO INTRODUCE KAREN, THE HOSPITAL PSYCHOLOGIST, WHO WILL BE SITTING IN AS PART OF HER RESEARCH
HELLO

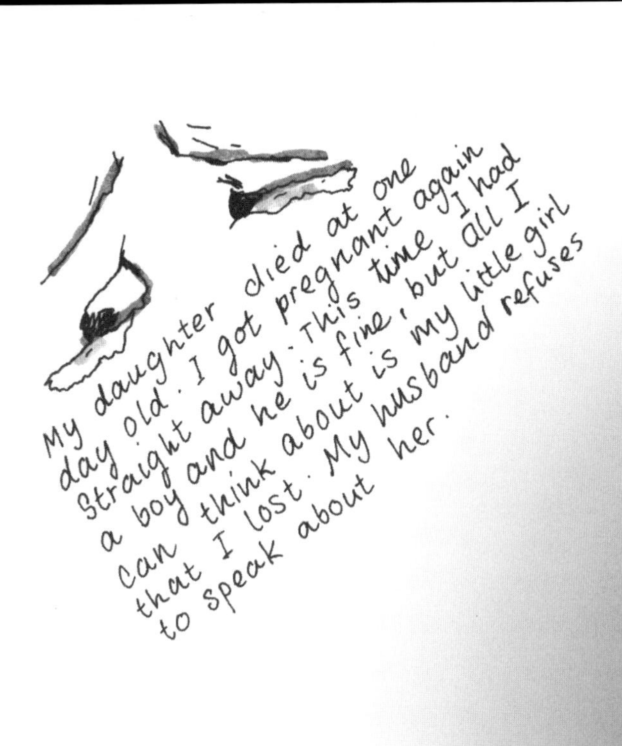

My daughter died at one
day old. I got pregnant again
straight away. This time I had
a boy and he is fine, but all I
can think about is my little girl
that I lost. My husband refuses
to speak about her.

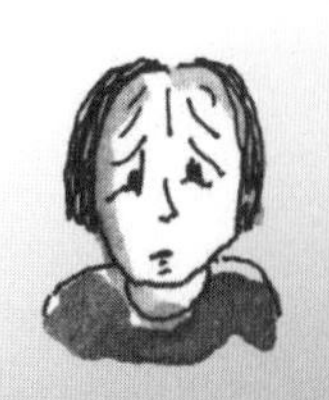

our baby girl died at two days old.
Then we had another baby...
...Also a girl...she
died when she was four
days old...

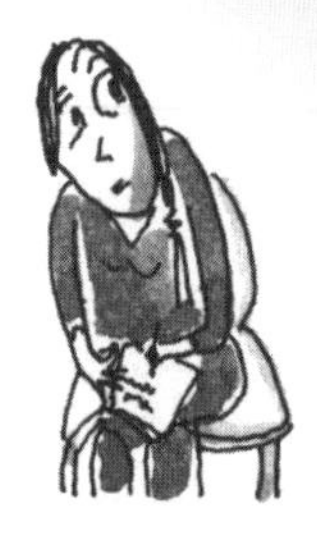

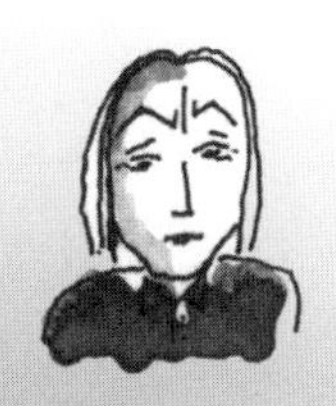

The tests I had during my
pregnancy showed very severe
deformities in my baby. I decided
to have a termination and because
my pregnancy was... advanced... I
had to give birth... and... when my son
was delivered... s... s... he had... s... no
deformities...

My son was born with
a number of heart abnormalities.
He spent a lot of his life here in
the hospital and died when
he was eight.

THEN... IT WAS OUR TURN

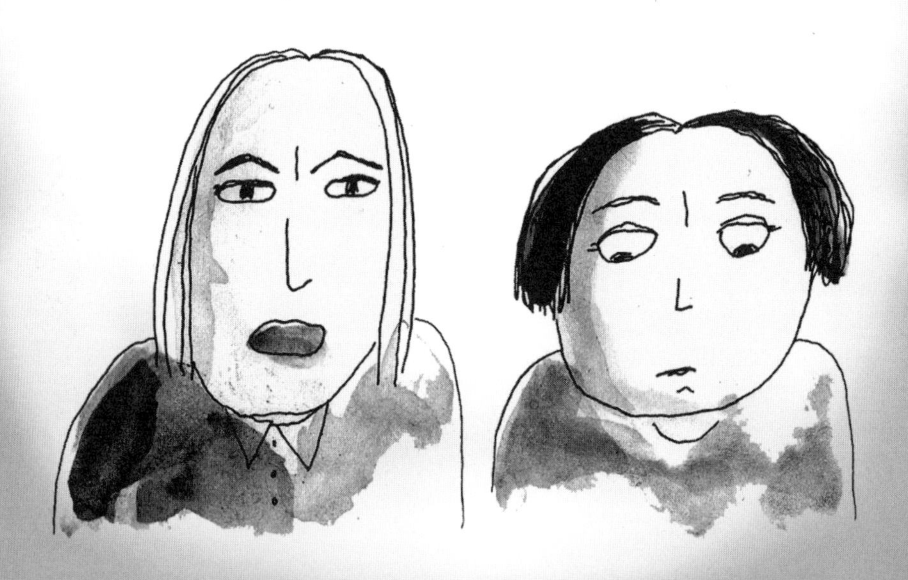
BILLY WAS TWO AND A BIT WHEN HE DIED. HE DIED FOLLOWING SURGERY TO CORRECT FOUR CONGENITAL HEART DEFORMITIES. THESE WERE DIAGNOSED TEN DAYS BEFORE HE DIED

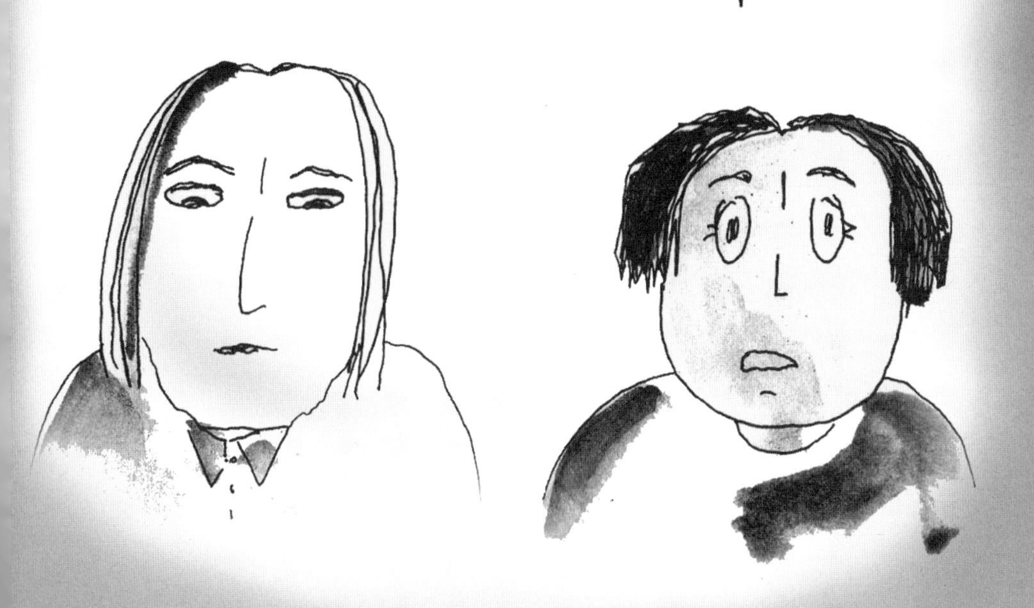
HE'D DEVELOPED ASTHMA-LIKE SYMPTOMS WHEN HE WAS ABOUT ONE. THE DOCTORS DID LOADS OF TESTS AND THEY ALL CAME BACK NEGATIVE... SO WE ALL THOUGHT IT MUST BE ASTHMA

AND THEN, FROM THIS INTENSE SHARING OF PAIN AND TEARS, THE MOOD CHANGED TO ONE OF HILARITY. OUR FOCUS TURNED TO THE COMIC ASPECTS OF OUR EXPERIENCES.

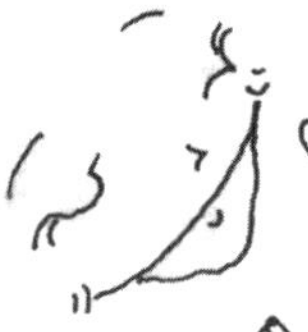

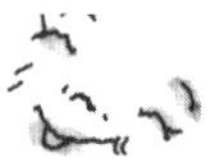

ho ho

we talked about having headstones and ashes in our living rooms while we decided what to do with them ... and forgetting they were there ...

ha ha ha ha

ha ha

... and people's confusion if they saw them and

DIDN'T KNOW

hee hee

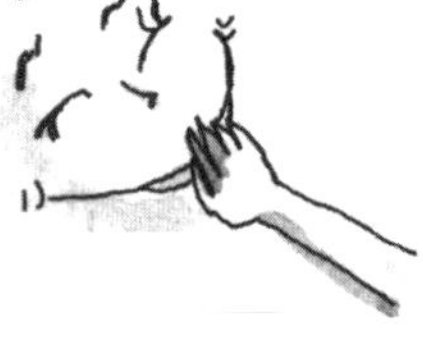

... and how often people who DIDN'T KNOW would make

OH hee hee YES

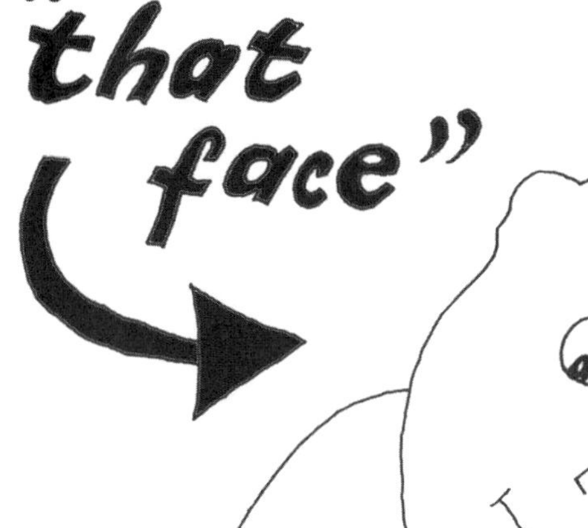

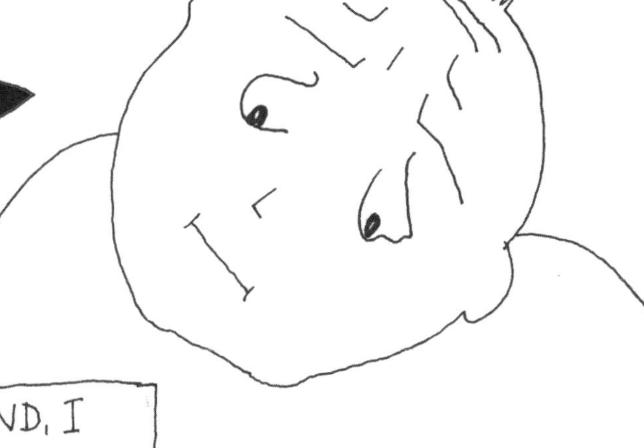

AT THE END, I ASKED THE PSYCHOLOGIST WHAT SHE'D THOUGHT OF THE MEETING.

IT WASN'T WHAT I'D EXPECTED

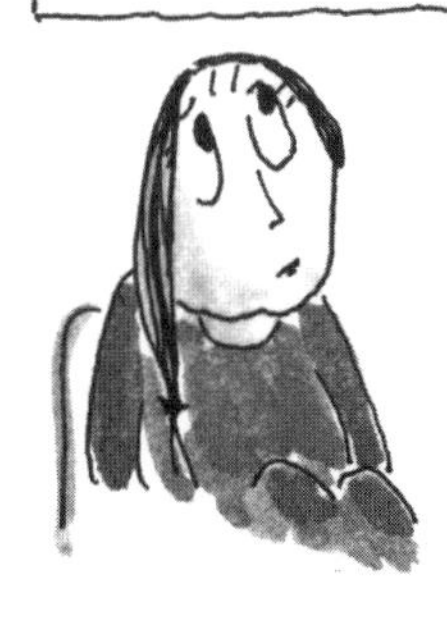

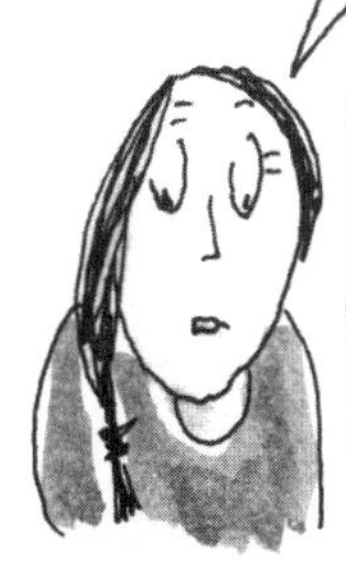

EVER SINCE, I HAVE WONDERED WHAT SHE **HAD** EXPECTED.

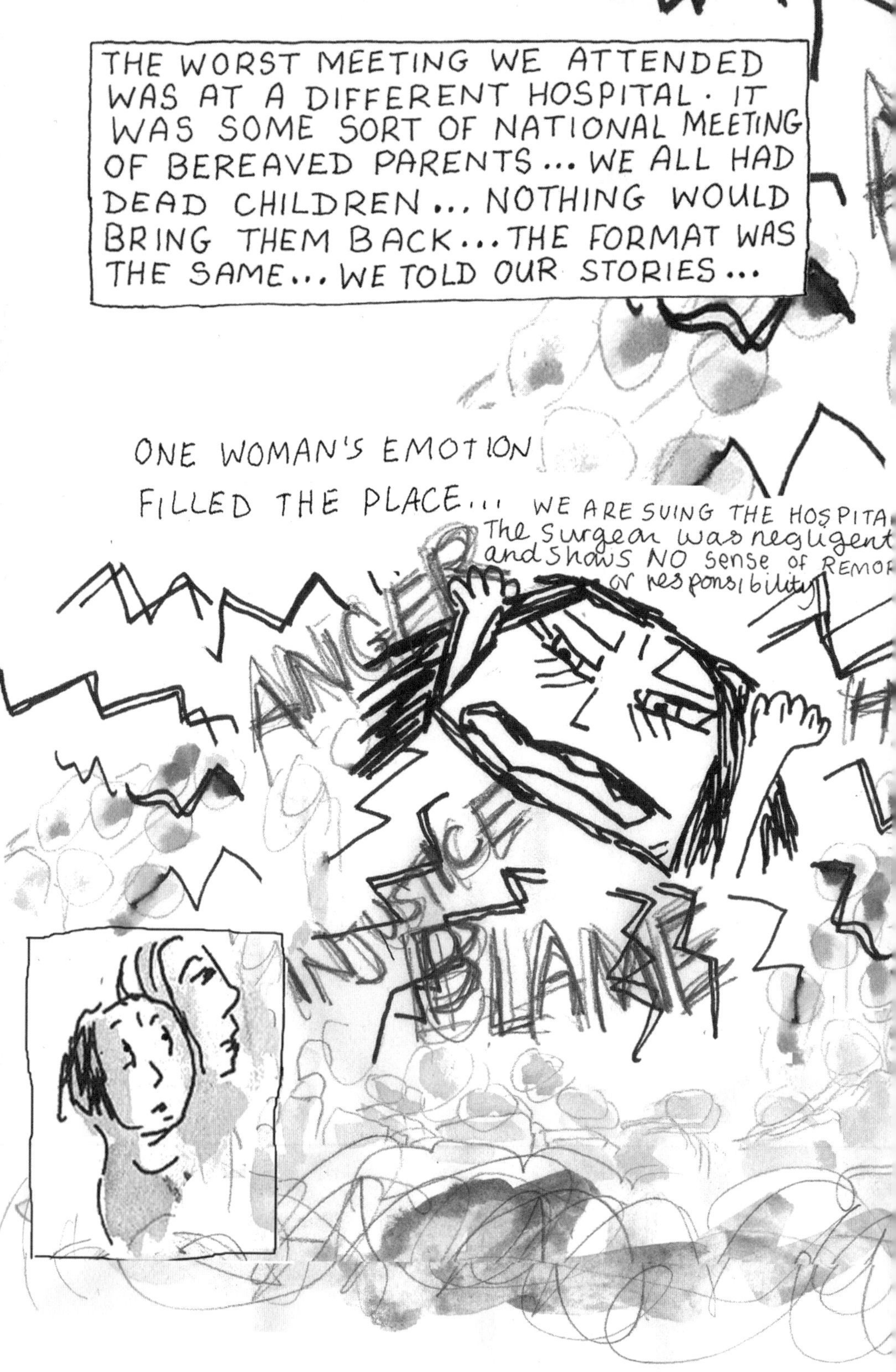
THE WORST MEETING WE ATTENDED WAS AT A DIFFERENT HOSPITAL. IT WAS SOME SORT OF NATIONAL MEETING OF BEREAVED PARENTS... WE ALL HAD DEAD CHILDREN... NOTHING WOULD BRING THEM BACK... THE FORMAT WAS THE SAME... WE TOLD OUR STORIES...
ONE WOMAN'S EMOTION FILLED THE PLACE...
WE ARE SUING THE HOSPITA
The surgeon was negligent and shows NO sense of REMOR or responsibility
ANGER
INJUSTICE
BLAME

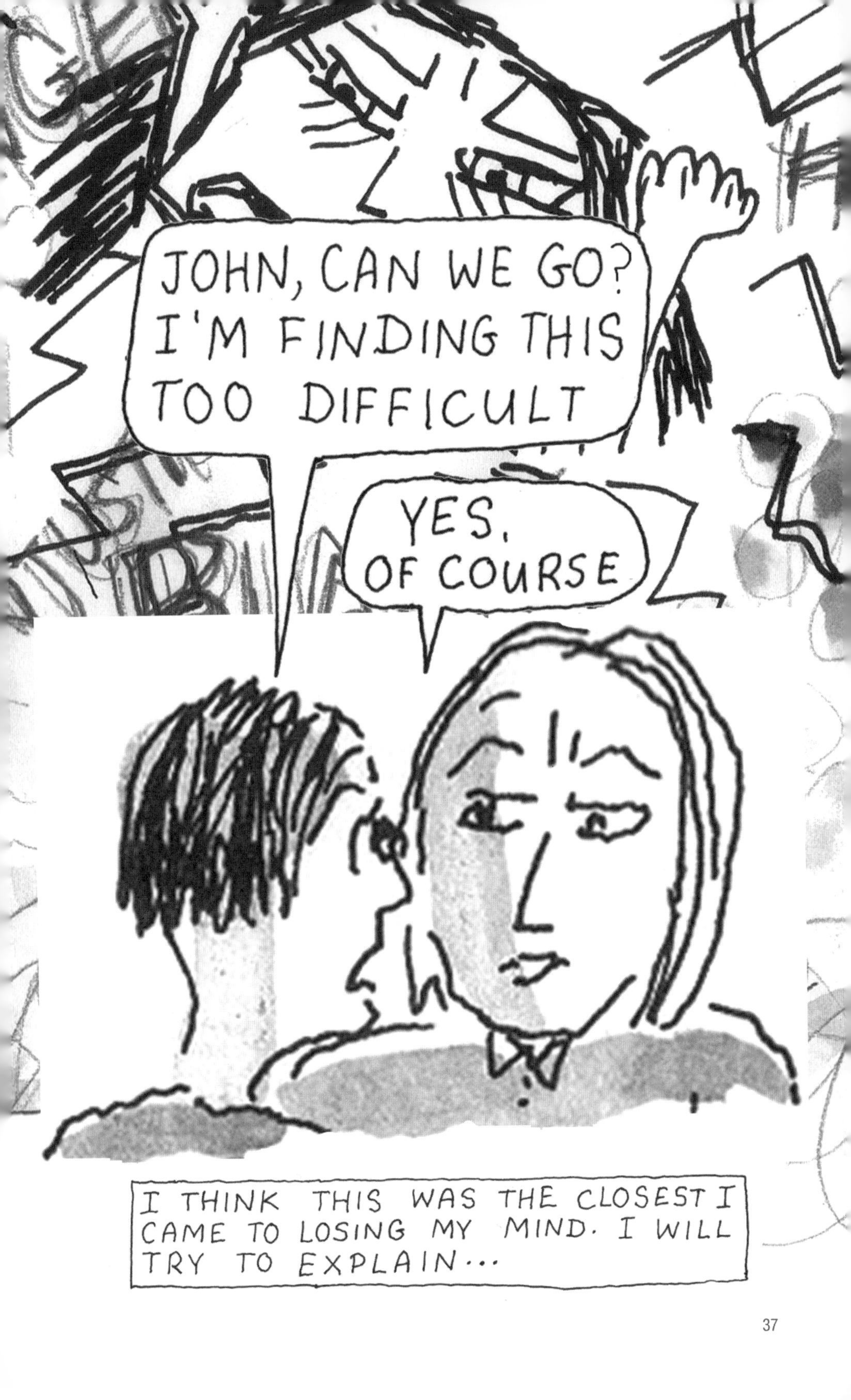
JOHN, CAN WE GO? I'M FINDING THIS TOO DIFFICULT
YES, OF COURSE
I THINK THIS WAS THE CLOSEST I CAME TO LOSING MY MIND. I WILL TRY TO EXPLAIN...

HER STORY THREATENED THE BASIC PREMISE OF MY "SOFT ZONE" WHICH WAS THAT PEOPLE ARE HONEST, KIND AND HELPFUL . . . YES, OF COURSE I WAS BLOCKING STUFF OUT, BUT . . .

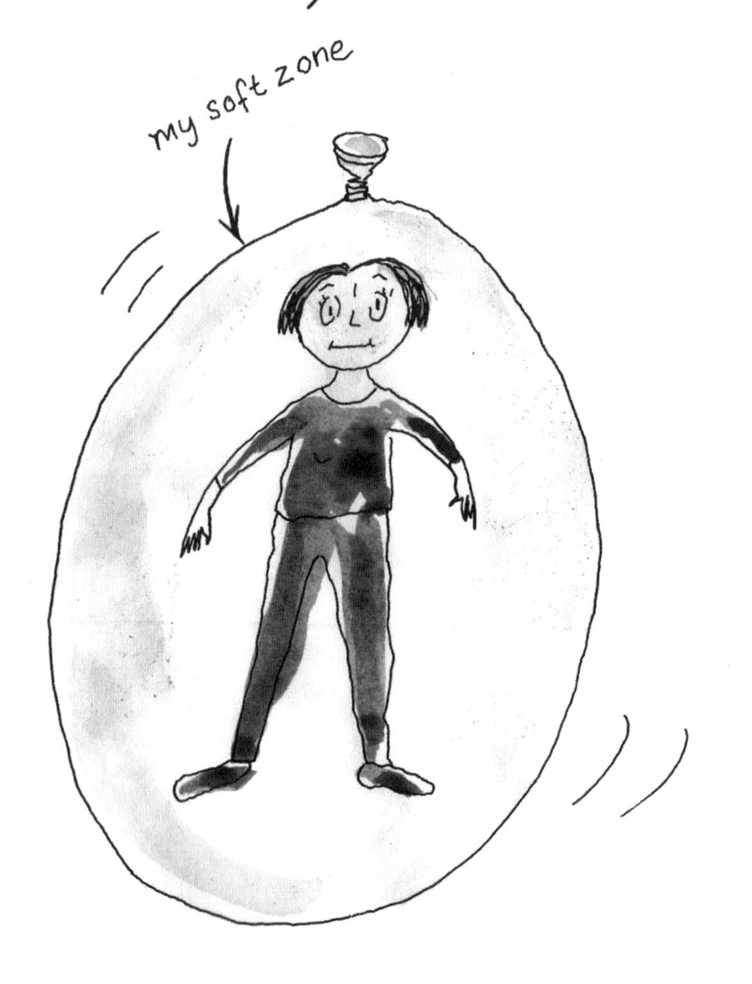

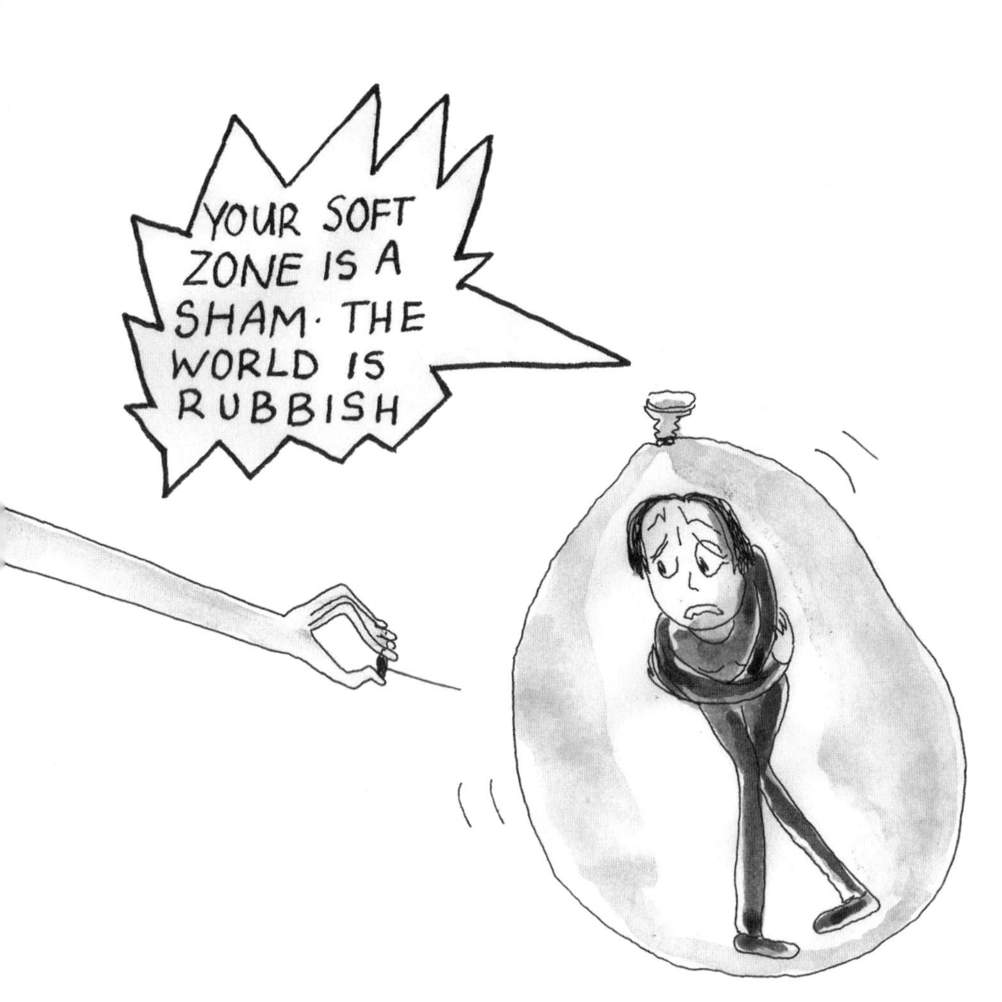
YOUR SOFT ZONE IS A SHAM. THE WORLD IS RUBBISH
... IF MY SOFT ZONE GOT DAMAGED I KNEW KILLING MYSELF WOULD HAVE TOO MUCH APPEAL

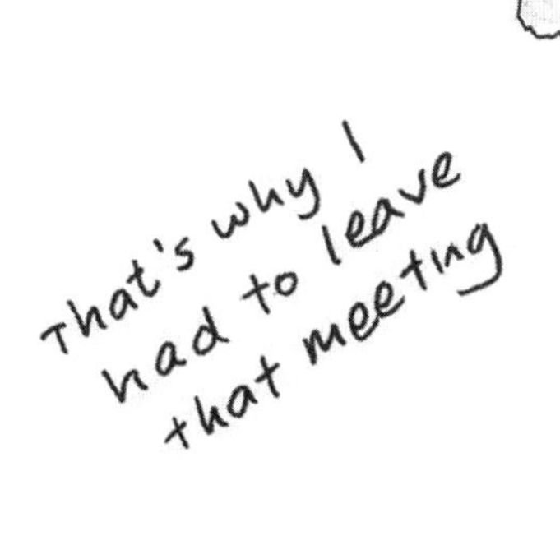
That's why I had to leave that meeting

MEANWHILE I CARRIED ON DOING MY JOB TEACHING NIGHT CLASSES. BUT MY WALK HOME WAS BECOMING INCREASINGLY DIFFICULT.

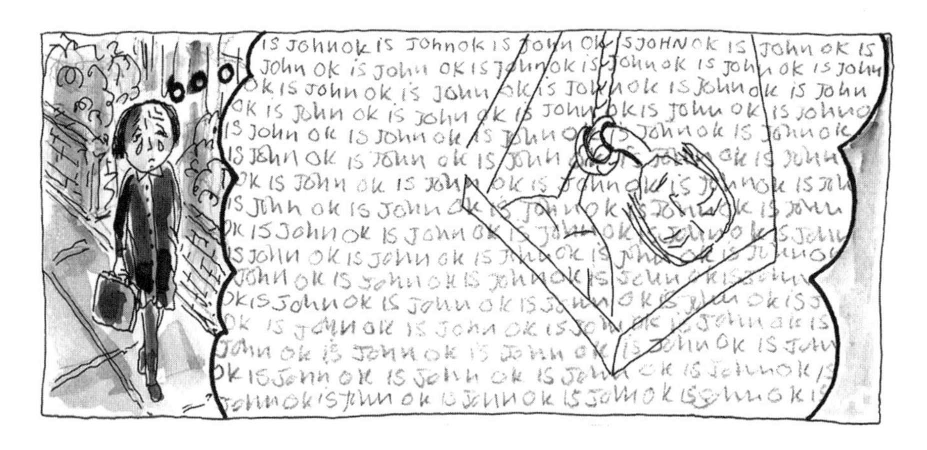

JOHN HAD FELT UNABLE TO RETURN TO HIS WORK OR STUDIO.

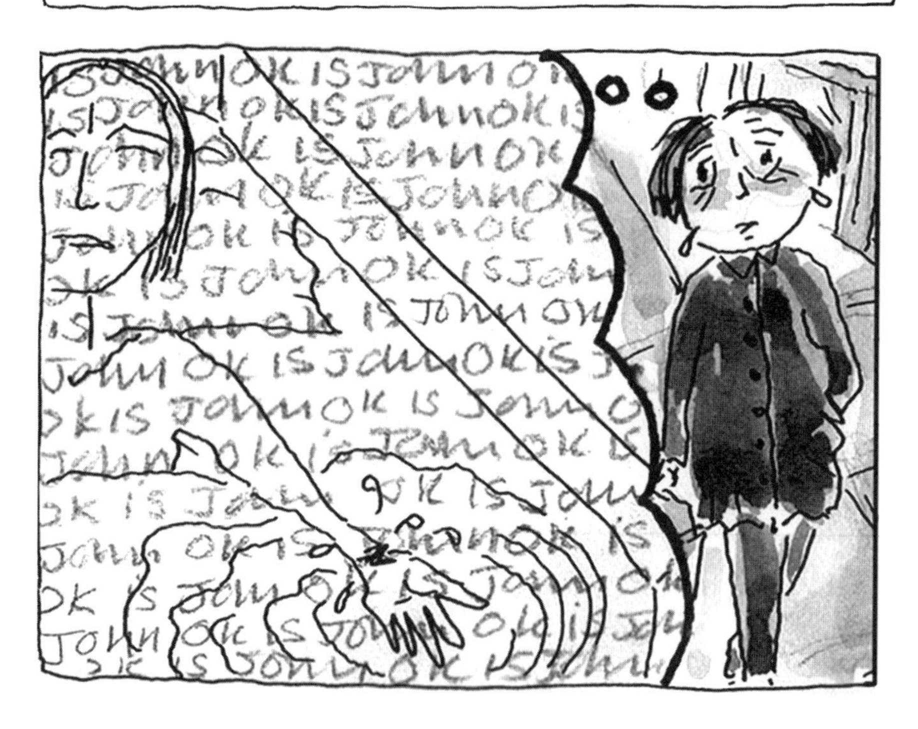

HE'D STARTED TO SPEND MORE AND MORE TIME IN BED...

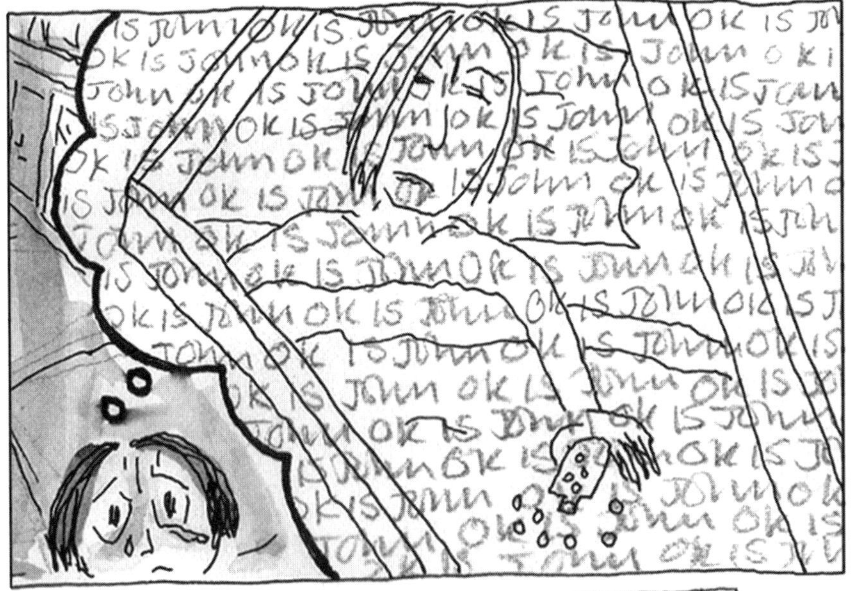
IS JOHN OK IS JOHN OK IS JOHN OK

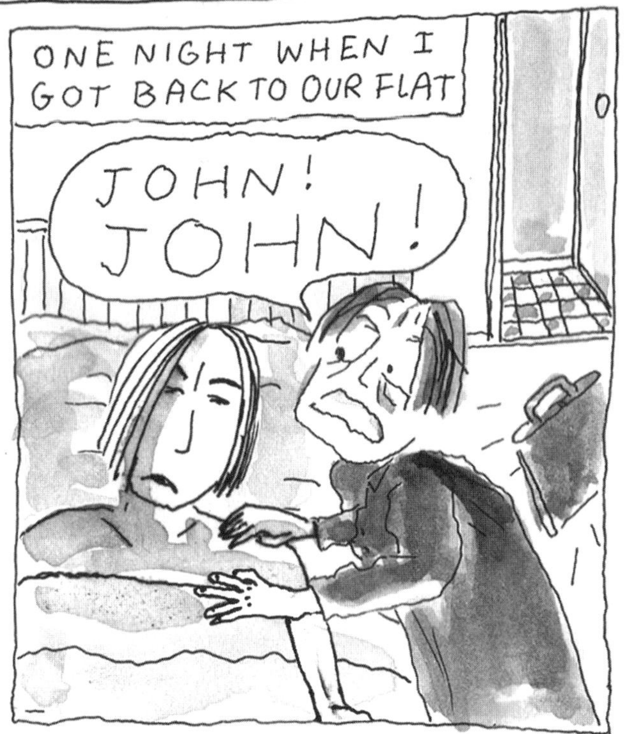
ONE NIGHT WHEN I GOT BACK TO OUR FLAT
JOHN! JOHN!

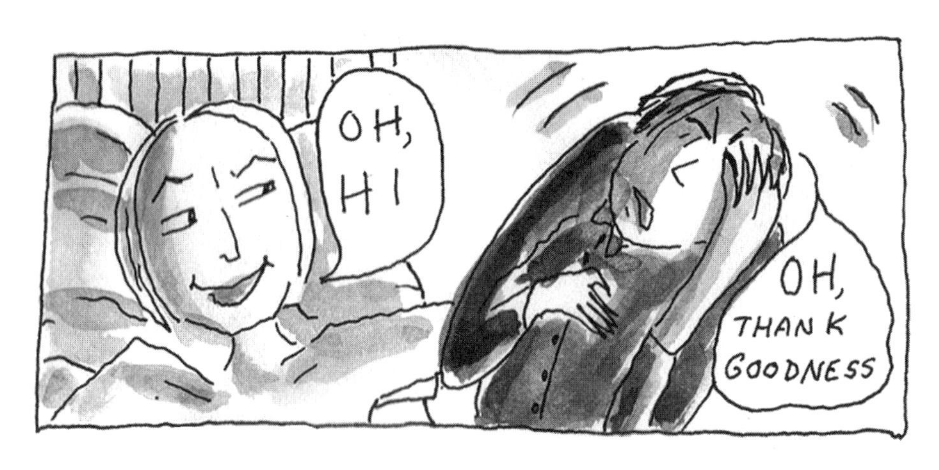
OH, HI
OH, THANK GOODNESS

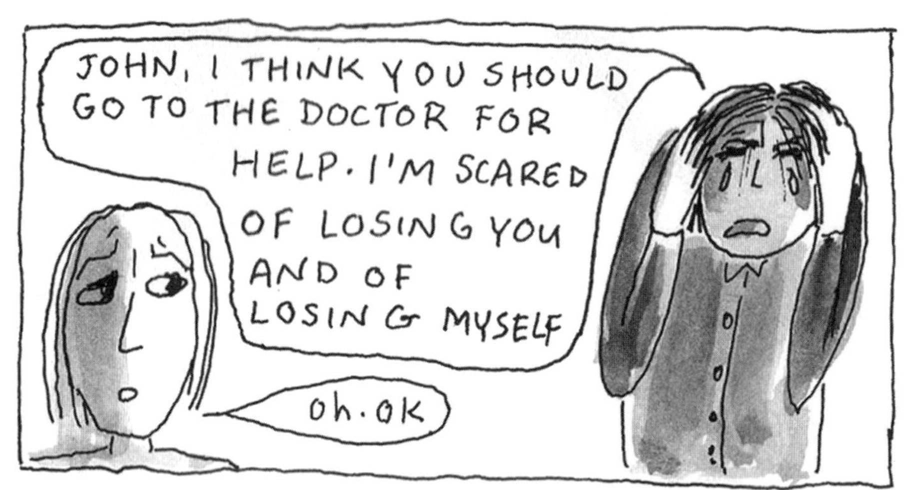
JOHN, I THINK YOU SHOULD GO TO THE DOCTOR FOR HELP. I'M SCARED OF LOSING YOU AND OF LOSING MYSELF
oh. OK

THAT NIGHT I DREAMED...

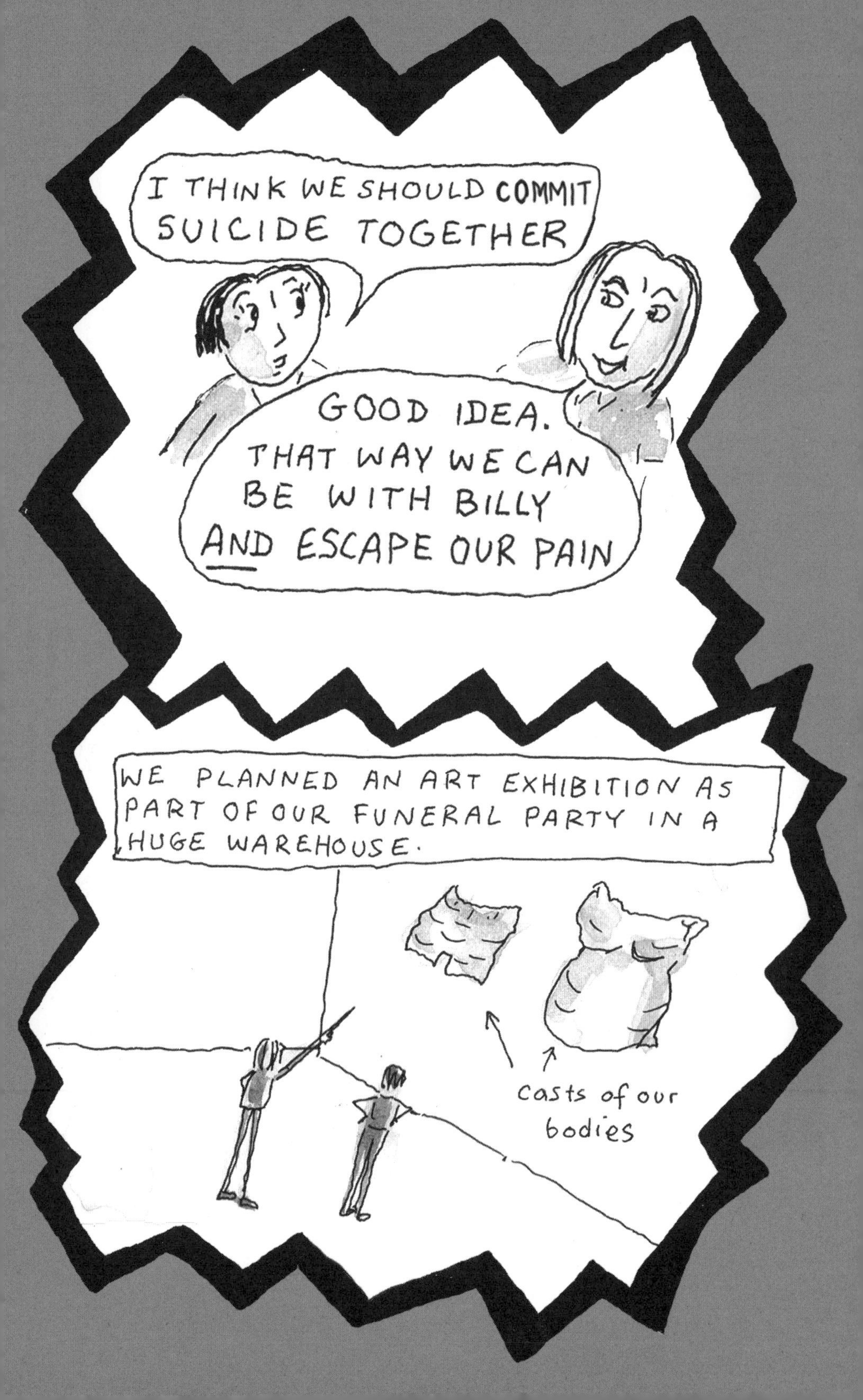
I THINK WE SHOULD COMMIT SUICIDE TOGETHER
GOOD IDEA. THAT WAY WE CAN BE WITH BILLY AND ESCAPE OUR PAIN
WE PLANNED AN ART EXHIBITION AS PART OF OUR FUNERAL PARTY IN A HUGE WAREHOUSE.
casts of our bodies

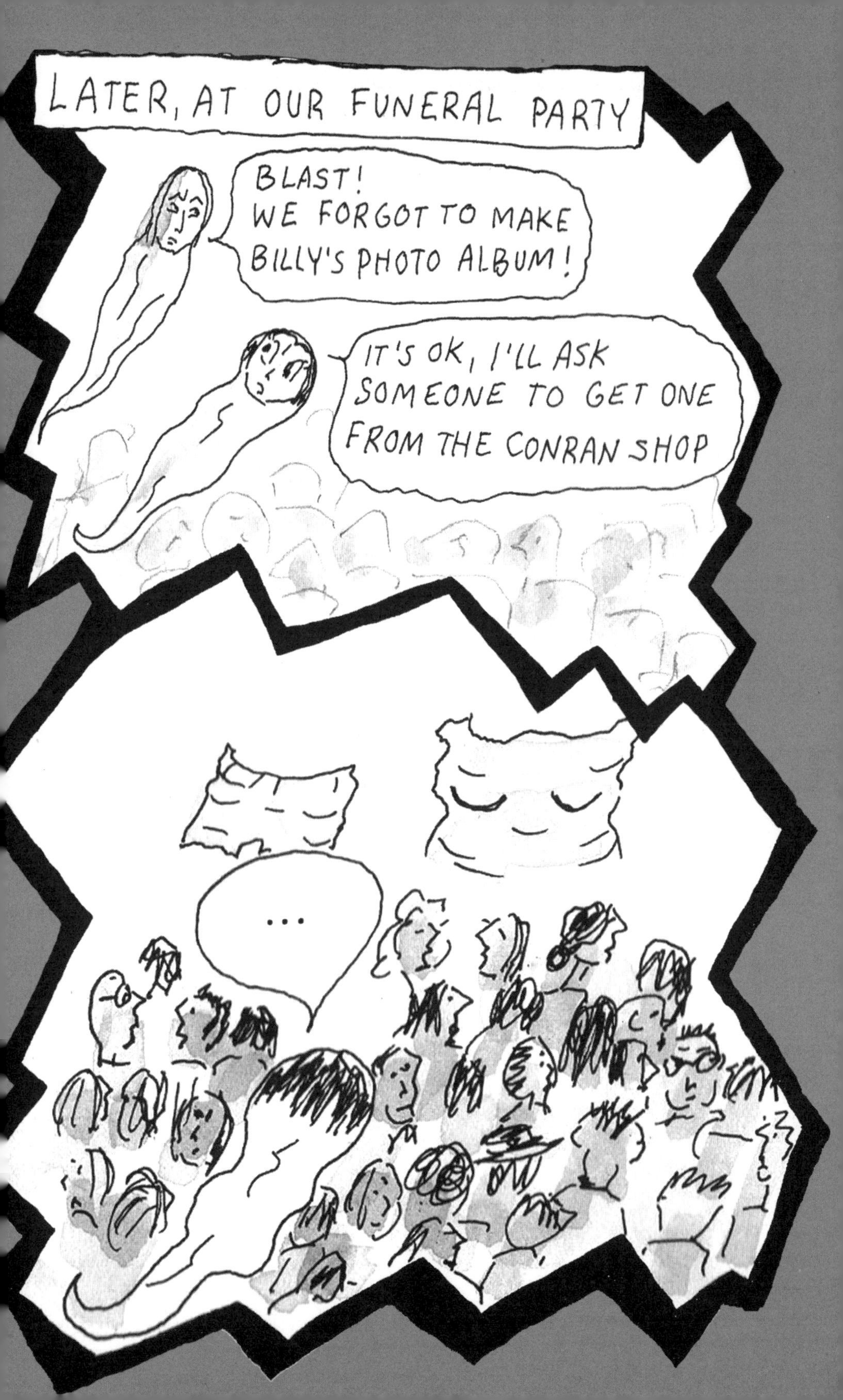
LATER, AT OUR FUNERAL PARTY
BLAST! WE FORGOT TO MAKE BILLY'S PHOTO ALBUM!
IT'S OK, I'LL ASK SOMEONE TO GET ONE FROM THE CONRAN SHOP
...

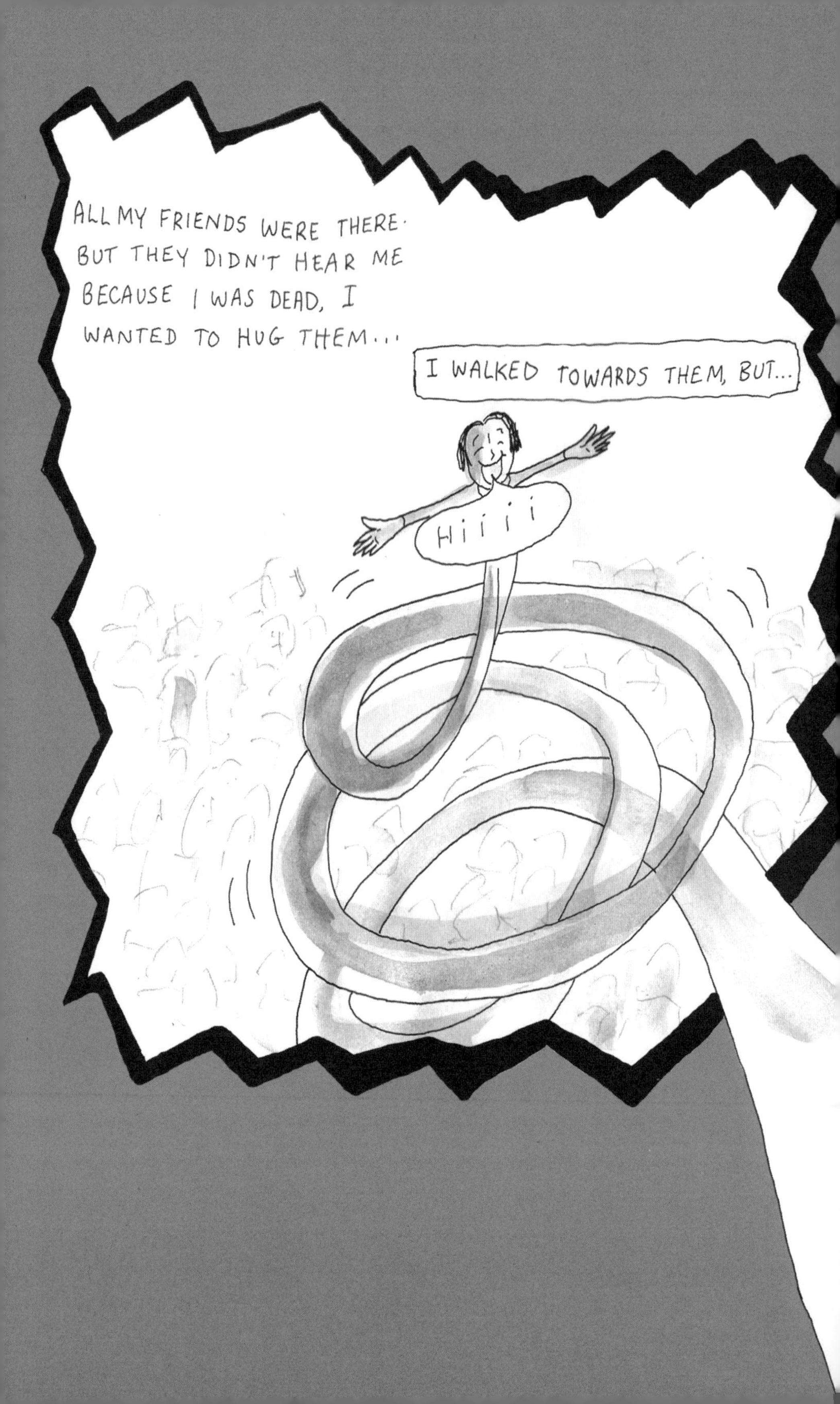
ALL MY FRIENDS WERE THERE. BUT THEY DIDN'T HEAR ME BECAUSE I WAS DEAD, I WANTED TO HUG THEM...
I WALKED TOWARDS THEM, BUT...
Hiiii

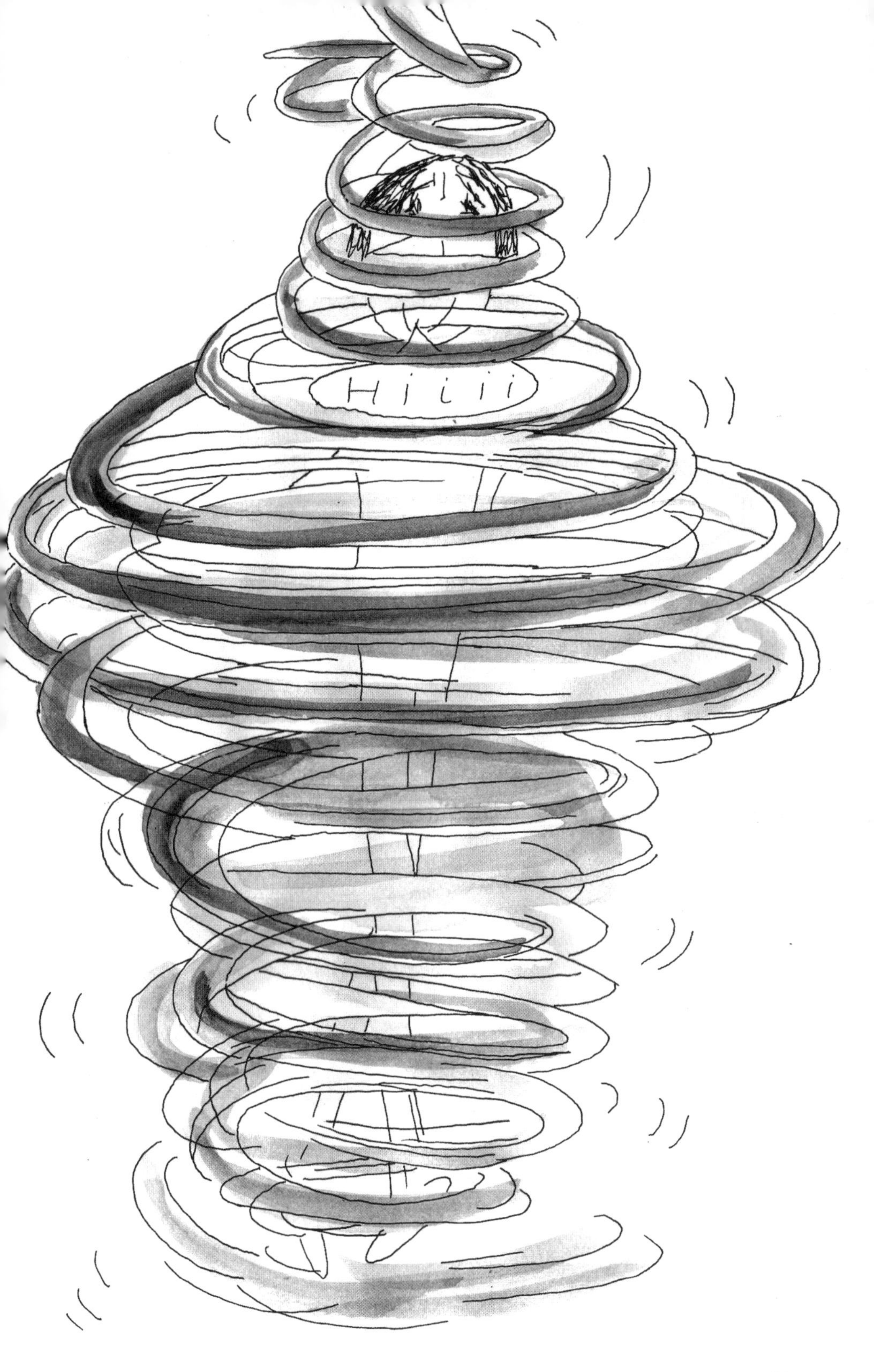
Hiiii

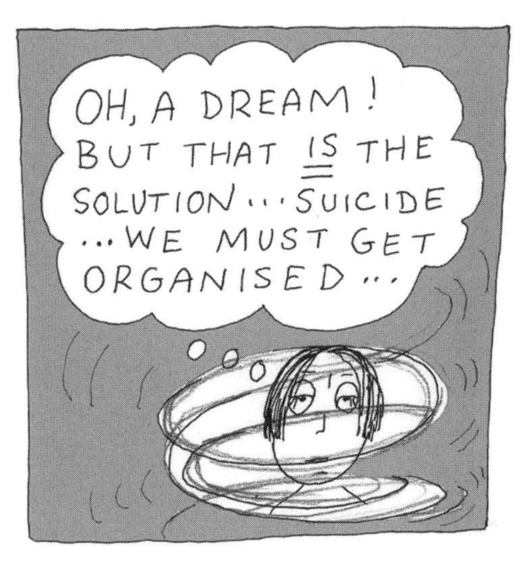
OH, A DREAM! BUT THAT IS THE SOLUTION ... SUICIDE ... WE MUST GET ORGANISED ...

!

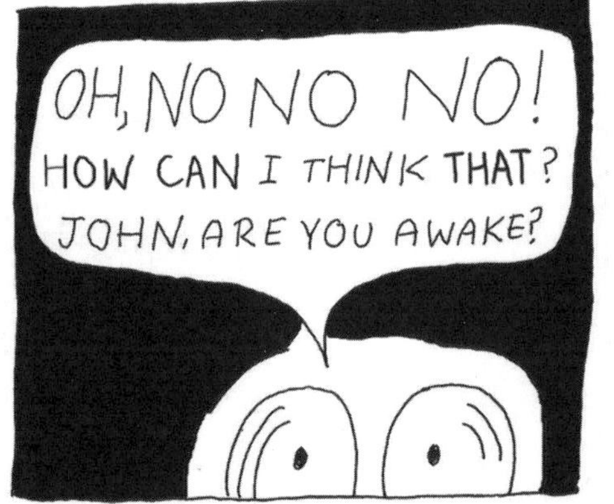
OH, NO NO NO! HOW CAN I THINK THAT? JOHN, ARE YOU AWAKE?

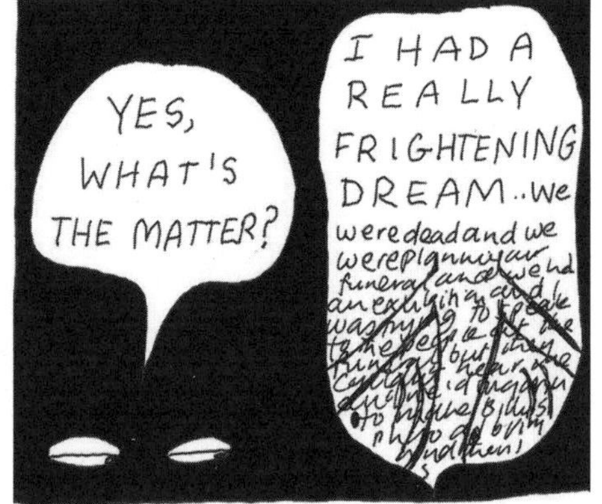
YES, WHAT'S THE MATTER?
I HAD A REALLY FRIGHTENING DREAM..we were dead and we

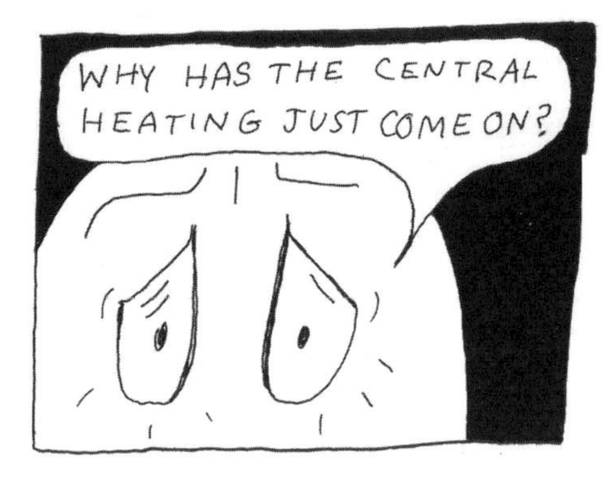
WHY HAS THE CENTRAL HEATING JUST COME ON?

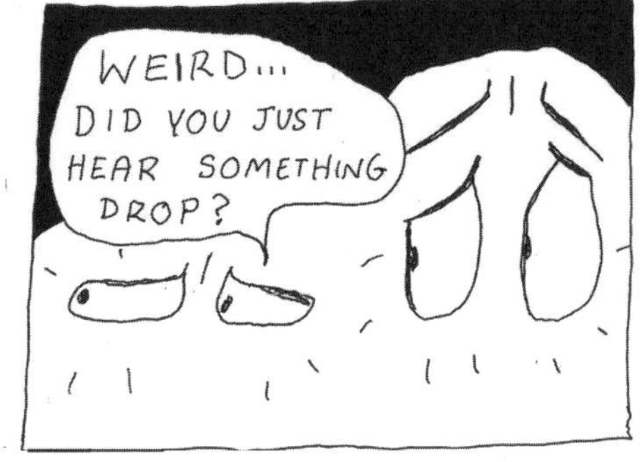
WEIRD... DID YOU JUST HEAR SOMETHING DROP?

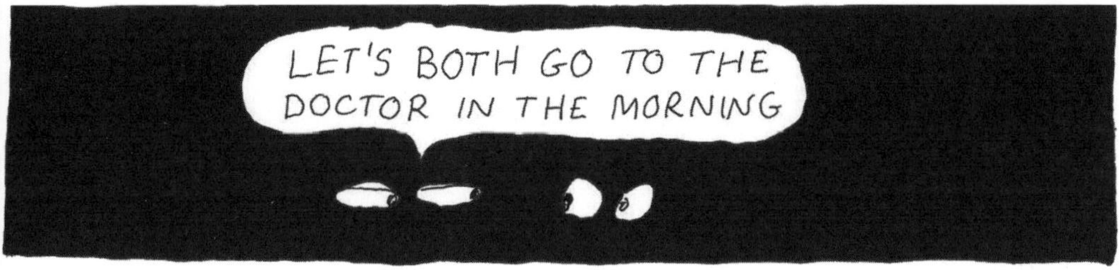

LET'S BOTH GO TO THE
DOCTOR IN THE MORNING

I CONTINUED TO TALK OPENLY TO FRIENDS ABOUT MY EXPERIENCE, SO I SUPPOSE I SHOULDN'T HAVE BEEN SURPRISED BY **THEM** TALKING OPENLY TO ME ABOUT MY EXPERIENCE ... BUT SOMETIMES I WAS...

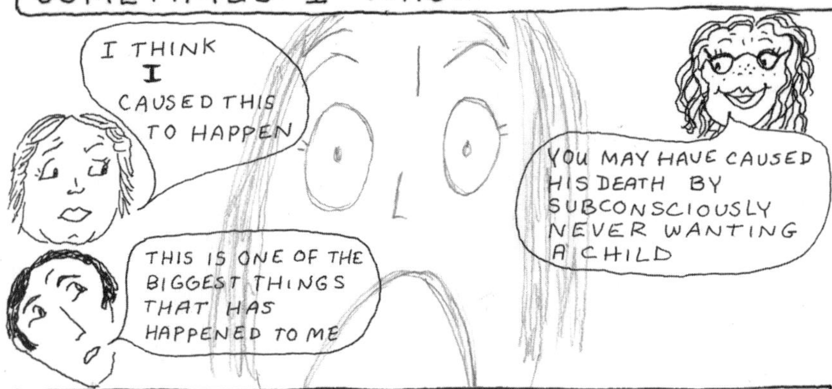
I THINK **I** CAUSED THIS TO HAPPEN
THIS IS ONE OF THE BIGGEST THINGS THAT HAS HAPPENED TO ME
YOU MAY HAVE CAUSED HIS DEATH BY SUBCONSCIOUSLY NEVER WANTING A CHILD

SO WHEN I STARTED TO SEE "MY" THERAPIST, I HAD PLENTY TO UNLOAD.

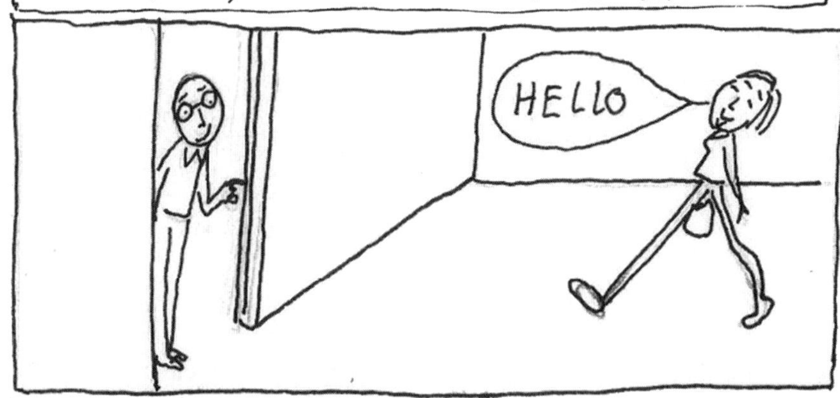
HELLO

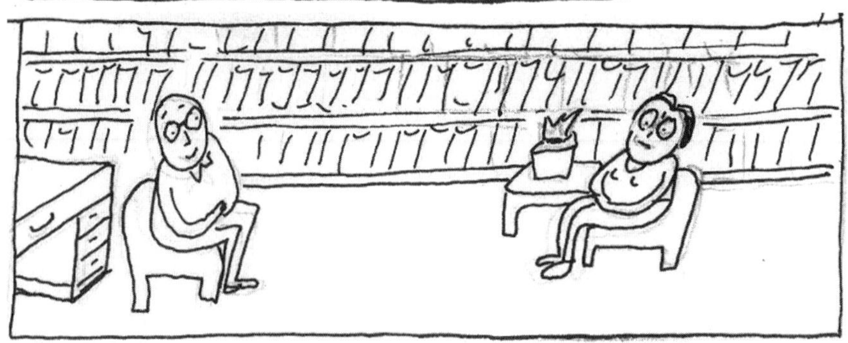

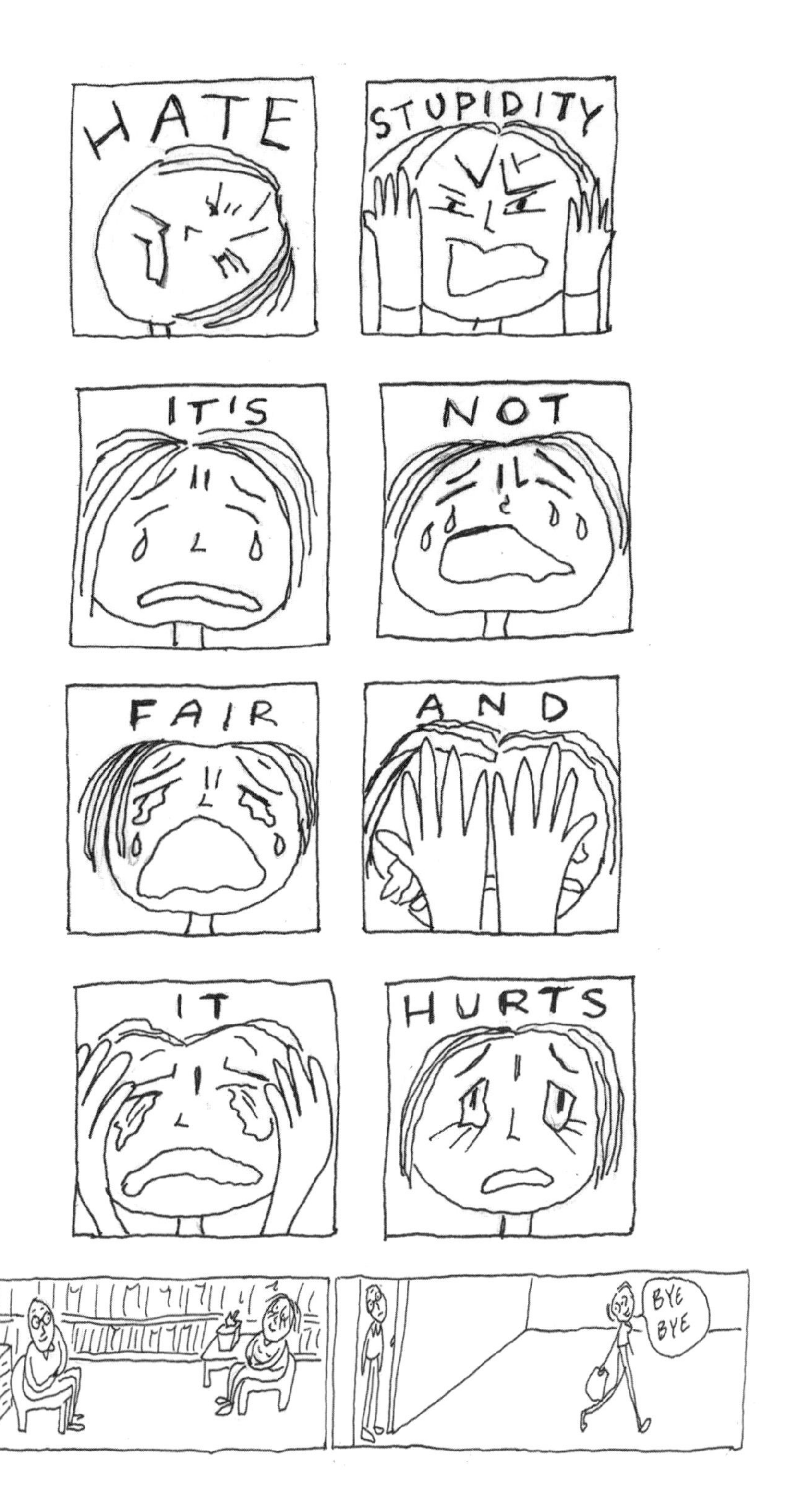
HATE
STUPIDITY
IT'S
NOT
FAIR
AND
IT
HURTS
BYE BYE

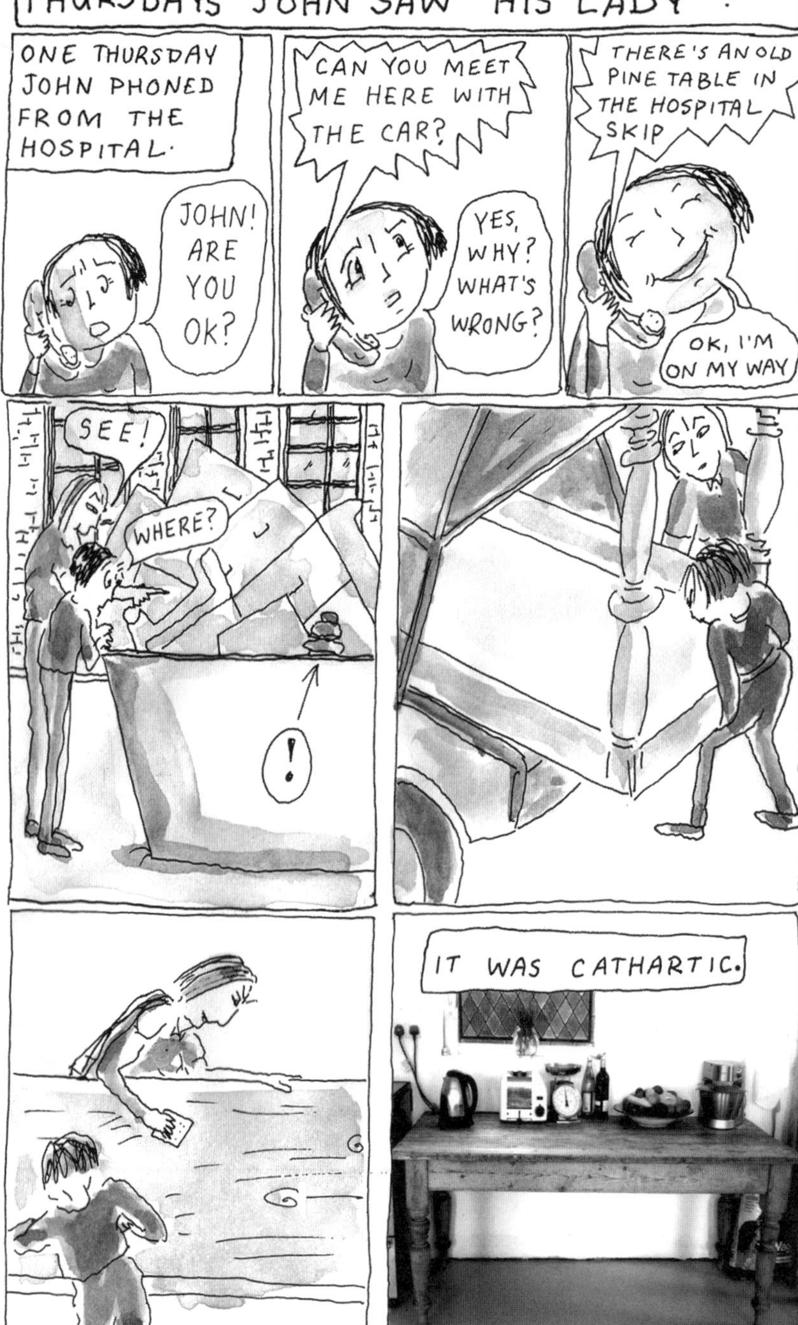
ON TUESDAYS I SAW "MY MAN" AND ON THURSDAYS JOHN SAW "HIS LADY".
ONE THURSDAY JOHN PHONED FROM THE HOSPITAL.
JOHN! ARE YOU OK?
CAN YOU MEET ME HERE WITH THE CAR?
YES, WHY? WHAT'S WRONG?
THERE'S AN OLD PINE TABLE IN THE HOSPITAL SKIP
OK, I'M ON MY WAY
SEE!
WHERE?
!
IT WAS CATHARTIC.

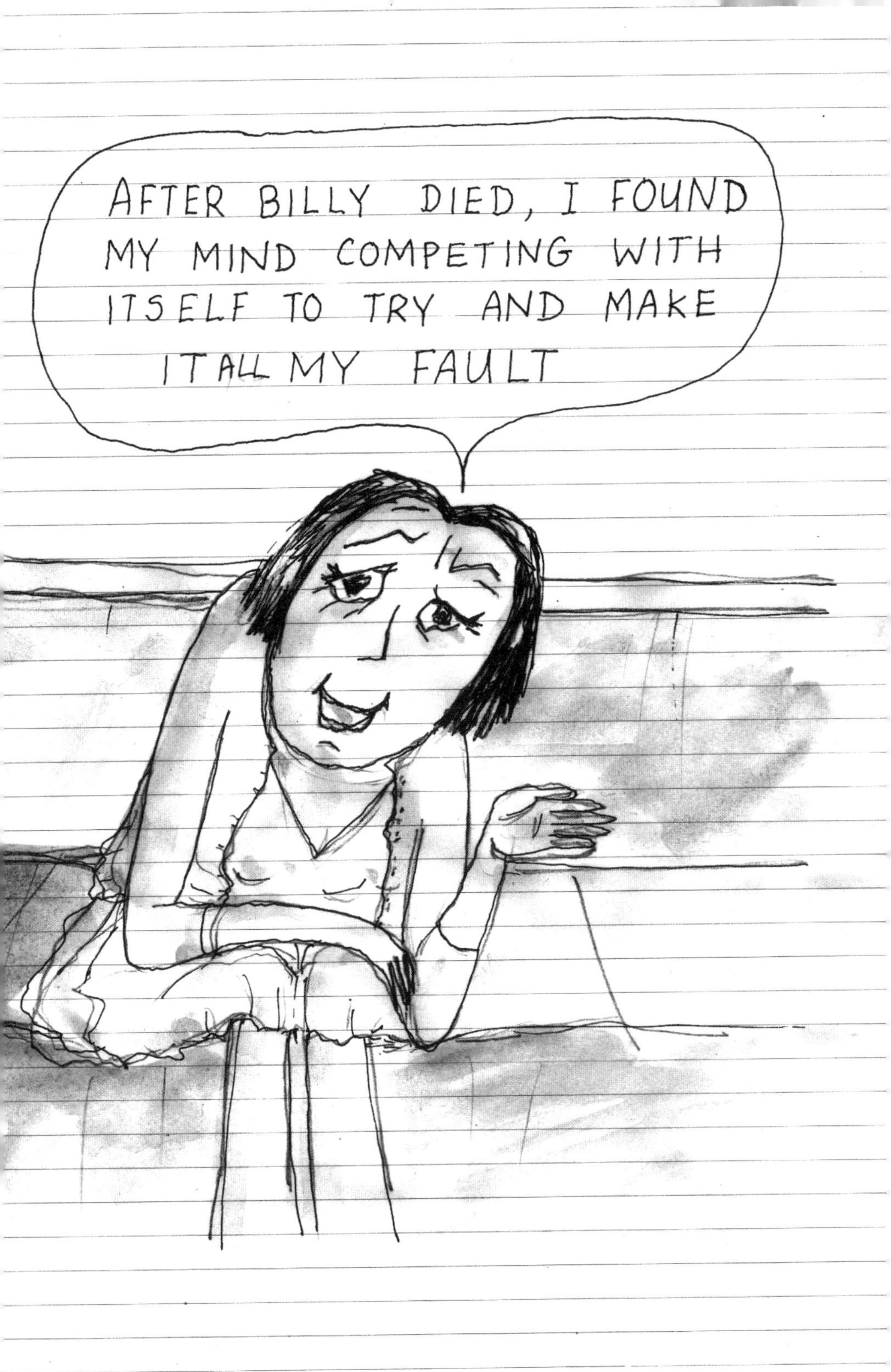
AFTER BILLY DIED, I FOUND MY MIND COMPETING WITH ITSELF TO TRY AND MAKE IT ALL MY FAULT

Wed	Thu	Fri	Sat	Sun	Mon	Tue	Wed	Thu	Fri	Sat	Sun	Mon	Tue	Wed	Thu	Fri	Sat	Sun	Mon	Tue	Wed	Thu	Fri	Sat	Sun	Mon
1	2	3	4	5	6	7	8	9	10	11	12	13	14	15	16	17	18	19	20	21	22	23	24	25	26	27

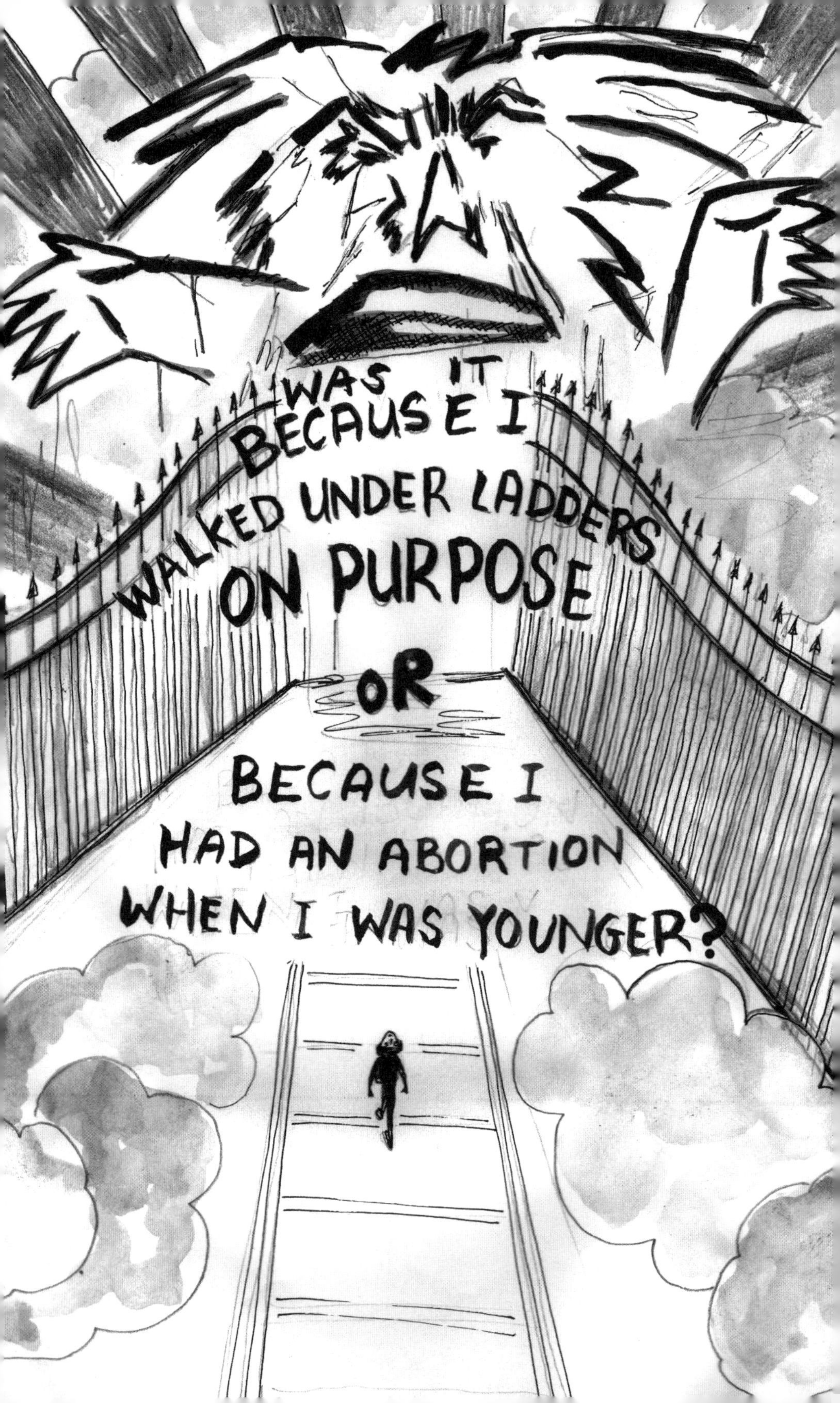
WAS IT
BECAUSE I
WALKED UNDER LADDERS
ON PURPOSE
OR
BECAUSE I
HAD AN ABORTION
WHEN I WAS YOUNGER?

IT MUST BE RETRIBUTION FOR MY SMUGNESS AND FOR NOT SEEING HOW **LUCKY I WAS.**

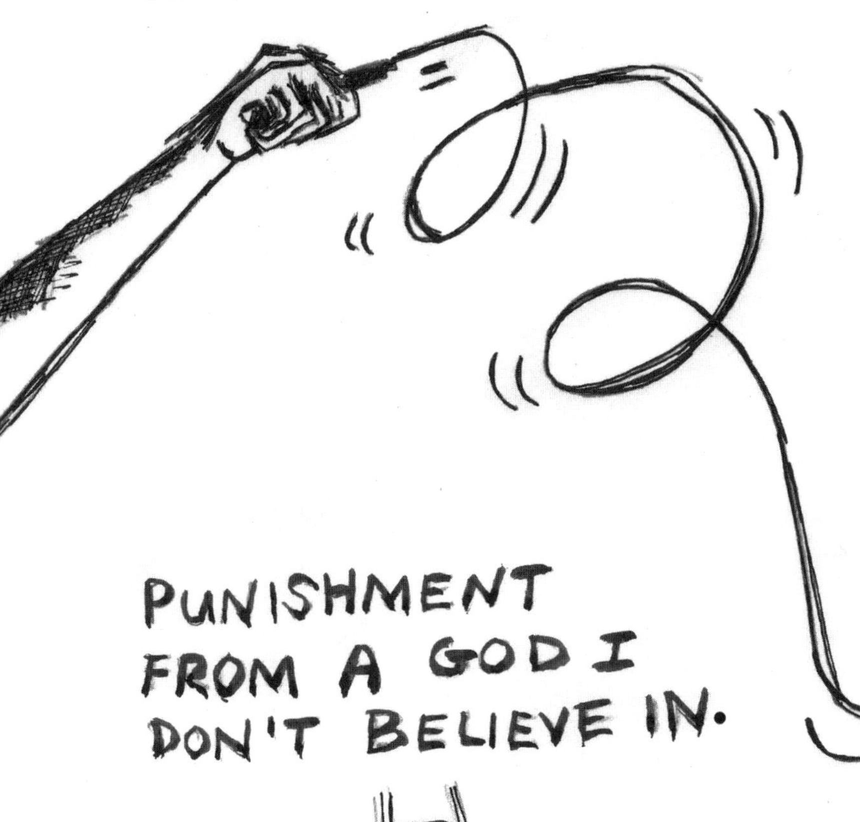

PUNISHMENT FROM A GOD I DON'T BELIEVE IN.

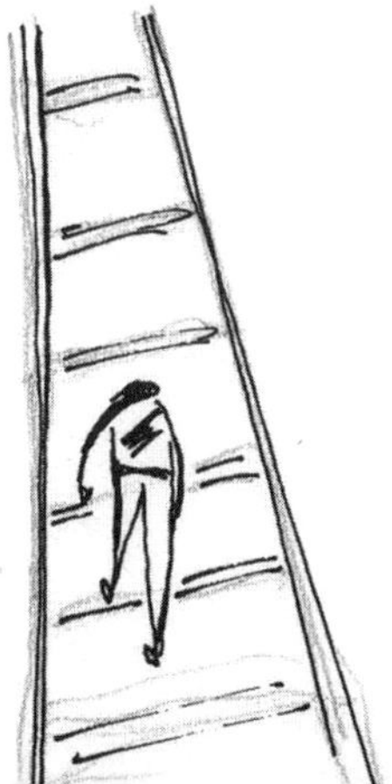

SOON AFTER BILLY DIED, JOHN AND I WENT TO MARIE'S PARTY.
IT SEEMED LIKE EVERYONE WAS PREGNANT.

I'M 8 WEEKS! I'VE BOOKED A PLACE IN THE NURSERY AT WORK

CONGRATULATIONS

SHE CAN'T—IT'S NOT FAIR! MAYBE IF HER BABY COULD DIE JUST FOR A BIT...OH, WHAT AM I THINKING?

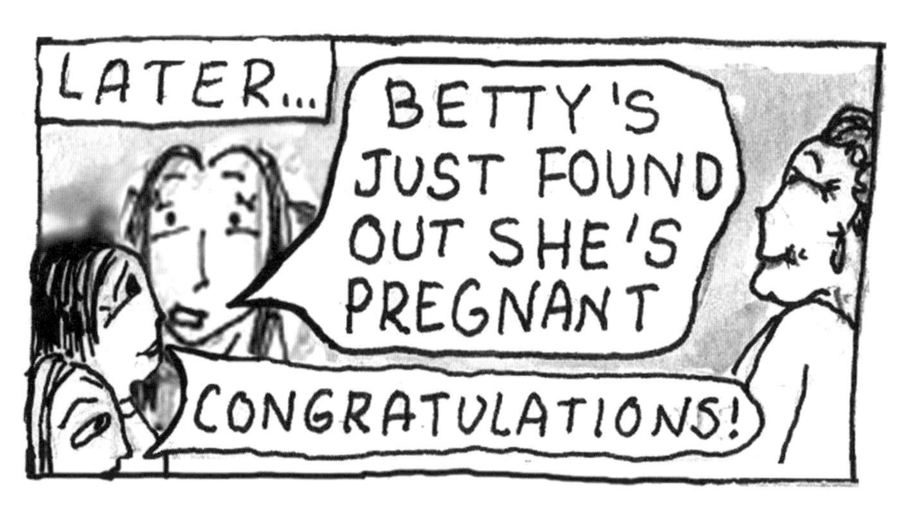
LATER...
BETTY'S JUST FOUND OUT SHE'S PREGNANT
CONGRATULATIONS!

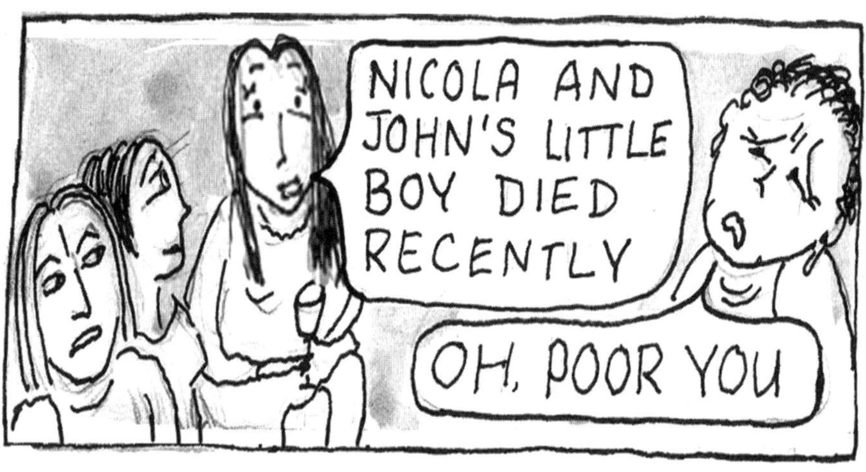
NICOLA AND JOHN'S LITTLE BOY DIED RECENTLY
OH, POOR YOU

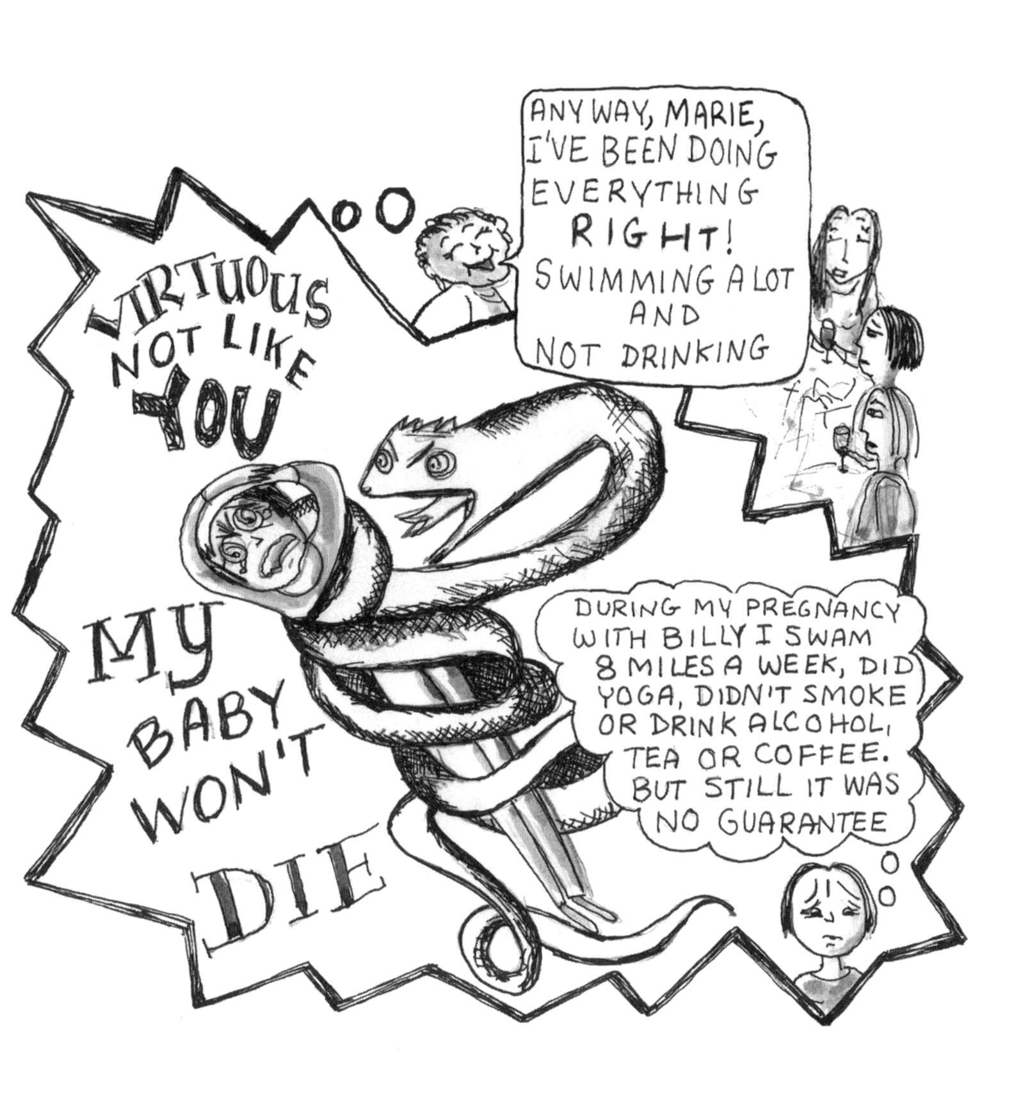

ANY WAY, MARIE, I'VE BEEN DOING EVERYTHING RIGHT! SWIMMING A LOT AND NOT DRINKING
VIRTUOUS NOT LIKE YOU
MY BABY WON'T DIE
DURING MY PREGNANCY WITH BILLY I SWAM 8 MILES A WEEK, DID YOGA, DIDN'T SMOKE OR DRINK ALCOHOL, TEA OR COFFEE. BUT STILL IT WAS NO GUARANTEE

HAD I BEEN A BAD PARENT? WAS THAT IT?

I REMEMBERED HOW MY LIFE HAD BEEN.

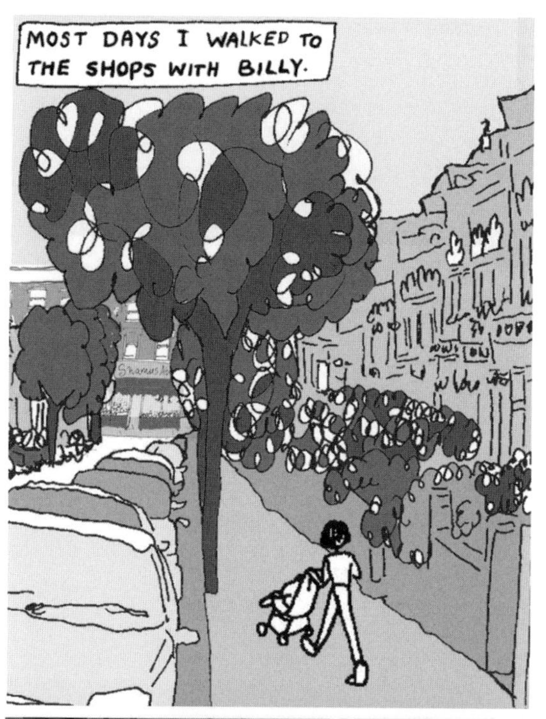
MOST DAYS I WALKED TO THE SHOPS WITH BILLY.

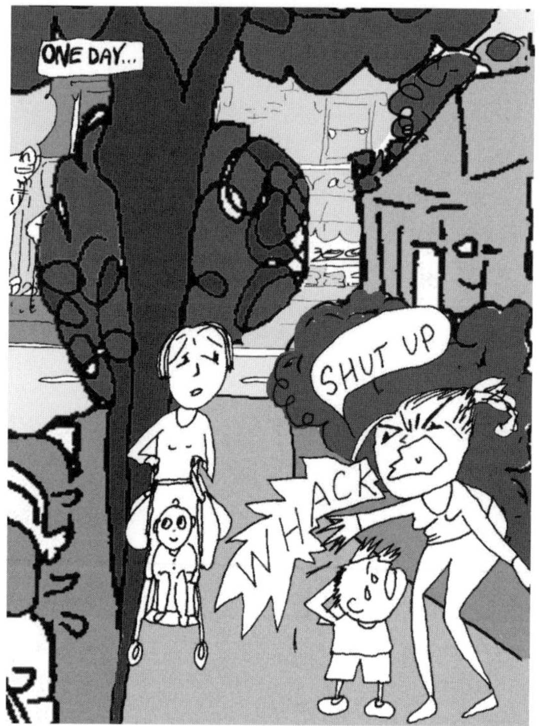
ONE DAY...
SHUT UP
WHACK

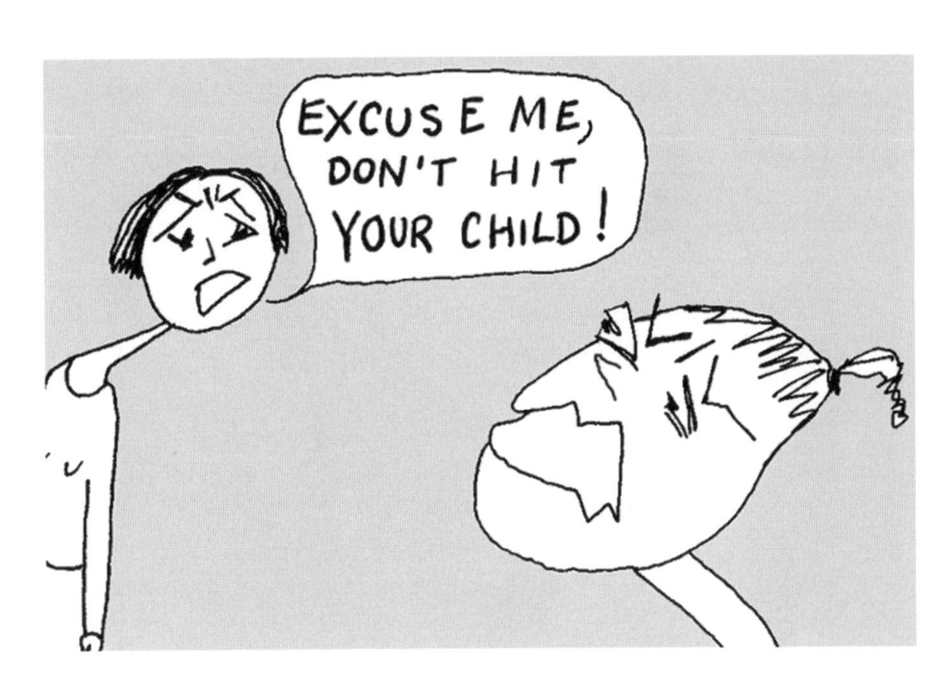
EXCUSE ME, DON'T HIT YOUR CHILD!

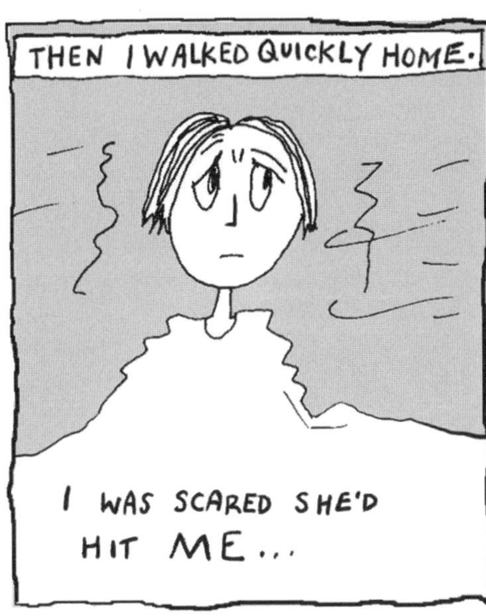
THEN I WALKED QUICKLY HOME.
I WAS SCARED SHE'D HIT ME...

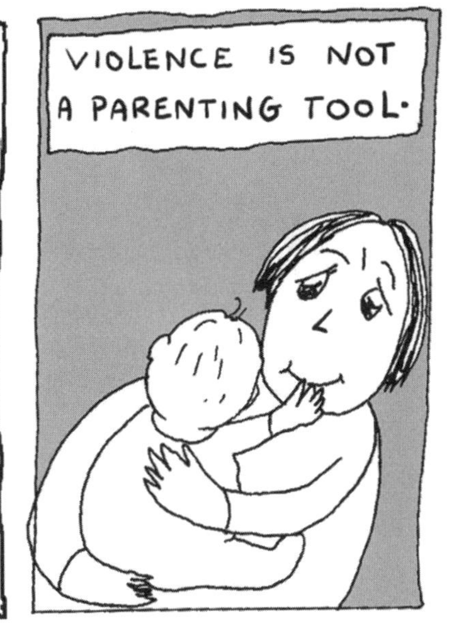
VIOLENCE IS NOT A PARENTING TOOL.

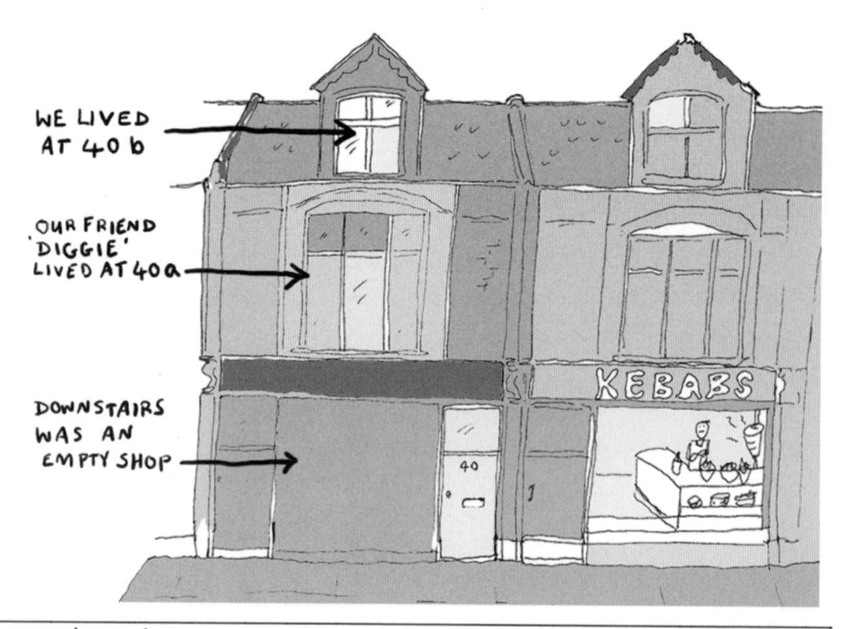
WE LIVED AT 40b
OUR FRIEND 'DIGGIE' LIVED AT 40a
DOWNSTAIRS WAS AN EMPTY SHOP
KEBABS
40

OUR LANDLORD WAS KIND AND FAIR. HE GOT DEPRESSION AND OFTEN SKIPPED HIS MEDICATION BECAUSE IT NUMBED HIM TOO MUCH.

HE DECIDED TO TURN THE EMPTY SHOP DOWNSTAIRS INTO A CHARITY SHOP.

ON HIS GOOD DAYS HE ENJOYED DRESSING UP IN THE DONATED CLOTHES.

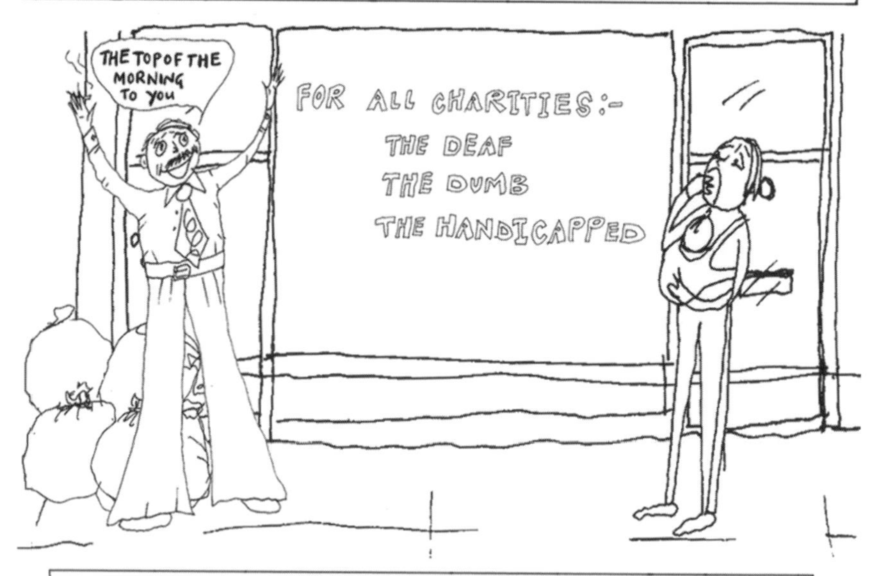
THE TOP OF THE MORNING TO YOU
FOR ALL CHARITIES:-
THE DEAF
THE DUMB
THE HANDICAPPED

SUDDENLY HE WENT TO VISIT FAMILY IN IRELAND AND NEVER RETURNED.

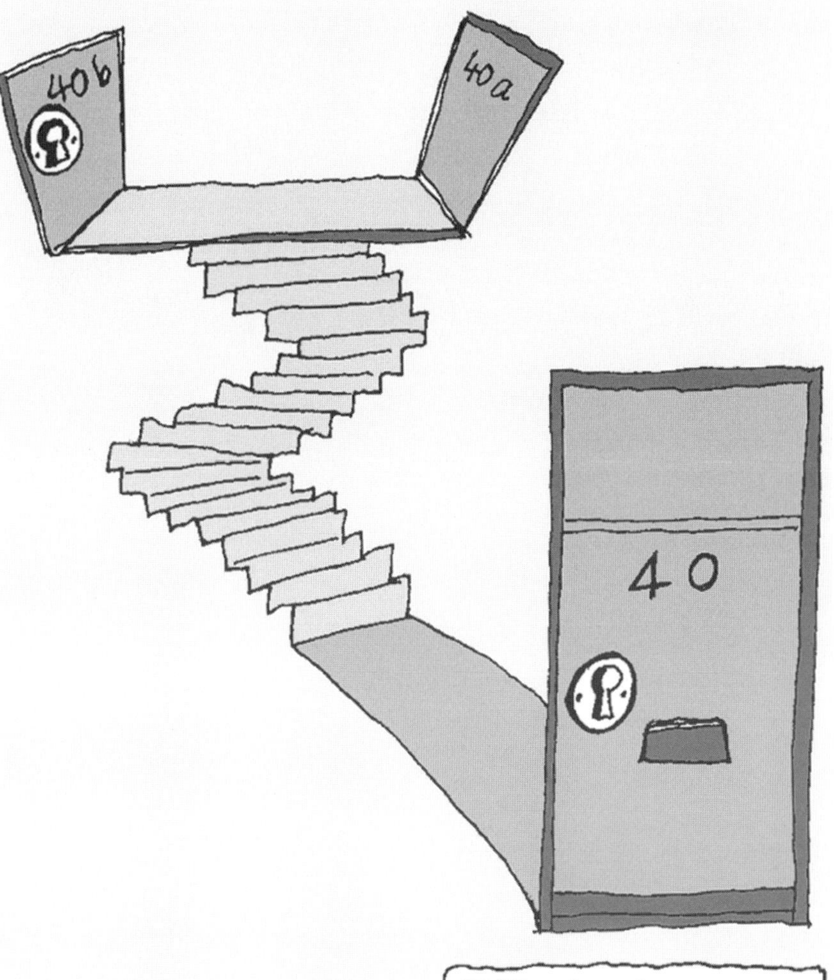
TO LEAVE THE BUILDING WE HAD TO UNLOCK TWO DOORS FROM THE INSIDE.
40b
40a
40
ONE DAY I FORGOT MY KEYS...

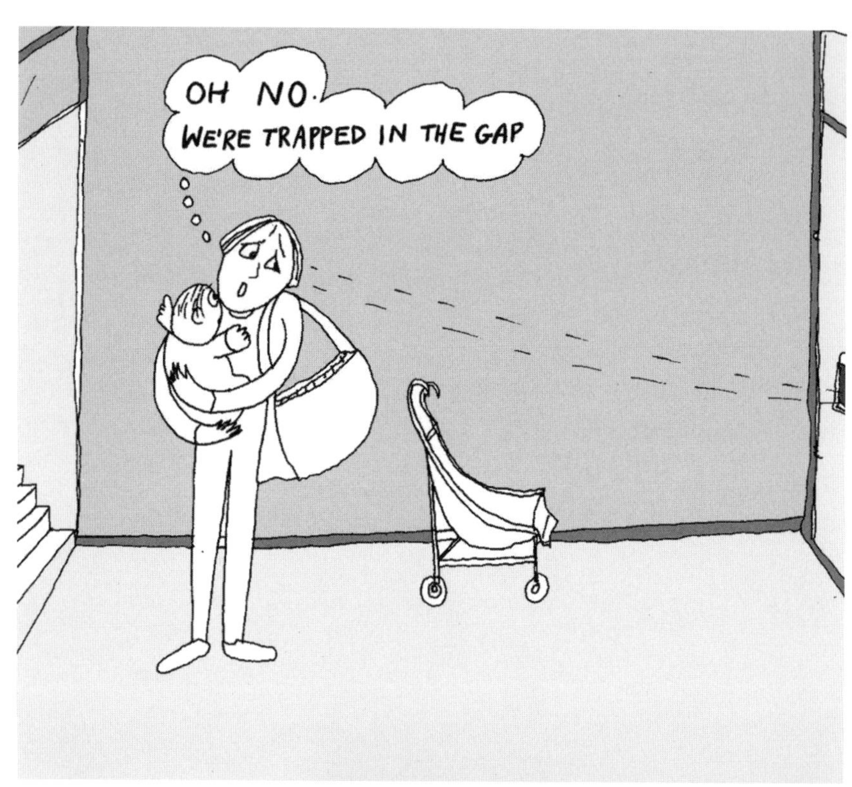
OH NO.
WE'RE TRAPPED IN THE GAP

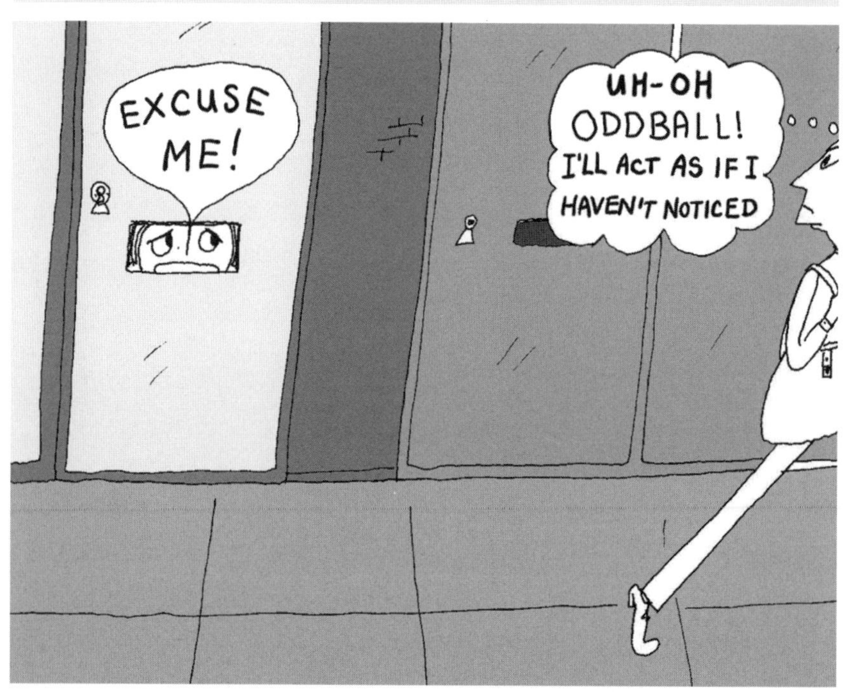
EXCUSE ME!
UH-OH ODDBALL! I'LL ACT AS IF I HAVEN'T NOTICED

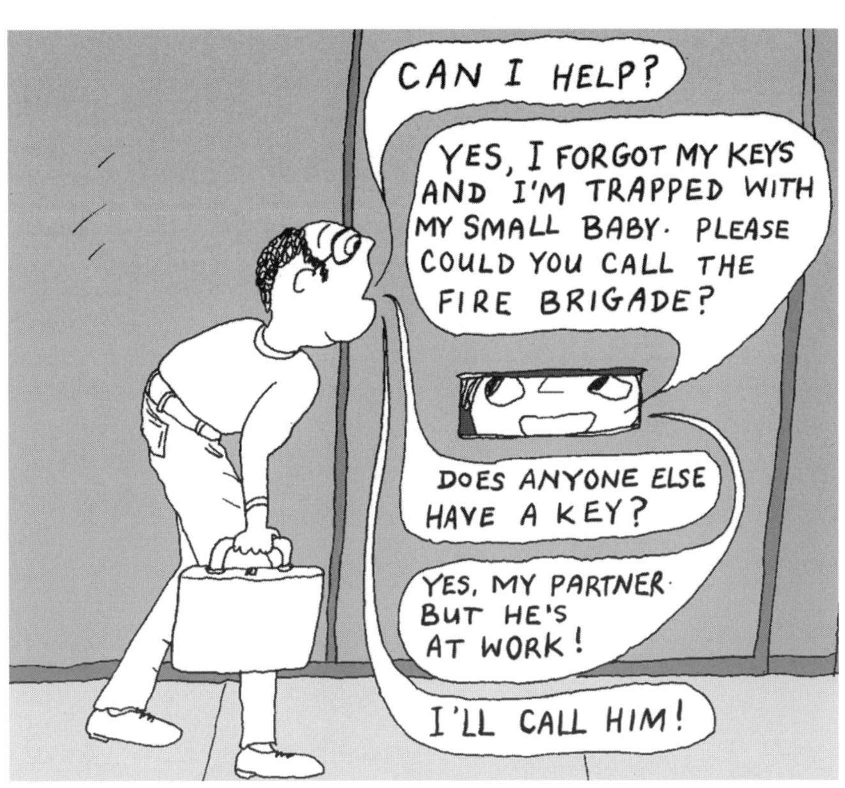
CAN I HELP?
YES, I FORGOT MY KEYS AND I'M TRAPPED WITH MY SMALL BABY. PLEASE COULD YOU CALL THE FIRE BRIGADE?
DOES ANYONE ELSE HAVE A KEY?
YES, MY PARTNER. BUT HE'S AT WORK!
I'LL CALL HIM!

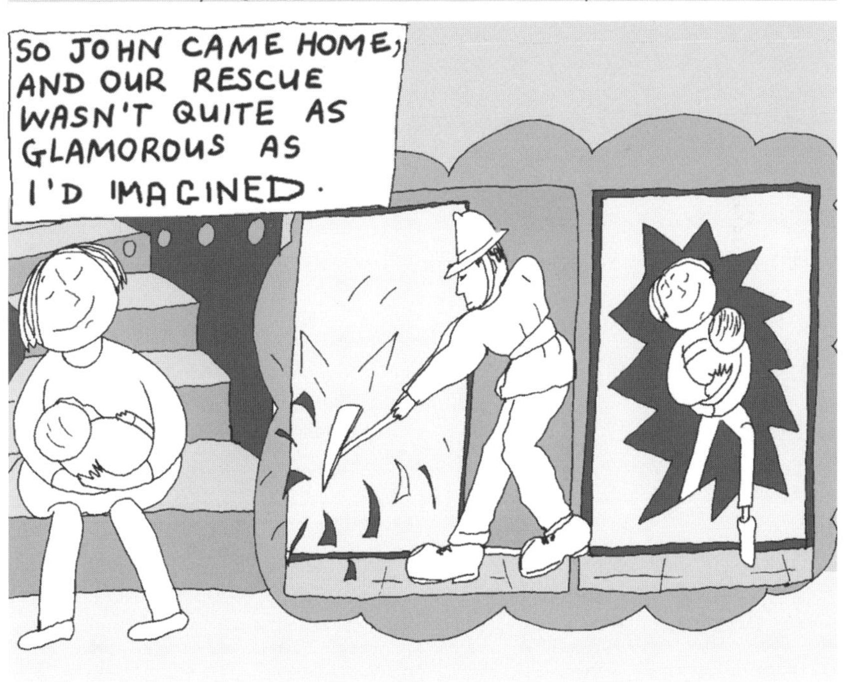
SO JOHN CAME HOME, AND OUR RESCUE WASN'T QUITE AS GLAMOROUS AS I'D IMAGINED.

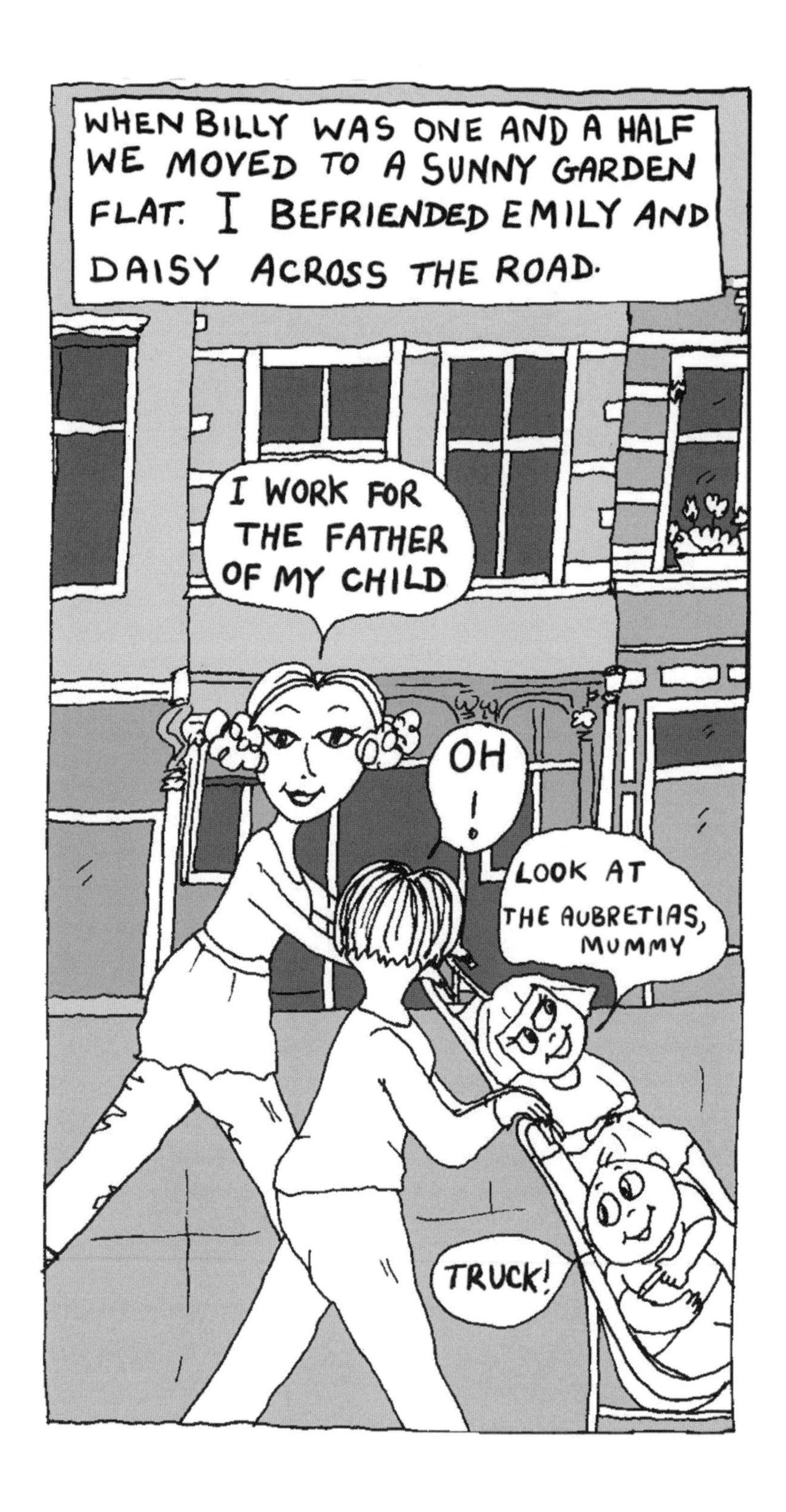
WHEN BILLY WAS ONE AND A HALF WE MOVED TO A SUNNY GARDEN FLAT. I BEFRIENDED EMILY AND DAISY ACROSS THE ROAD.
I WORK FOR THE FATHER OF MY CHILD
OH!
LOOK AT THE AUBRETIAS, MUMMY
TRUCK!

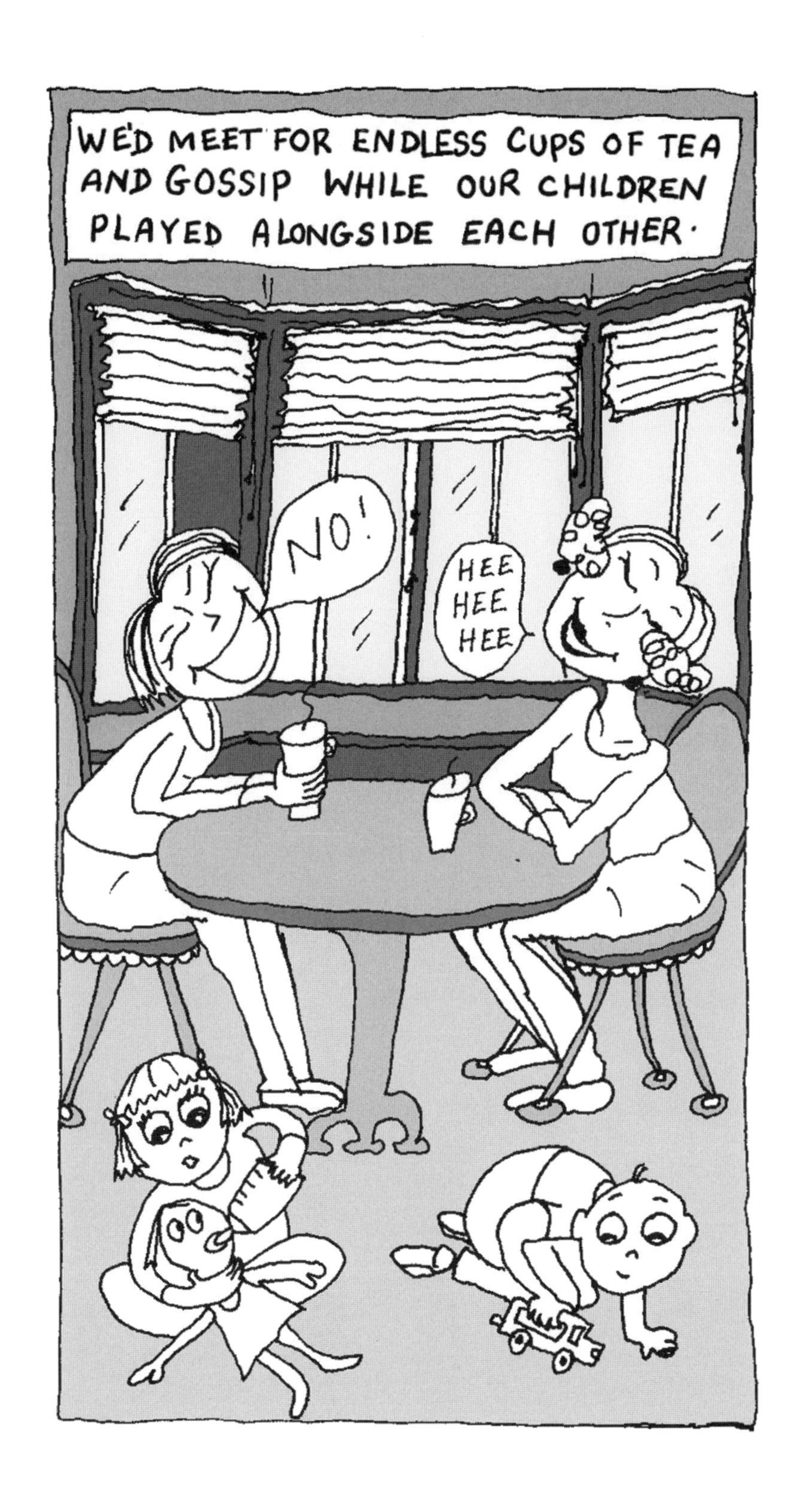
WE'D MEET FOR ENDLESS CUPS OF TEA AND GOSSIP WHILE OUR CHILDREN PLAYED ALONGSIDE EACH OTHER.
NO!
HEE HEE HEE

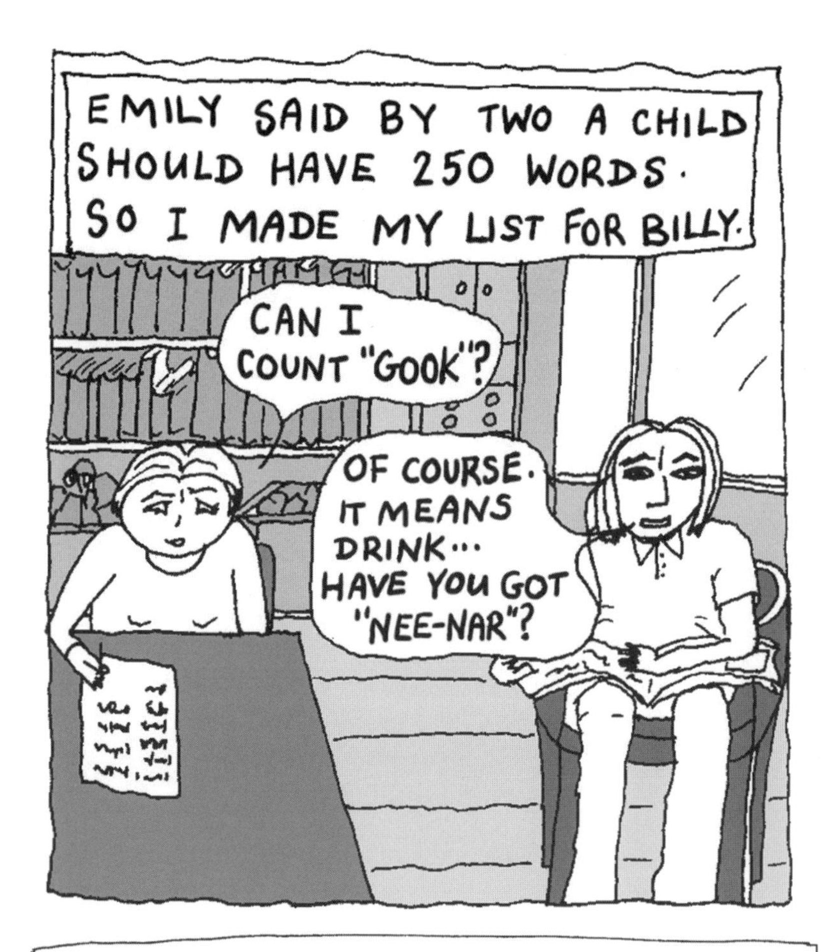
EMILY SAID BY TWO A CHILD SHOULD HAVE 250 WORDS. SO I MADE MY LIST FOR BILLY.
CAN I COUNT "GOOK"?
OF COURSE. IT MEANS DRINK... HAVE YOU GOT "NEE-NAR"?

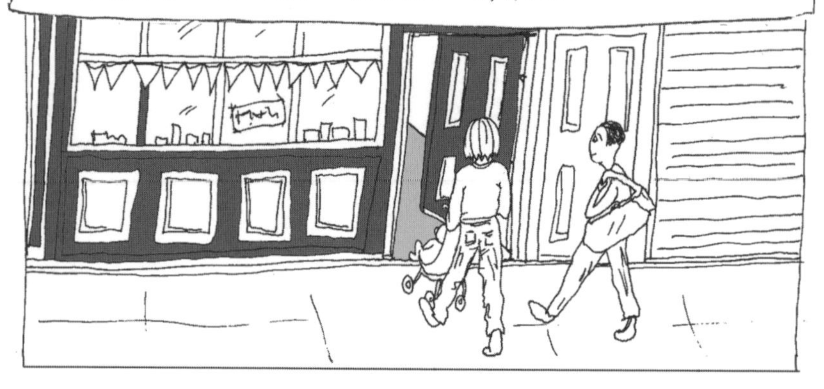
AT WEEKENDS WE WENT TO ART GALLERIES. ONE SUNDAY WE WENT TO SEE A TEMPORARY "ART SHOP" SET UP BY TWO ARTISTS NEAR BRICK LANE.

The Calling of St Anthony

Integrity
Dignity
Humour
Teeth
Hair
Heart
Love
Temper
Grip
Life
Vision
Souls
Kidneys
Eyes
Limbs
Mind
Sight
Truth
Fortune
Faith
Friendship
Health
Home
Confidence
Taste
Smell
Way
Strength
Skill
Passion
Honour
White cells
Red cells
Self respect
Magic
Cool
Marbles
etc. etc.

The patron saint of all things lost

THEY WERE SELLING THEIR WORKS FOR JUST A FEW POUNDS. WE BOUGHT THIS TEXT PIECE BY TRACEY EMIN.

THE NEXT TIME I CAME ACROSS THAT ARTWORK WAS ON THE DAY BILLY DIED.

I arrived home with a splitting headache...

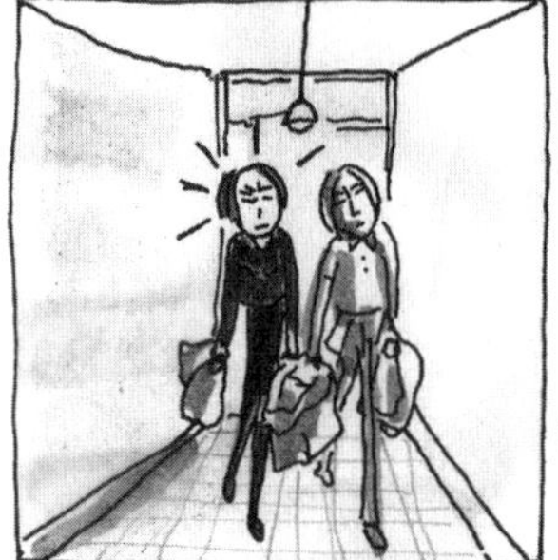

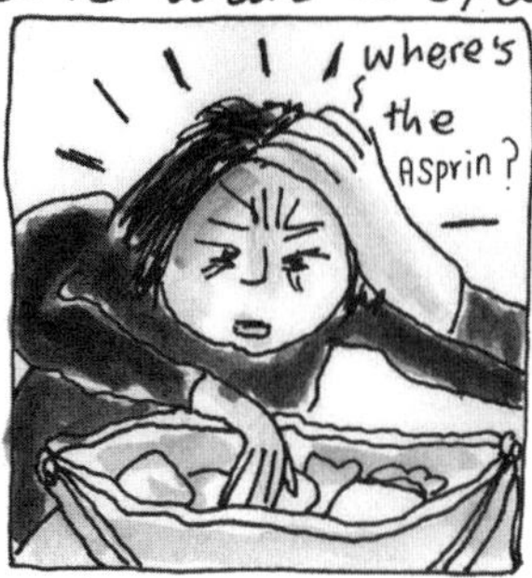

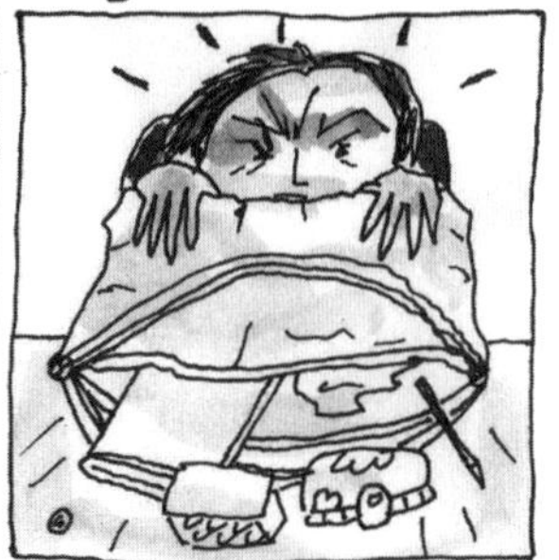

... why do some people say they've "lost" someone...

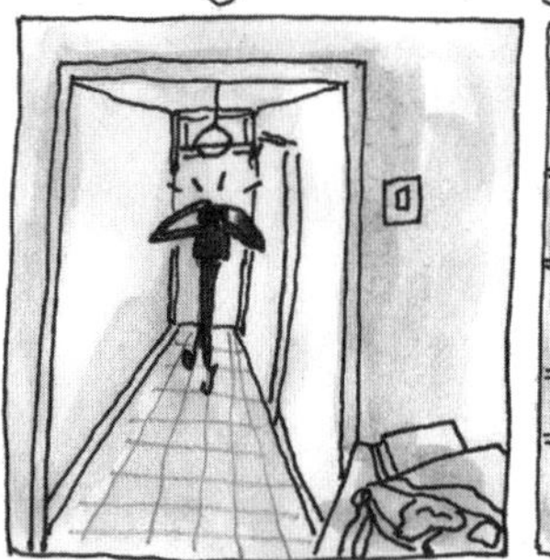

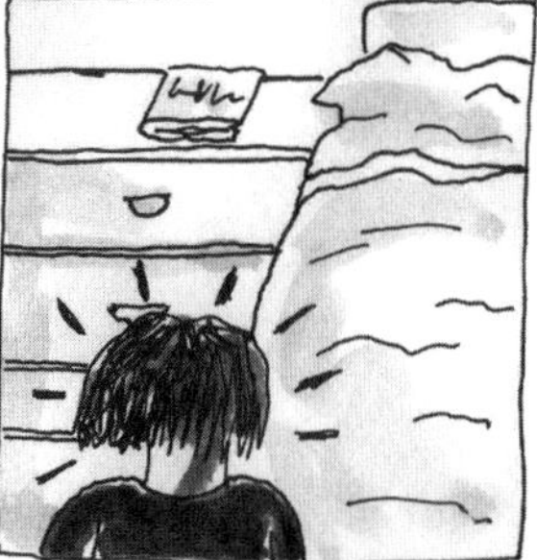

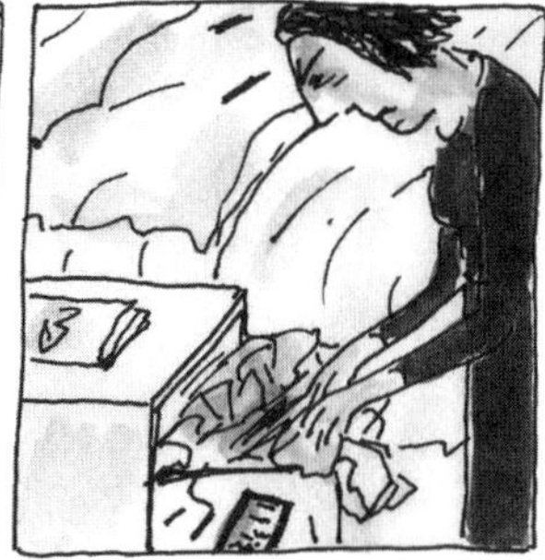

when they mean that person is DEAD?

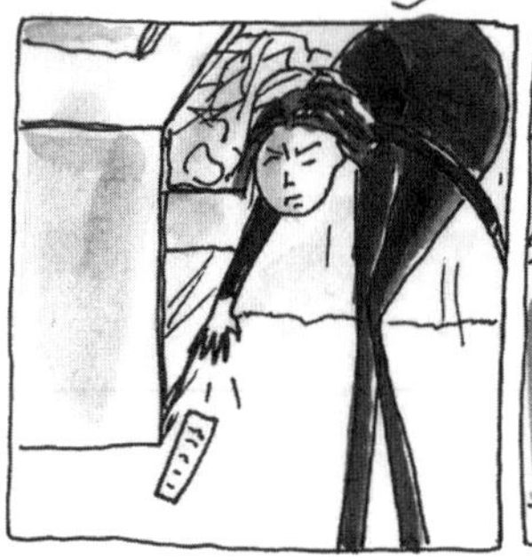

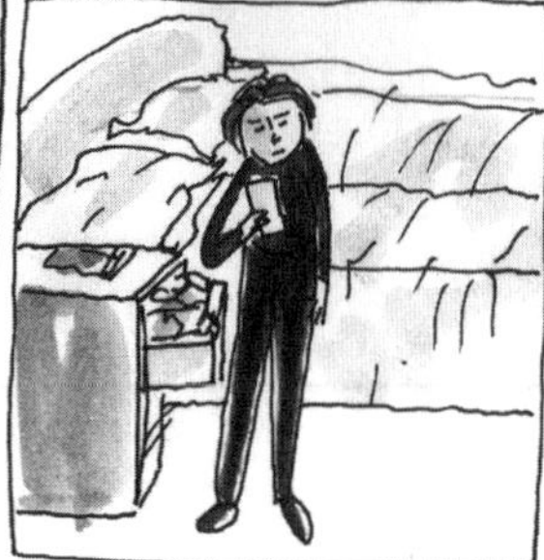

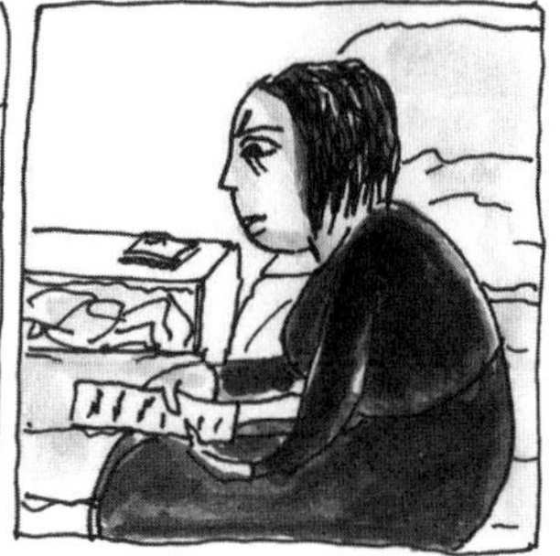

BILLY WASN'T "LOST", HE WAS
DEAD. IT WAS JOHN AND I... AS
THE PEOPLE WE'D BEEN
JUST ONE DAY BEFORE...
WHO WERE NOW LOST
FOR EVER (but not dead)

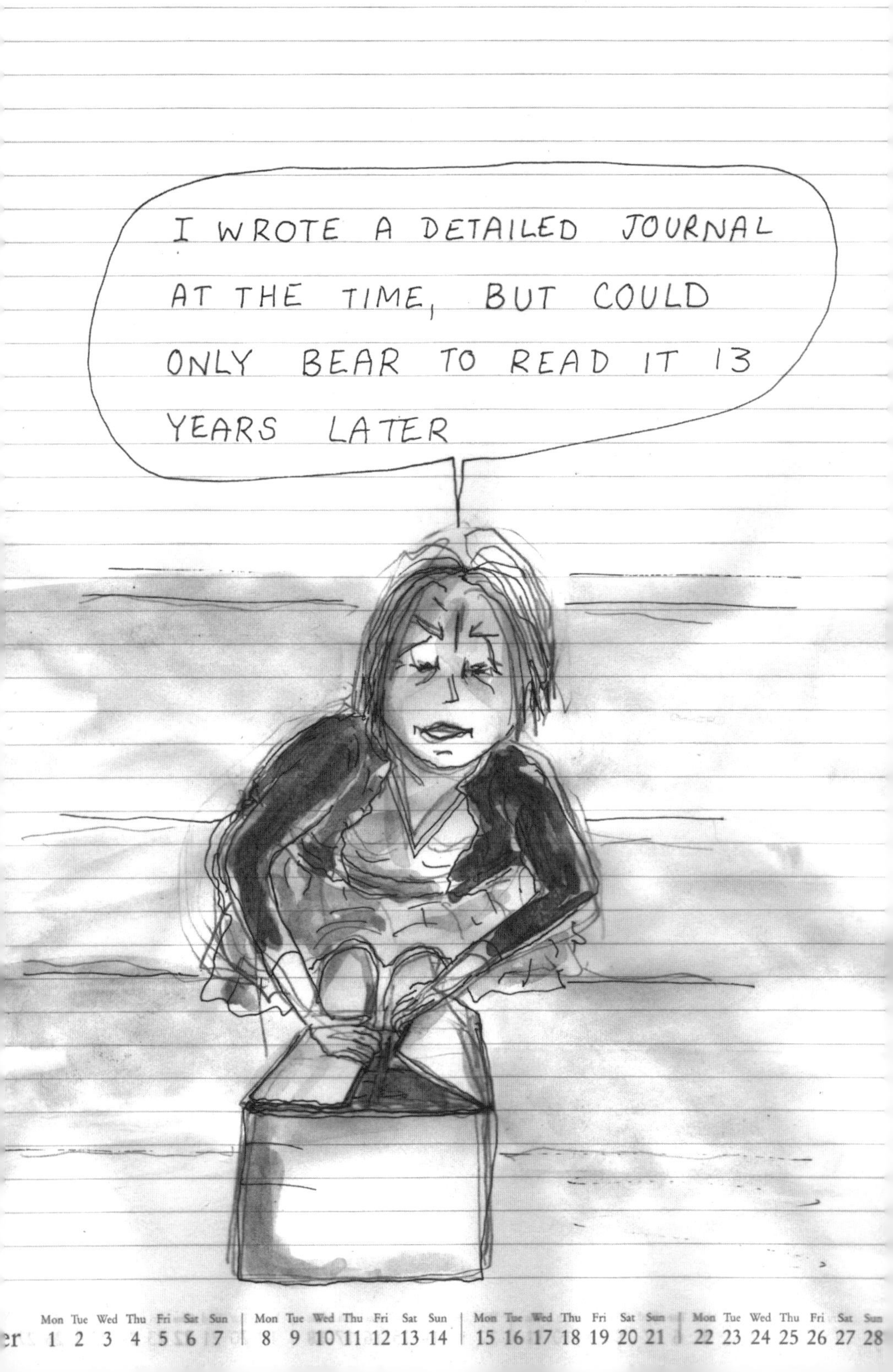
I WROTE A DETAILED JOURNAL AT THE TIME, BUT COULD ONLY BEAR TO READ IT 13 YEARS LATER
Mon Tue Wed Thu Fri Sat Sun Mon Tue Wed Thu Fri Sat Sun Mon Tue Wed Thu Fri Sat Sun Mon Tue Wed Thu Fri Sat Sun
1 2 3 4 5 6 7 8 9 10 11 12 13 14 15 16 17 18 19 20 21 22 23 24 25 26 27 28

IT WASN'T JUST THE JOURNAL. WE HAD CREATED AN ARCHIVE OF OBJECTS AND WRITINGS. LATER THESE BECAME PROMPTS FOR THE TELLING OF OUR STORY.

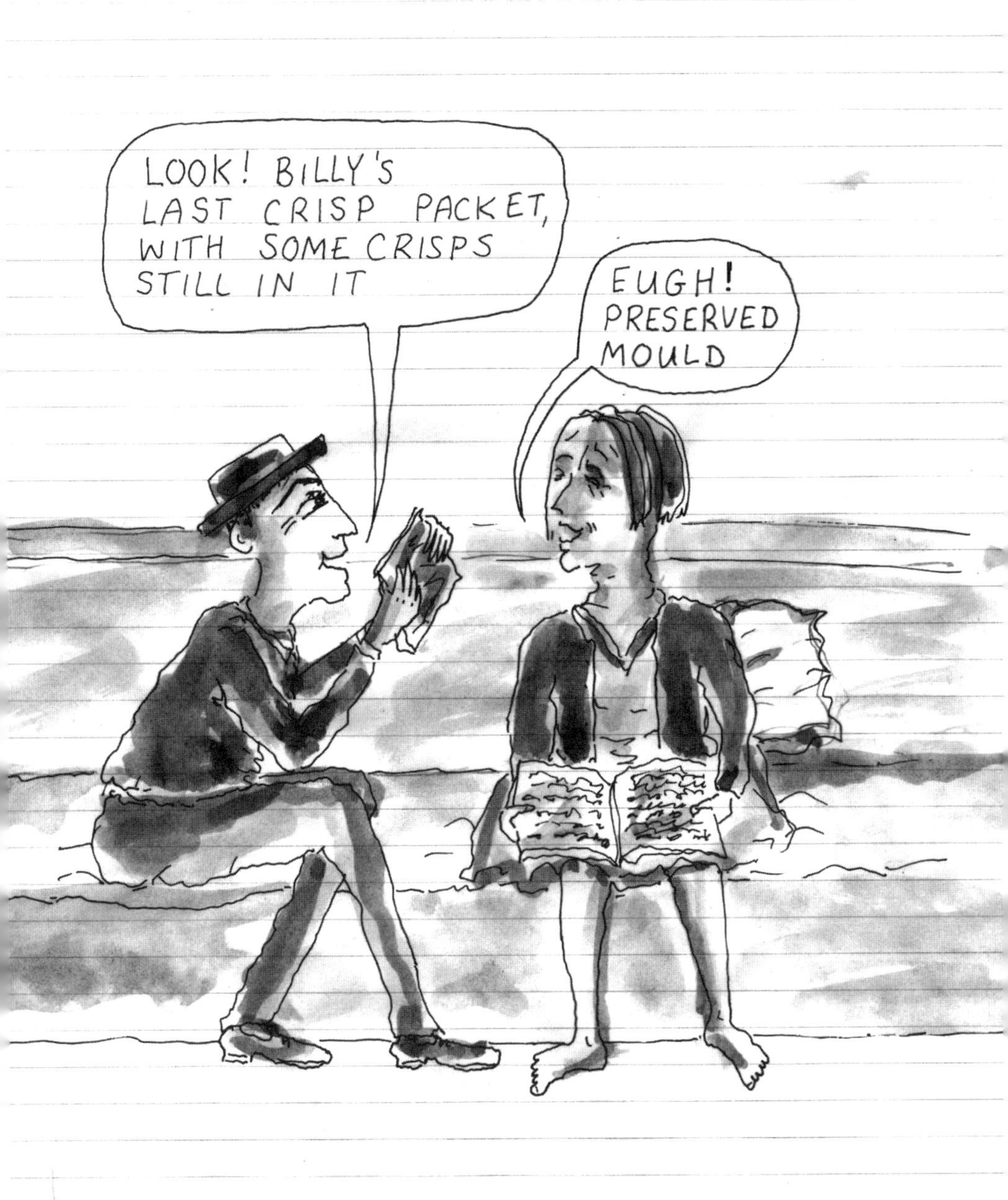
LOOK! BILLY'S LAST CRISP PACKET, WITH SOME CRISPS STILL IN IT
EUGH! PRESERVED MOULD

Wed Thu Fri Sat Sun | Mon Tue Wed Thu Fri Sat Sun | Mon Tue Wed Thu Fri Sat Sun | Mon Tue Wed Thu Fri Sat Sun | Mon Tue We
3 4 5 6 7 | 8 9 10 11 12 13 14 | 15 16 17 18 19 20 21 | 22 23 24 25 26 27 28 | 29 30 31

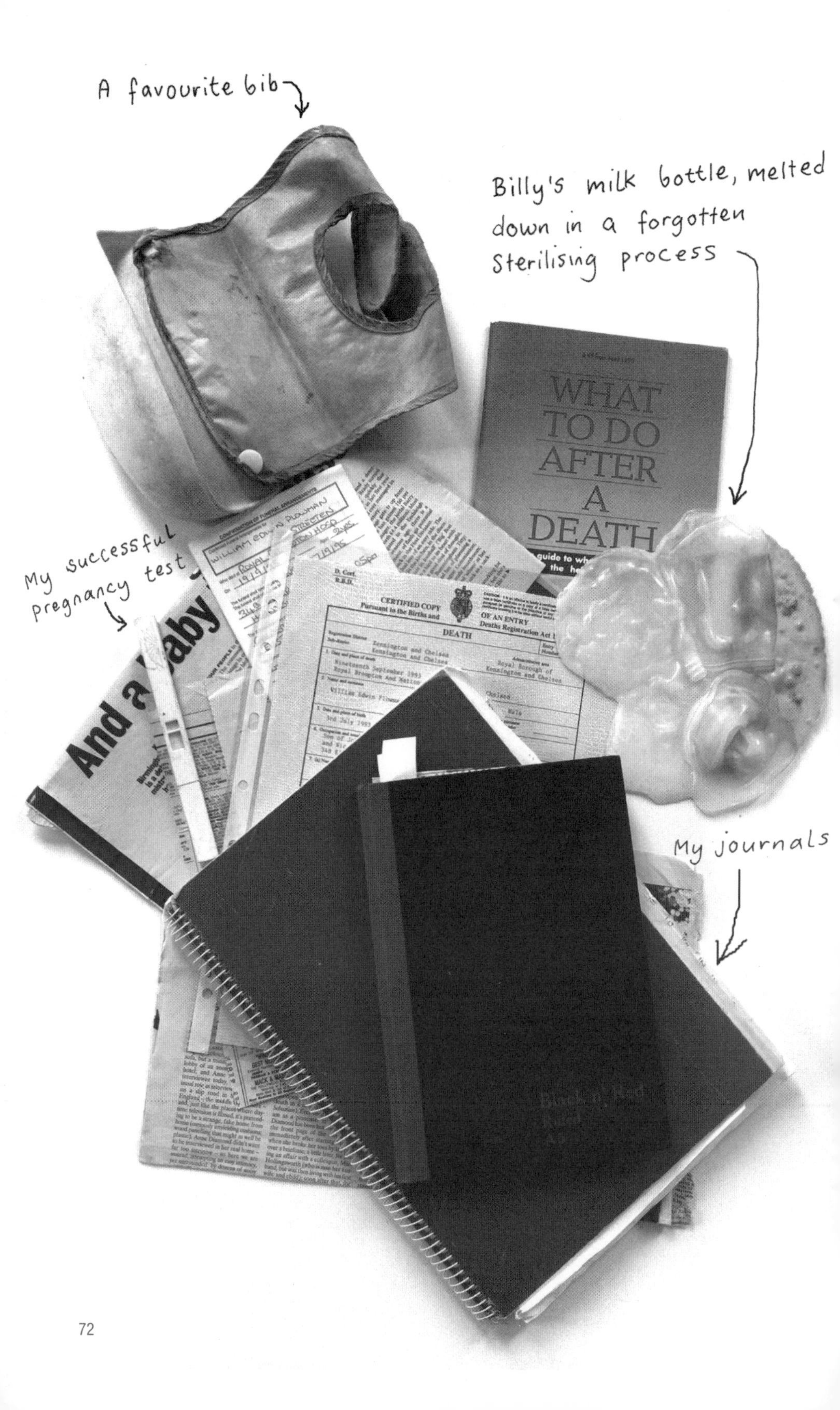

A favourite bib
Billy's milk bottle, melted down in a forgotten sterilising process
WHAT TO DO AFTER A DEATH
My successful pregnancy test
CERTIFIED COPY
DEATH
My journals

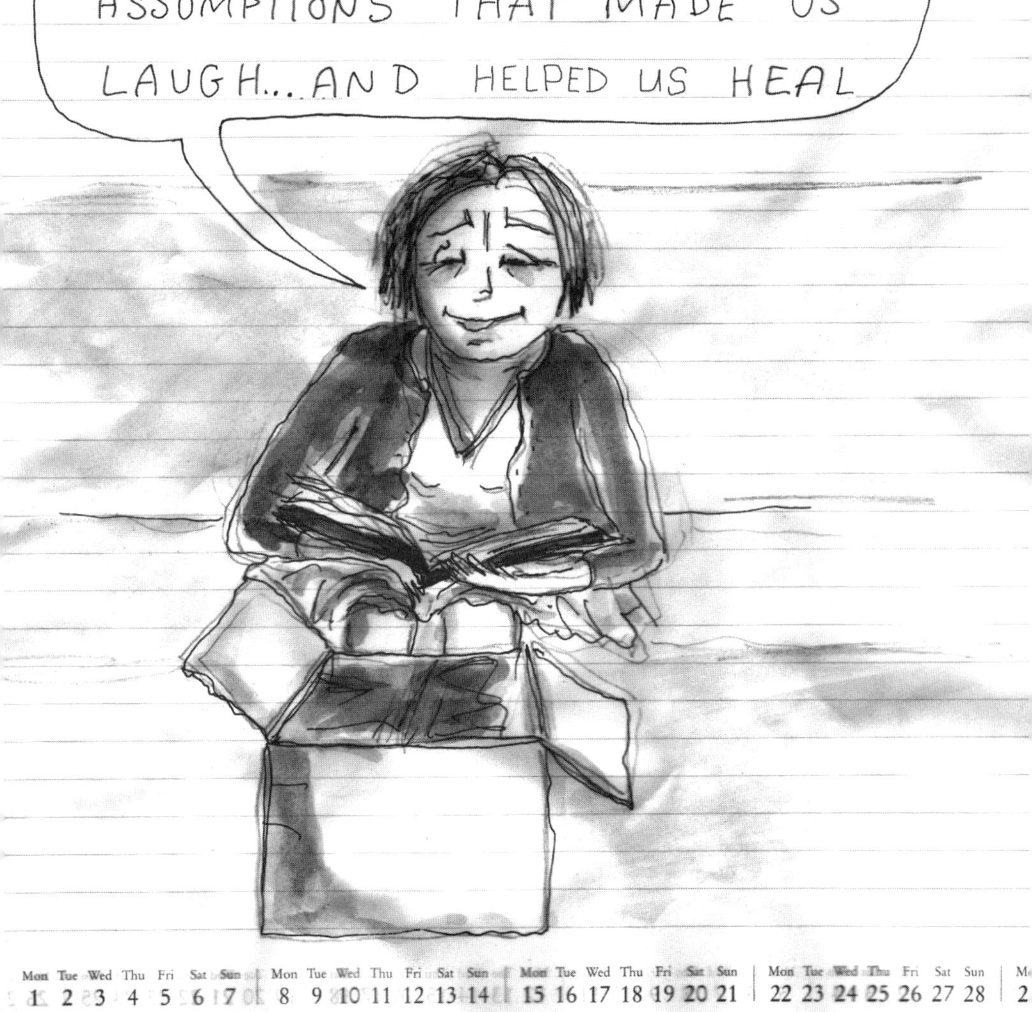
SOME THINGS I REMEMBER. BUT IT IS THE FORGOTTEN DETAILS ... ABSURDITIES AND ASSUMPTIONS THAT MADE US LAUGH... AND HELPED US HEAL
Mon Tue Wed Thu Fri Sat Sun Mon Tue Wed Thu Fri Sat Sun Mon Tue Wed Thu Fri Sat Sun Mon Tue Wed Thu Fri Sat Sun
1 2 3 4 5 6 7 8 9 10 11 12 13 14 15 16 17 18 19 20 21 22 23 24 25 26 27 28

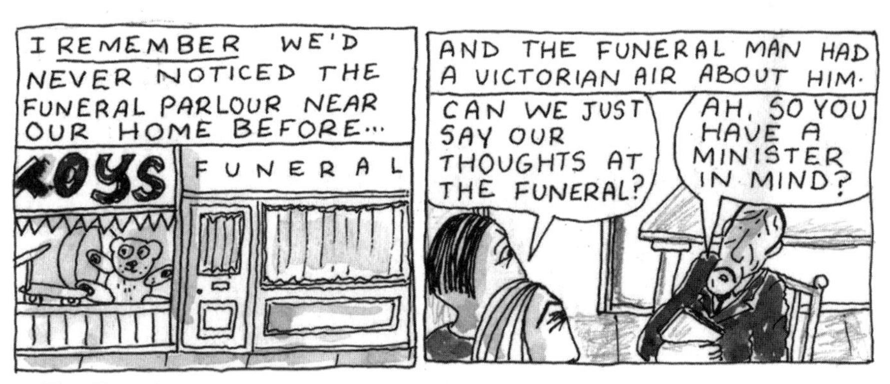
I REMEMBER WE'D NEVER NOTICED THE FUNERAL PARLOUR NEAR OUR HOME BEFORE...
FUNERAL
AND THE FUNERAL MAN HAD A VICTORIAN AIR ABOUT HIM.
CAN WE JUST SAY OUR THOUGHTS AT THE FUNERAL?
AH, SO YOU HAVE A MINISTER IN MIND?

I'D FORGOTTEN HIS CONFUSION OVER OUR NON-RELIGIOUS WISHES.

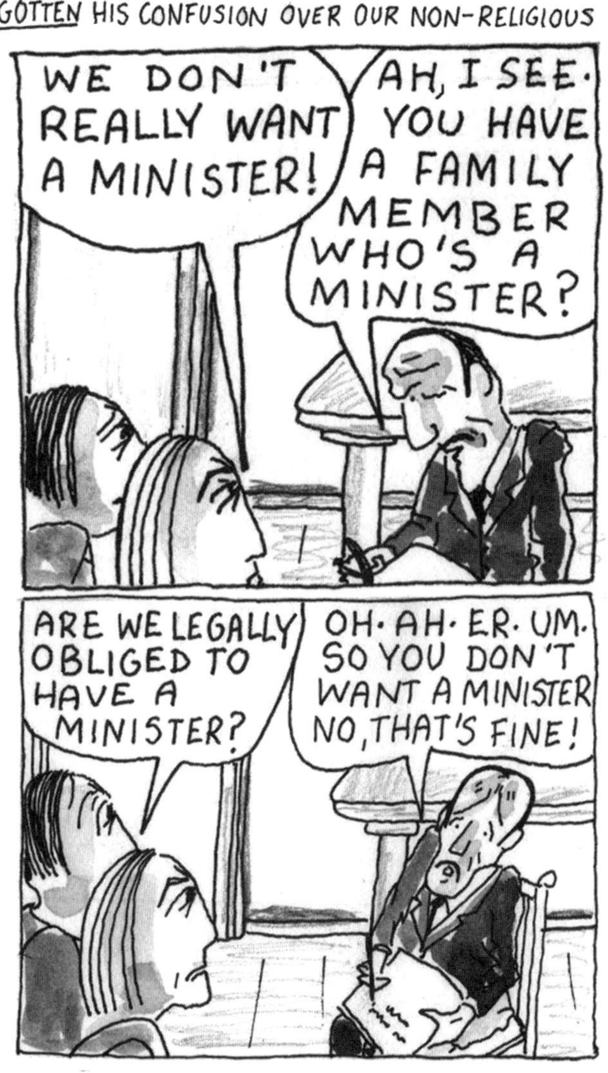
WE DON'T REALLY WANT A MINISTER!
AH, I SEE. YOU HAVE A FAMILY MEMBER WHO'S A MINISTER?
ARE WE LEGALLY OBLIGED TO HAVE A MINISTER?
OH. AH. ER. UM. SO YOU DON'T WANT A MINISTER NO, THAT'S FINE!

AND HIS ASSUMPTION THAT BILLY HADN'T COUNTED IN OUR LIVES QUITE SO MUCH, BEING "JUST A BABY"

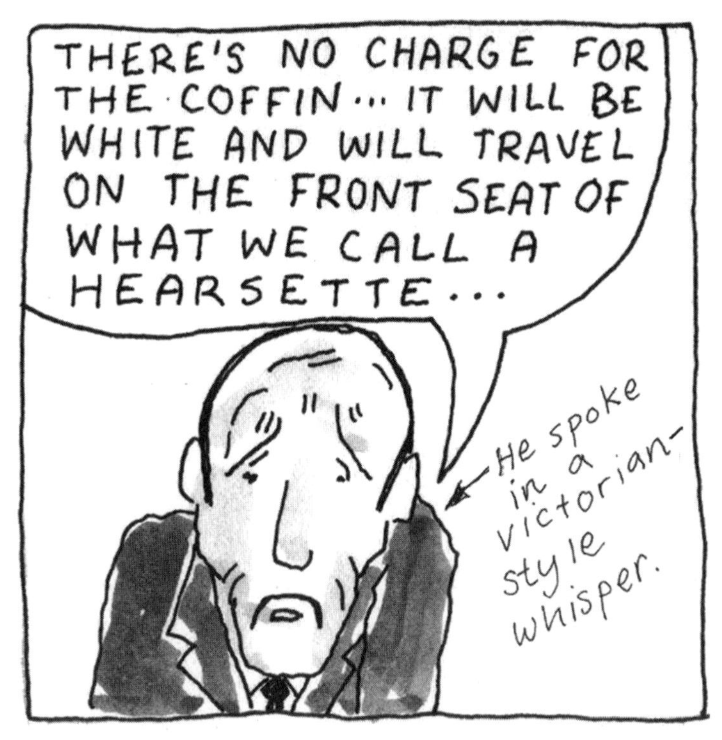
THERE'S NO CHARGE FOR THE COFFIN... IT WILL BE WHITE AND WILL TRAVEL ON THE FRONT SEAT OF WHAT WE CALL A HEARSETTE...
He spoke in a victorian-style whisper.

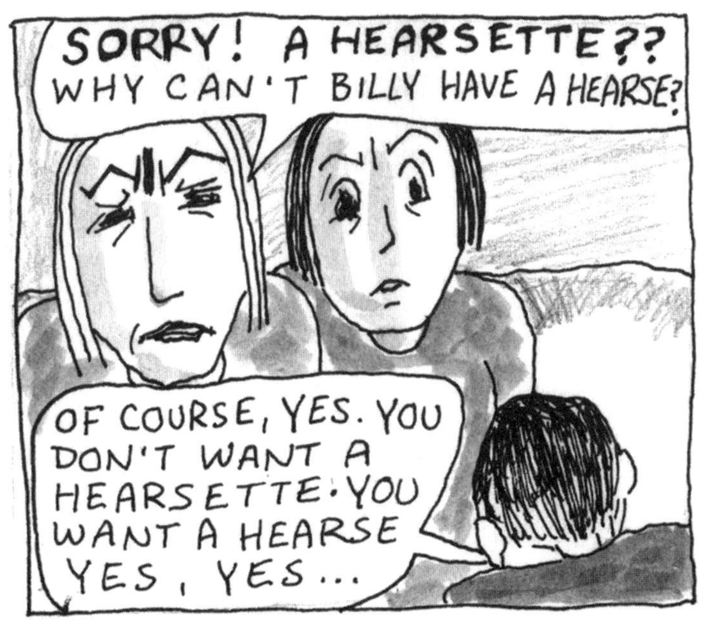
SORRY! A HEARSETTE?? WHY CAN'T BILLY HAVE A HEARSE?
OF COURSE, YES. YOU DON'T WANT A HEARSETTE. YOU WANT A HEARSE YES, YES...

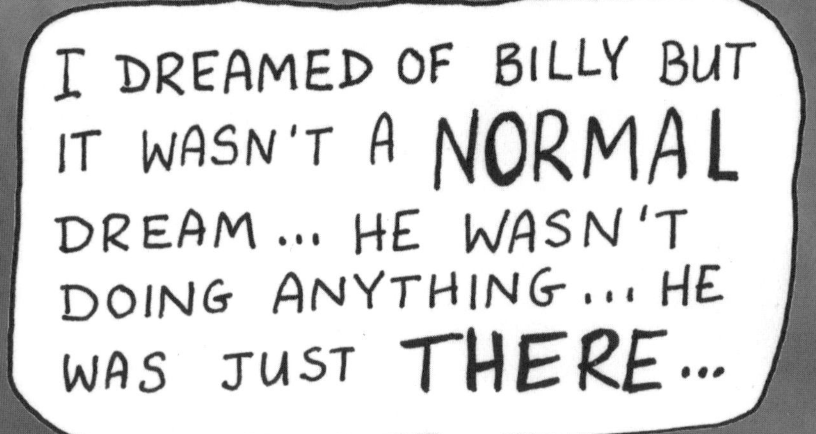
I DREAMED OF BILLY BUT IT WASN'T A NORMAL DREAM... HE WASN'T DOING ANYTHING... HE WAS JUST THERE...

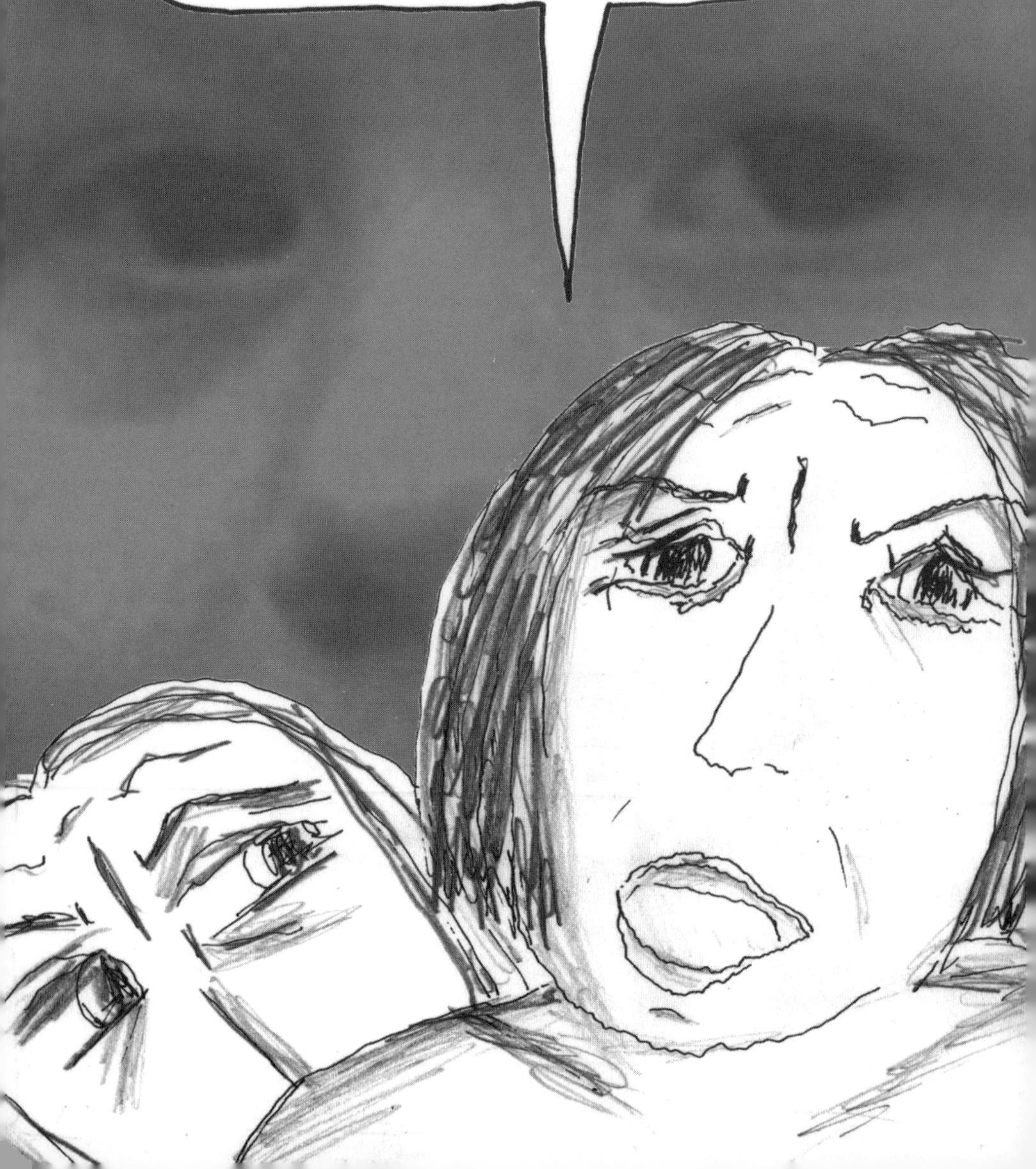

The Guardian Thursday September 21 1995

Private Lives

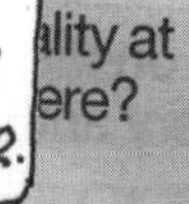

I REMEMBER
JOHN SHOWING ME A LETTER IN THE PAPER.

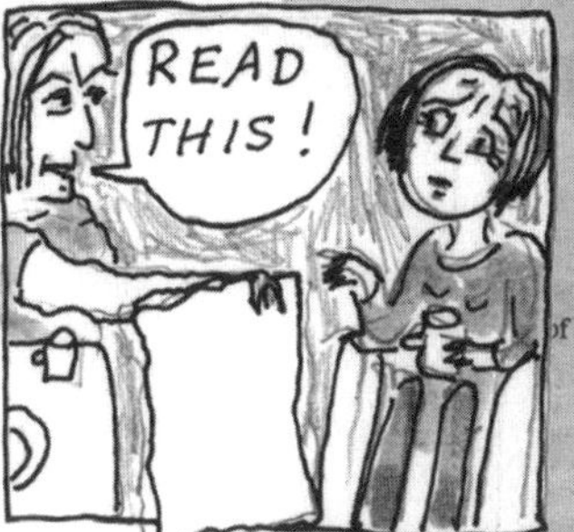

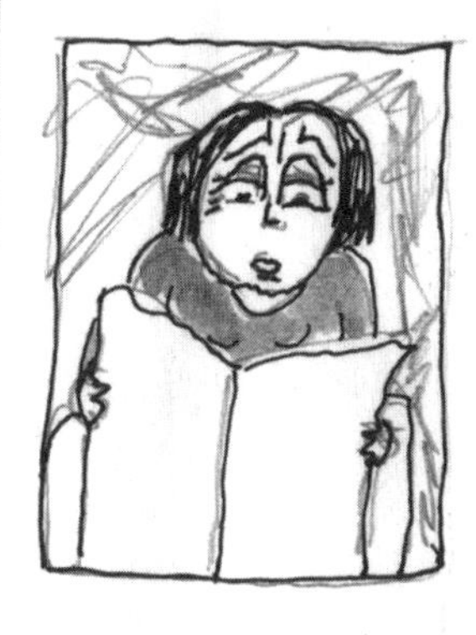

Next problem

Your baby girl seemed perfect when she was born – but she died at just three days old. How can you come to terms with your loss?

I AM 38 and have been married for four years. Our first child, a girl, was born three months ago — perfect and beautiful. She died when she was just three days old.

Initially, the registered cause of death was sudden infant death syndrome or "cot death". But then our local hospital notified us that her death was due to an "overwhelming infection" of a strain of bacteria, Streptococcus B.

We are managing to survive, but only just. I wonder if anyone can help? I have two problems.

The pragmatic consideration first: is there any support group for parents who have suffered a similar loss? Where can we find more information regarding this particular bacteria? There are so many questions I have that as yet the hospital seems unable to respond to.

Secondly, we are discovering that most people we know, in an effort to comfort us, turn to traditional Christian beliefs. Without doubt we have spiritual faith but personally I do not accept everything relating to Christianity as taught to me as a child.

People have attempted to comfort me by saying that my daughter and I will be reunited in heaven, or that she is an angel now, or even that God only takes the young . . . I do not find this any comfort. I just cannot accept a simplistic view of heaven and hell, with us being reunited, no doubt, with our family dog!

Has anyone answers to these questions?

Lesbian, Gay and
ety. It featured photos
, including the LGB
to of a hat with no face.
ficer had dropped out.
ll be your LGB Officer.
e few students who did
gs didn't want to be
tive" and were only
social gatherings. Fine,
nge discos.
of these discos (held in
J back room), I heard a
tside. In the stairwell,
ce for heterosexual
men were kissing.
complained to the
he men had been asked
is bouncer been
ing to the SU policy,
the complainant to
e had not been prop-
ecause the LGB group
cally active".
econd year (and I was
er, my smiley face in
, my partner and
oved from one hall to
threats of gang rape
in our hall. Note: we
ot them. We were
we took the matter
ld say goodbye to our
equal ops.
r stories include a
hurled downstairs by
of a house-mate,
her as a rival. In one
ersity had three
) male rapes and
s of women.
st each other.
around hall alone at
s go to parties with
n't know. Students
at university is just
s the real world.
stop talking
ook at facts.
to put anyone off
fer this advice. Fight
If there's no equal
policy, write and make
l. But still carry a
keep you head down
ecked out the
r fellow students.

I WROTE A REPLY AND THEN FORGOT ABOUT IT.

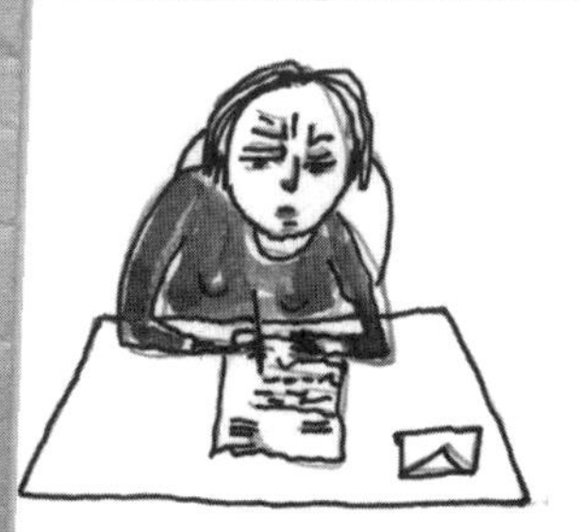

I REMEMBER JOHN AND I "KEPT BUSY" WITH DIY PROJECTS.

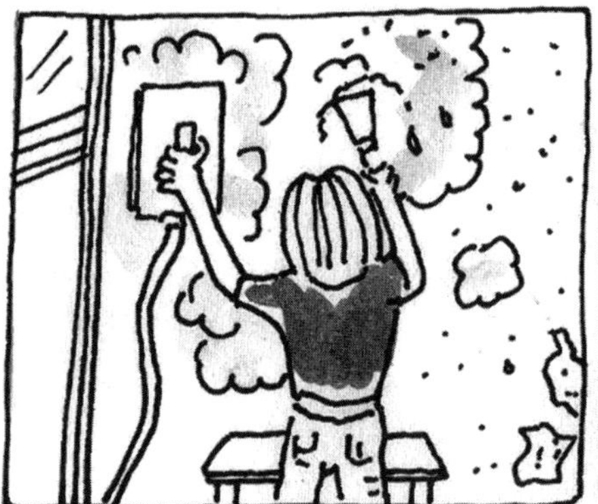

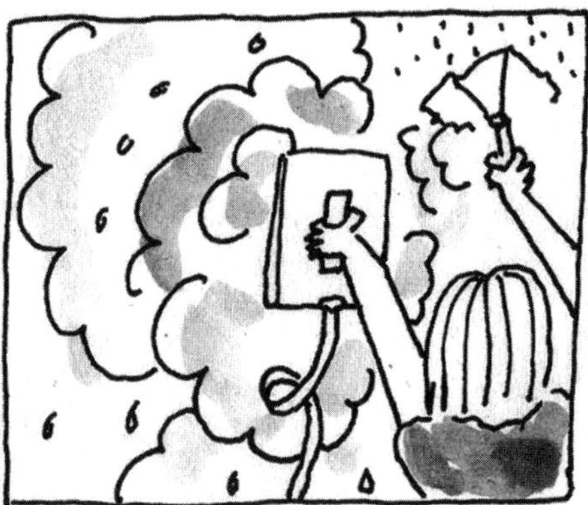

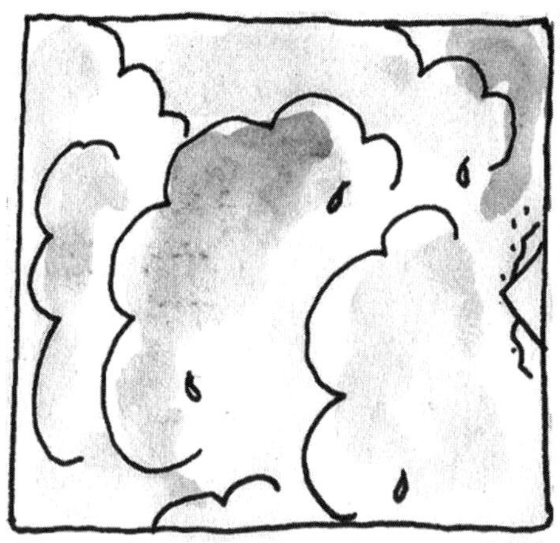

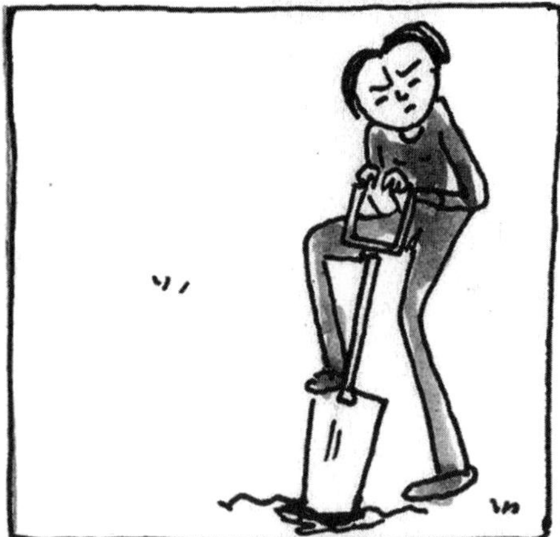

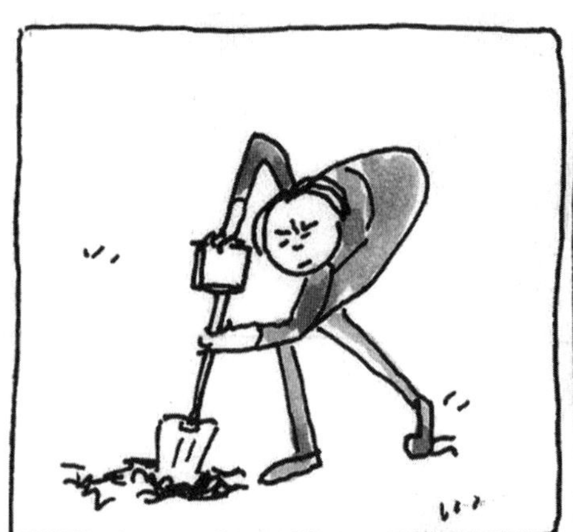

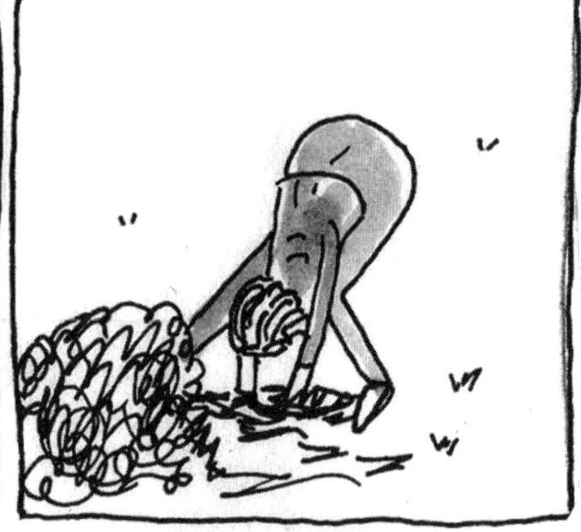

I REMEMBER HEARING A WINSTON CHURCHILL QUOTE THAT WENT SOMETHING LIKE, "WHEN YOU'RE WALKING IN HELL, WALK FASTER".

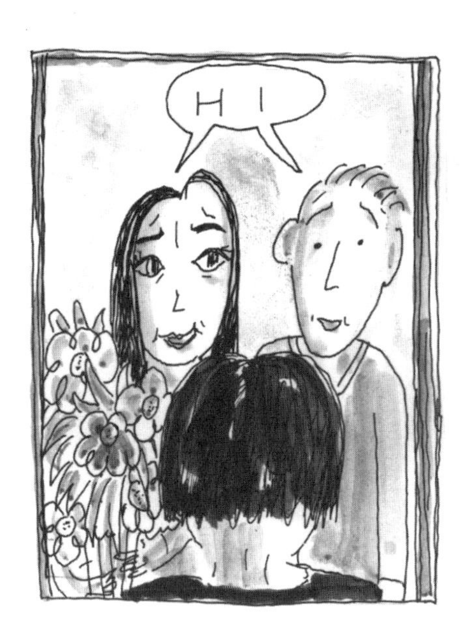

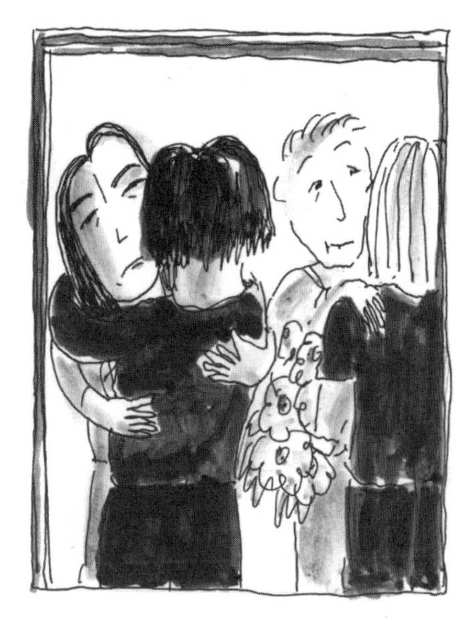

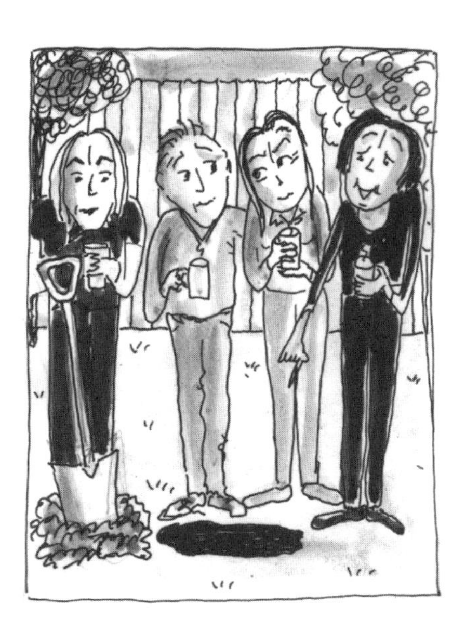

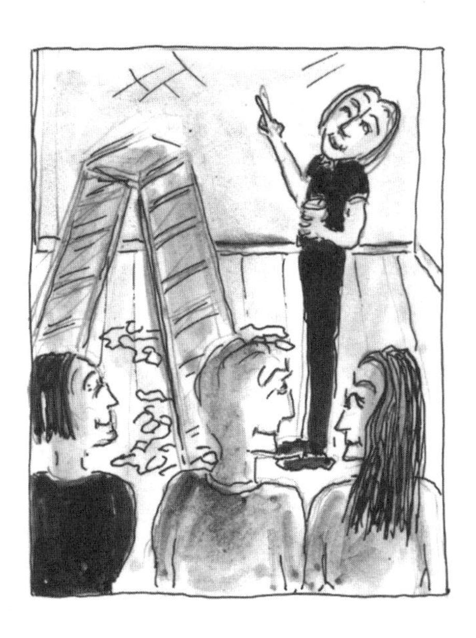

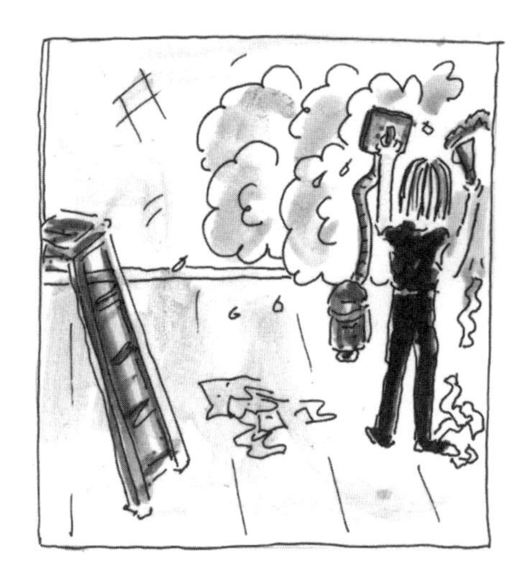
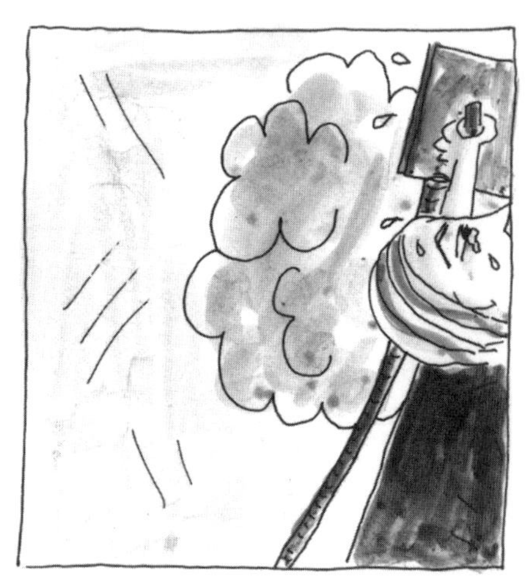
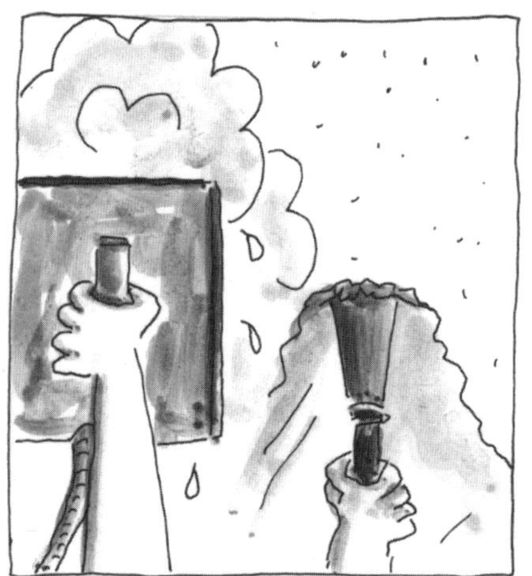
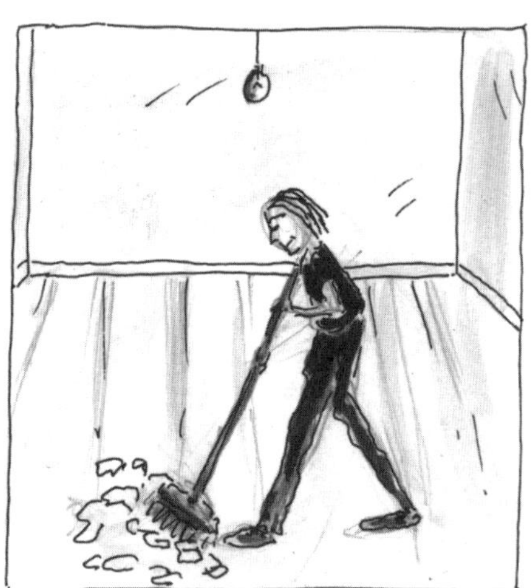
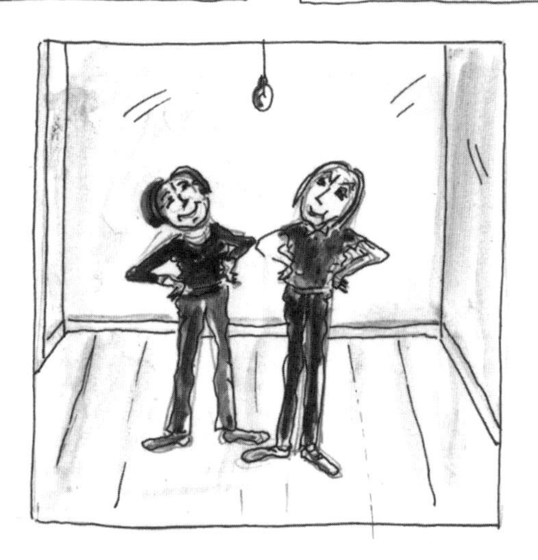

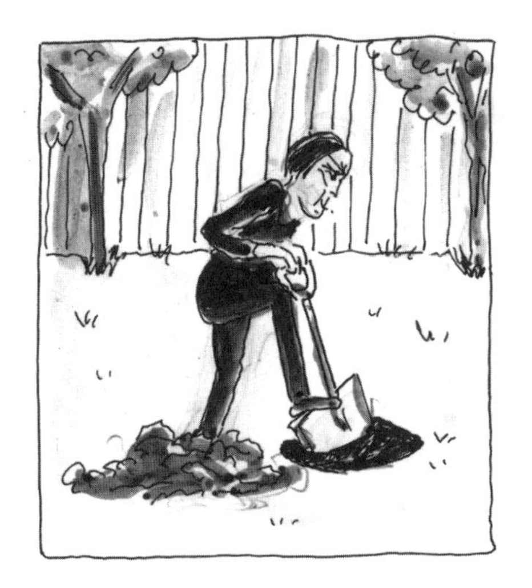

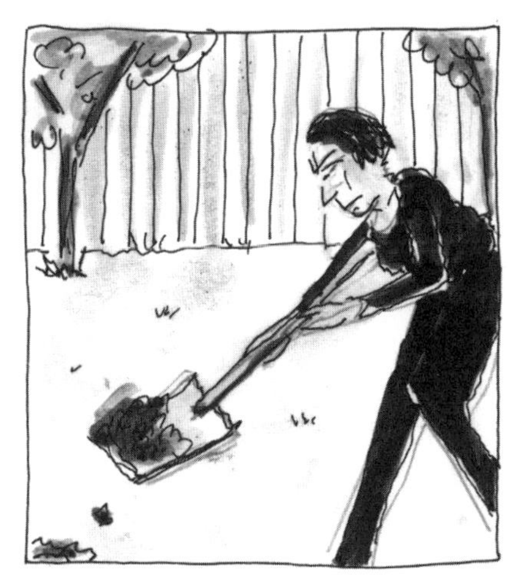

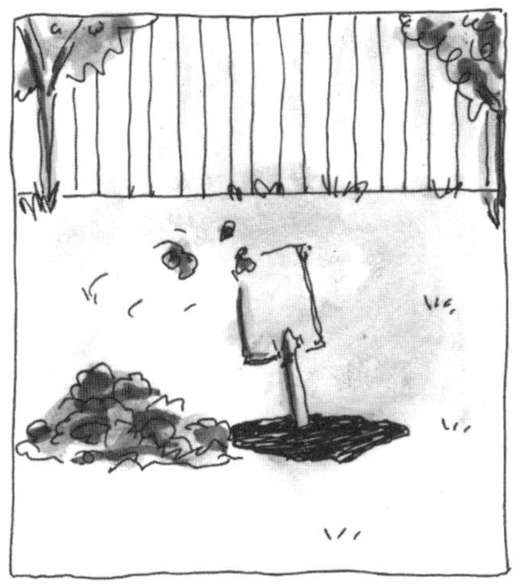

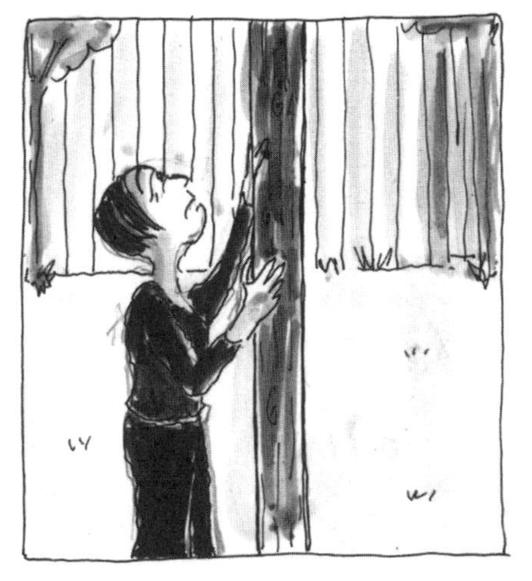

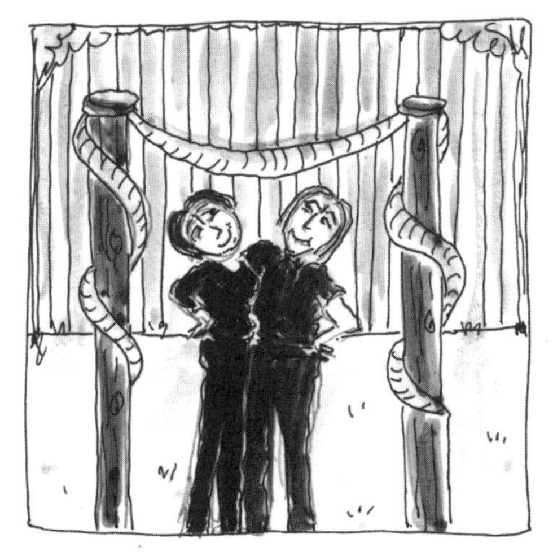

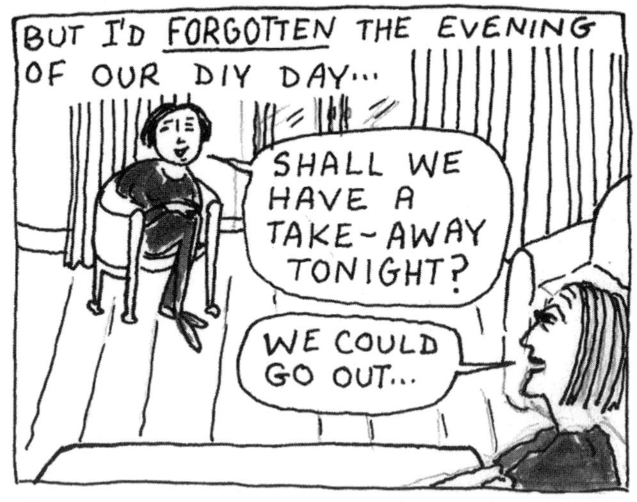
BUT I'D FORGOTTEN THE EVENING OF OUR DIY DAY...
SHALL WE HAVE A TAKE-AWAY TONIGHT?
WE COULD GO OUT...

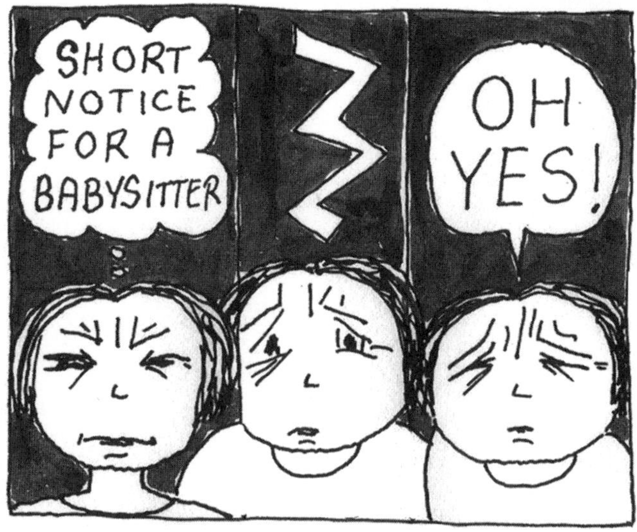
SHORT NOTICE FOR A BABYSITTER
OH YES!

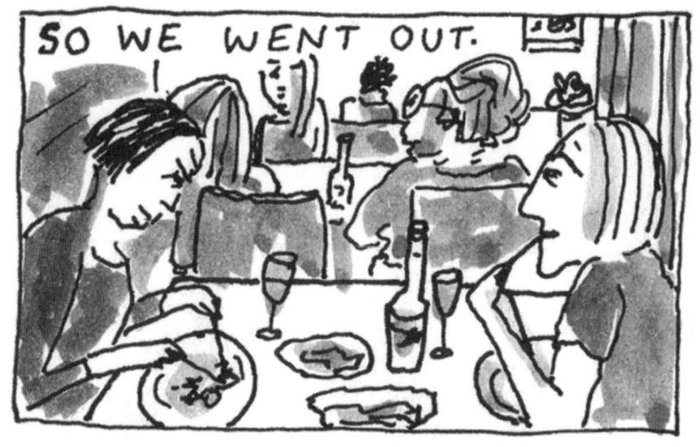
SO WE WENT OUT.

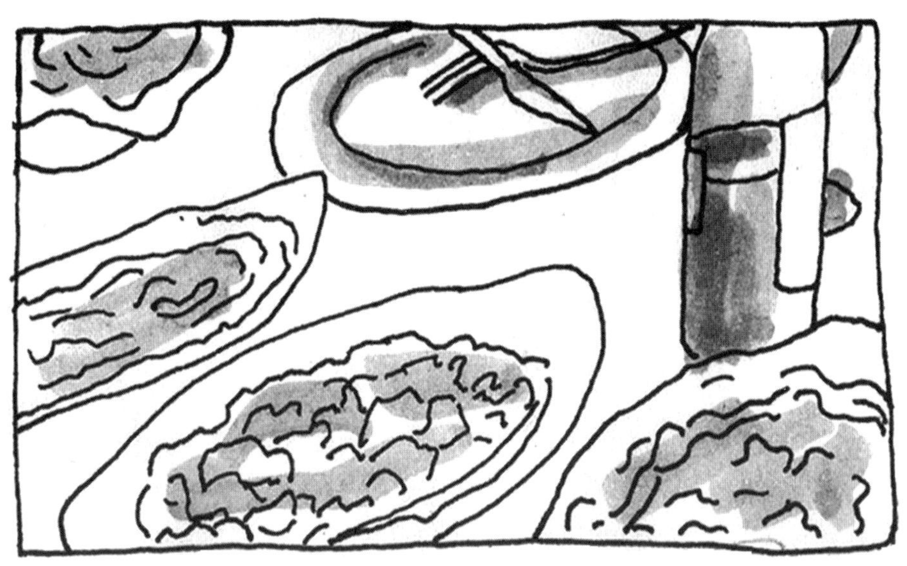

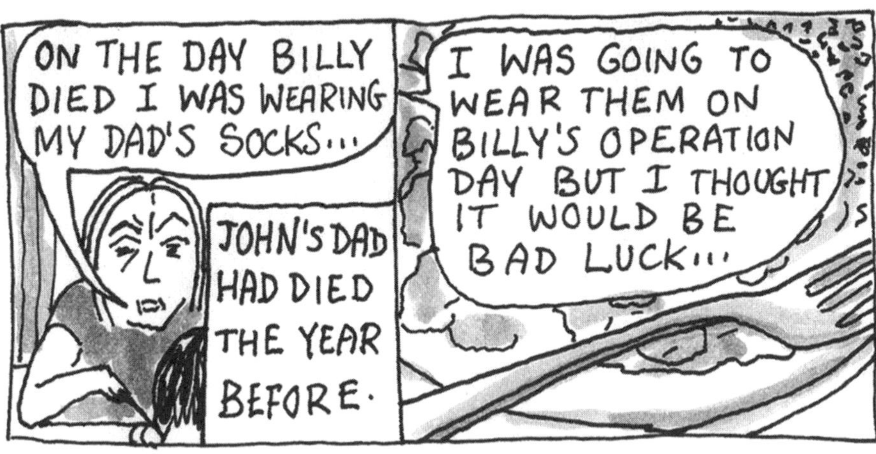
ON THE DAY BILLY DIED I WAS WEARING MY DAD'S SOCKS...
JOHN'S DAD HAD DIED THE YEAR BEFORE.
I WAS GOING TO WEAR THEM ON BILLY'S OPERATION DAY BUT I THOUGHT IT WOULD BE BAD LUCK...

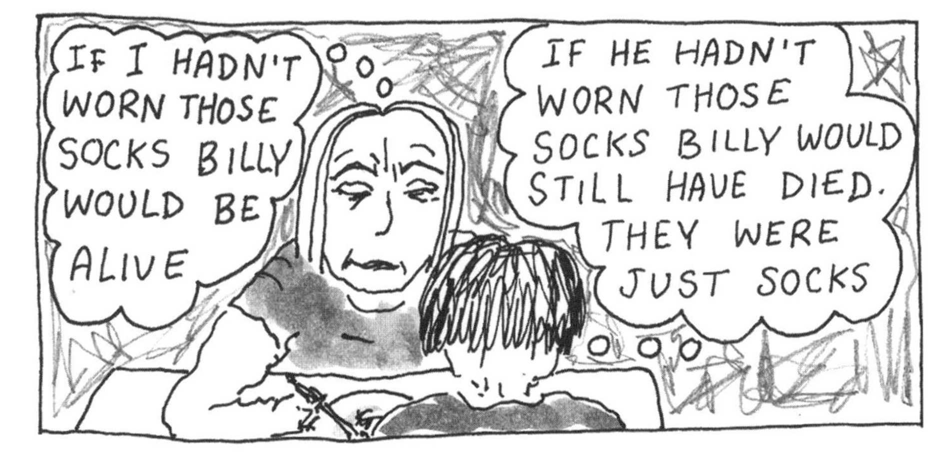
IF I HADN'T WORN THOSE SOCKS BILLY WOULD BE ALIVE
IF HE HADN'T WORN THOSE SOCKS BILLY WOULD STILL HAVE DIED. THEY WERE JUST SOCKS

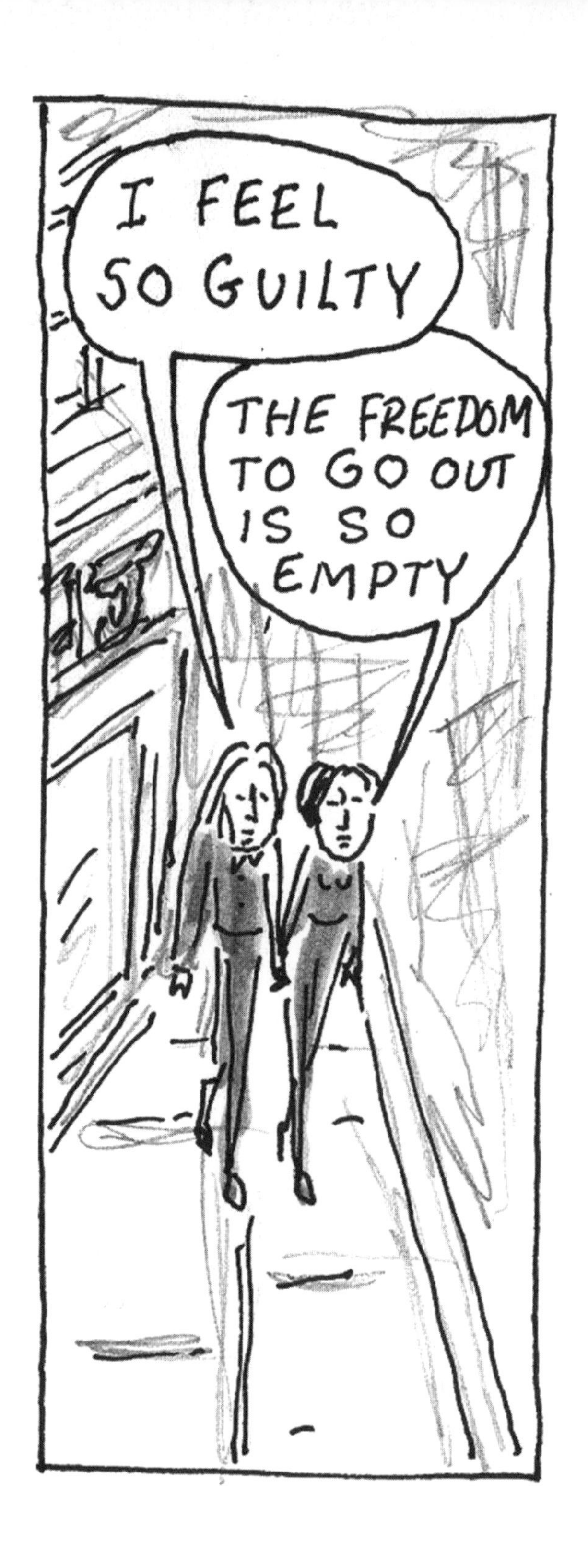
I FEEL SO GUILTY
THE FREEDOM TO GO OUT IS SO EMPTY

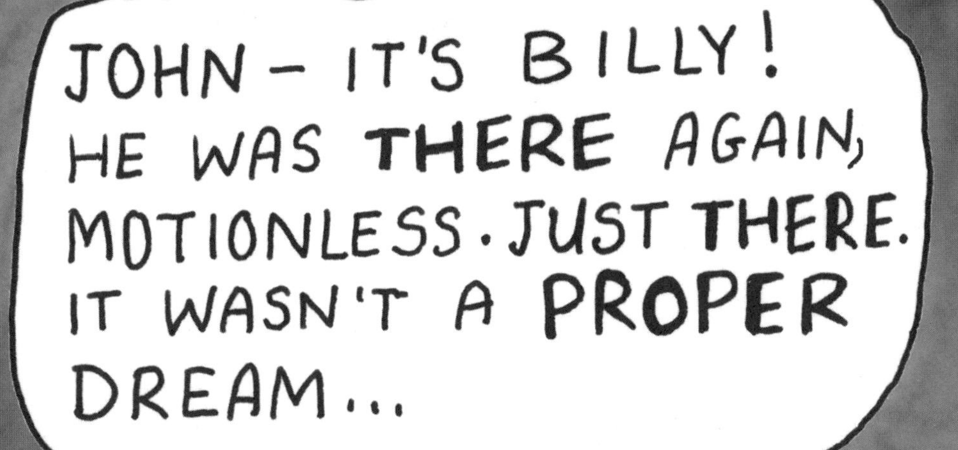
JOHN – IT'S BILLY! HE WAS **THERE** AGAIN, MOTIONLESS. JUST **THERE**. IT WASN'T A **PROPER** DREAM...

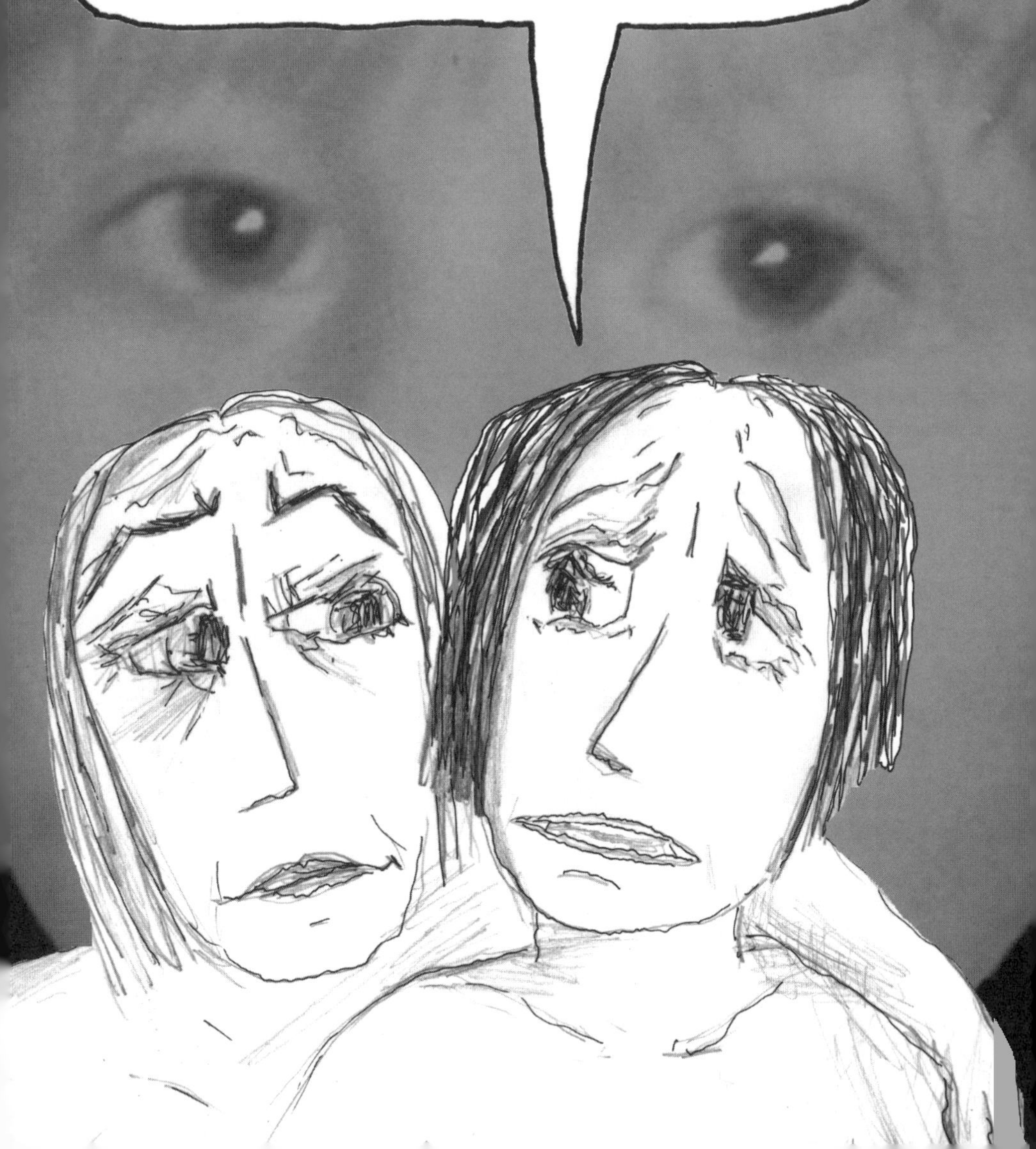

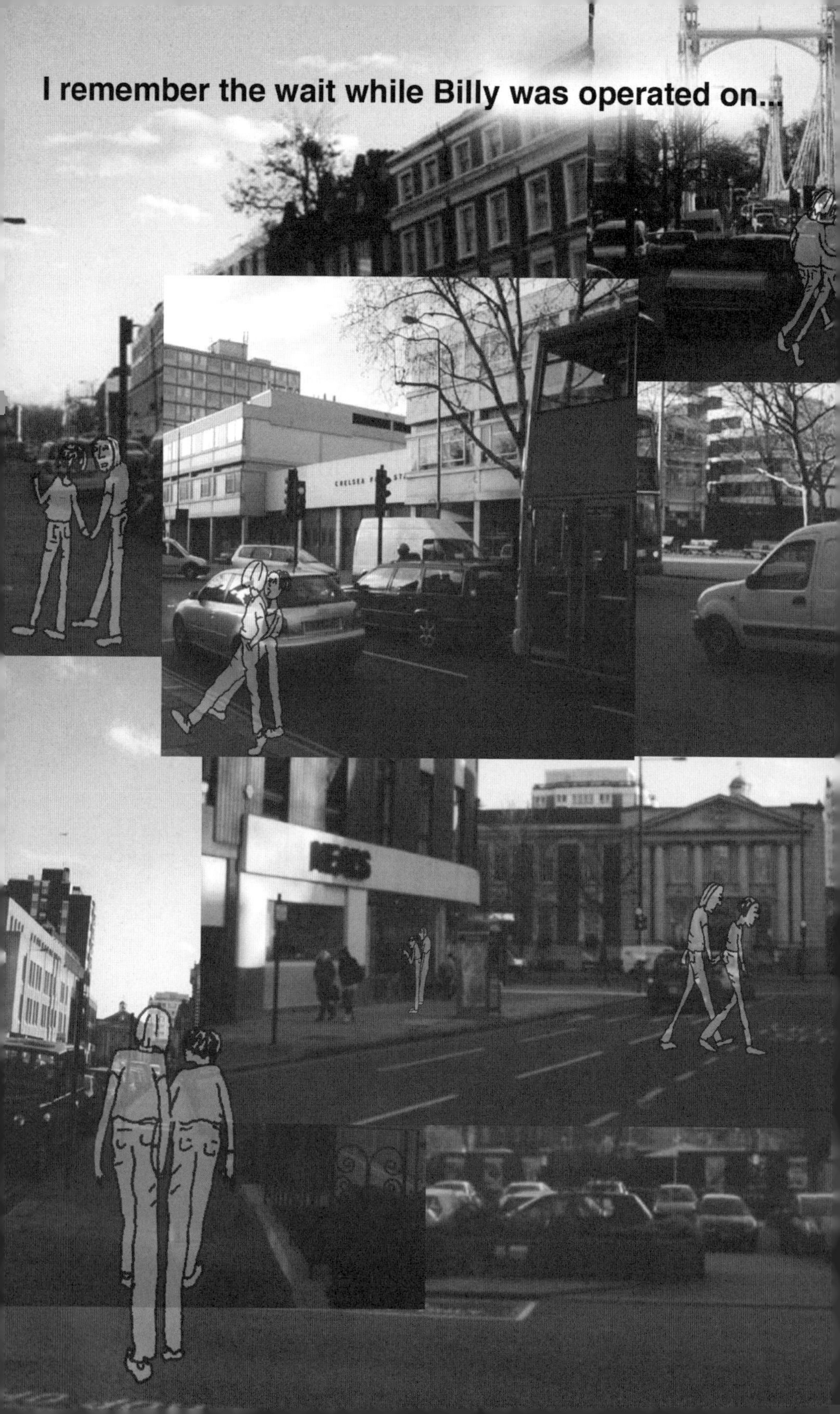
I remember the wait while Billy was operated on...

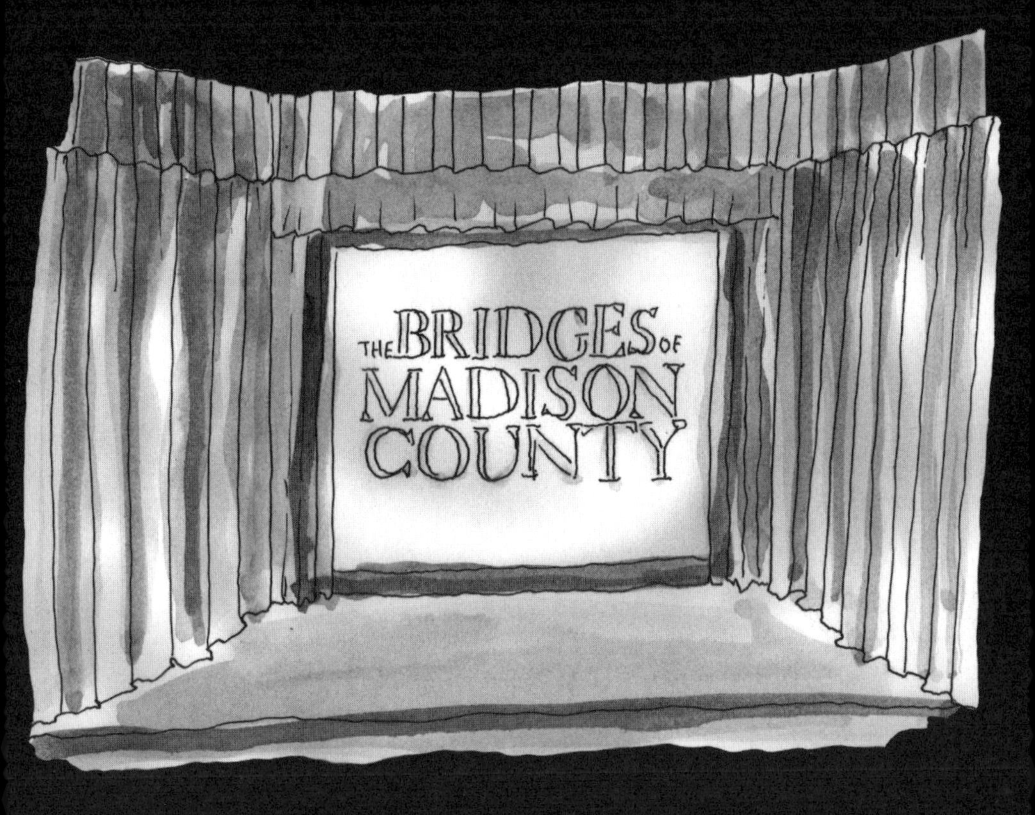
THE BRIDGES OF
MADISON
COUNTY

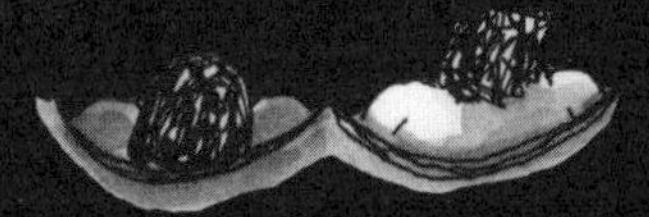

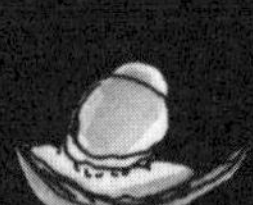

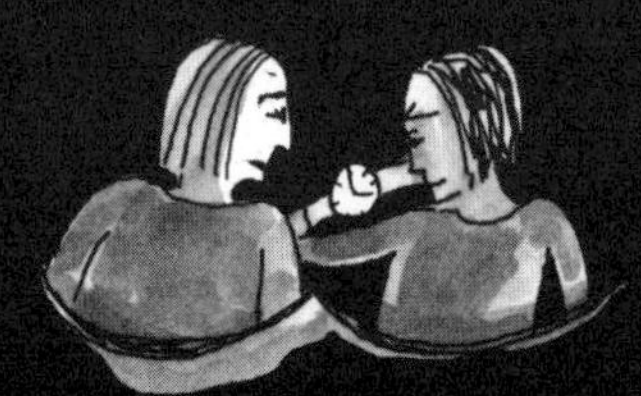

And the impotence time imposed on us

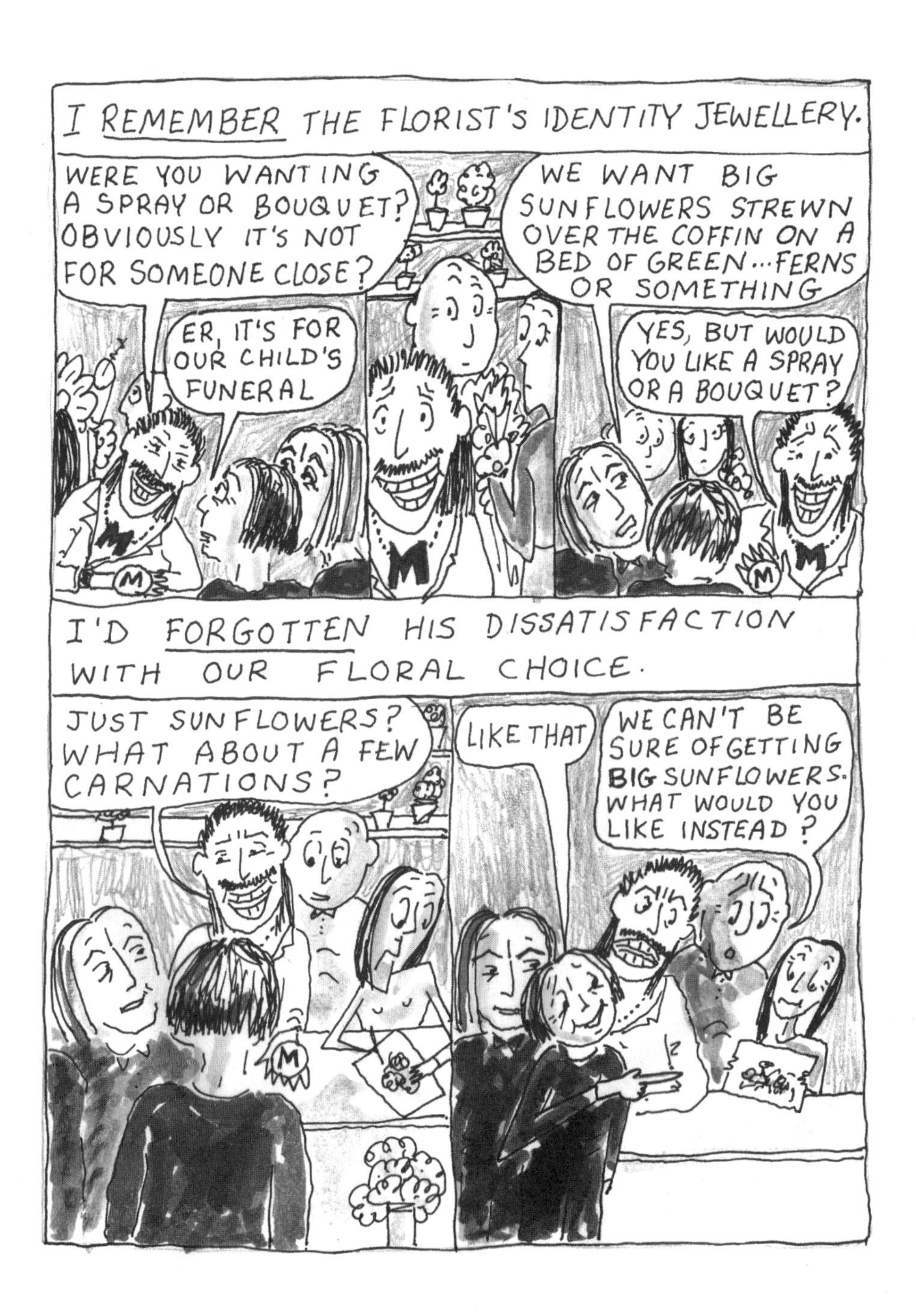
I REMEMBER THE FLORIST'S IDENTITY JEWELLERY.
WERE YOU WANTING A SPRAY OR BOUQUET? OBVIOUSLY IT'S NOT FOR SOMEONE CLOSE?
ER, IT'S FOR OUR CHILD'S FUNERAL
WE WANT BIG SUNFLOWERS STREWN OVER THE COFFIN ON A BED OF GREEN...FERNS OR SOMETHING
YES, BUT WOULD YOU LIKE A SPRAY OR A BOUQUET?
M
I'D FORGOTTEN HIS DISSATISFACTION WITH OUR FLORAL CHOICE.
JUST SUNFLOWERS? WHAT ABOUT A FEW CARNATIONS?
LIKE THAT
WE CAN'T BE SURE OF GETTING BIG SUNFLOWERS. WHAT WOULD YOU LIKE INSTEAD?

I REMEMBER EMILY'S THOUGHTFULNESS BUT HAD FORGOTTEN OUR CONVERSATIONS.

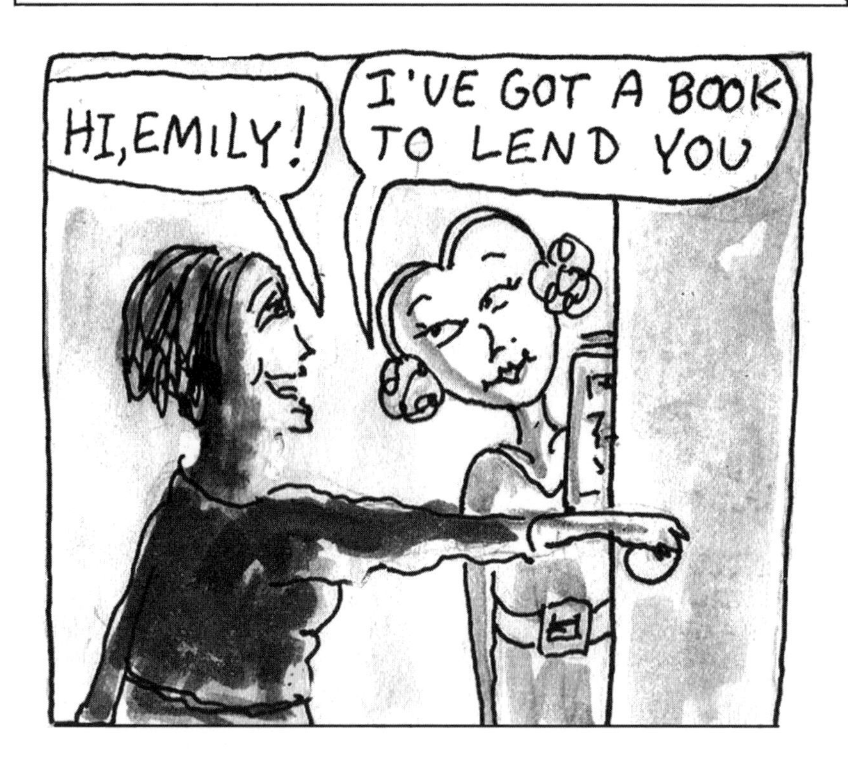
HI, EMILY!
I'VE GOT A BOOK TO LEND YOU

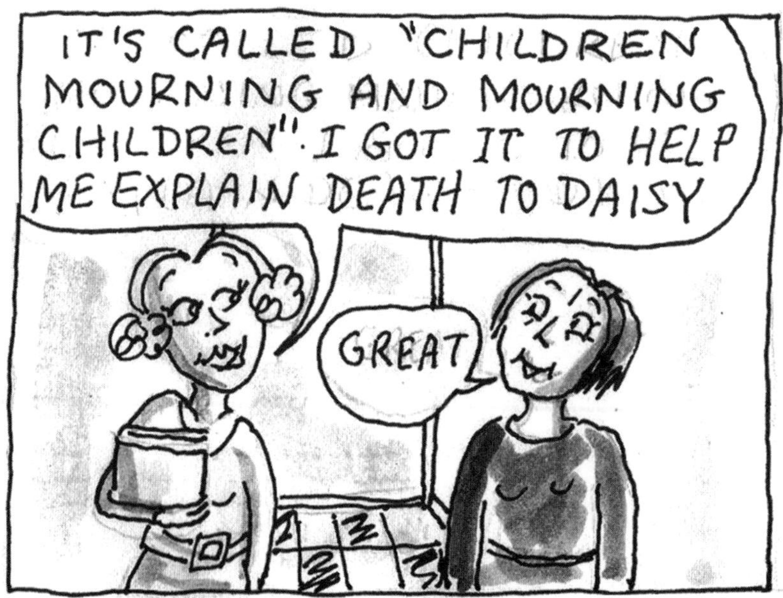
IT'S CALLED "CHILDREN MOURNING AND MOURNING CHILDREN". I GOT IT TO HELP ME EXPLAIN DEATH TO DAISY
GREAT

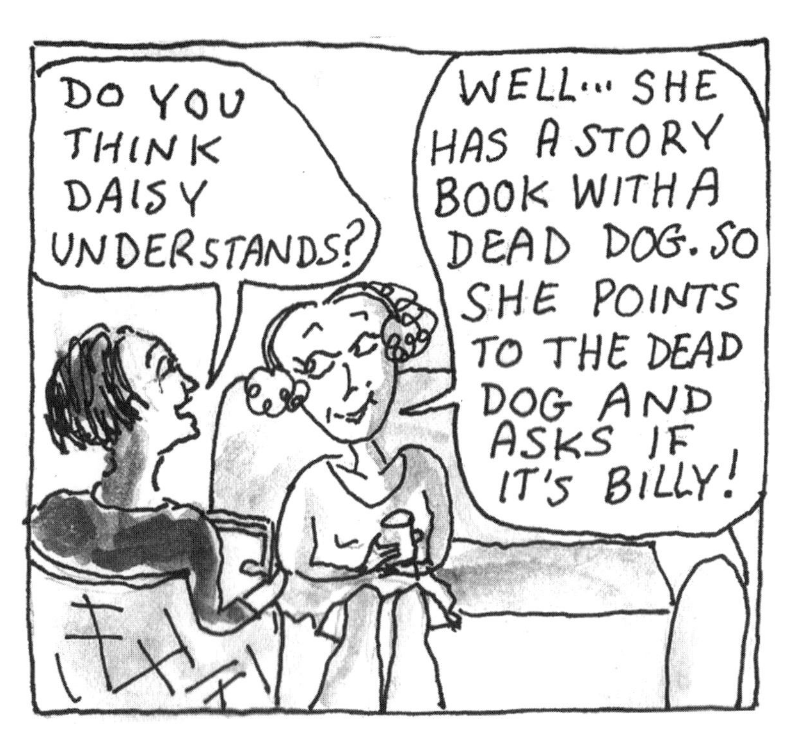
DO YOU THINK DAISY UNDERSTANDS?
WELL... SHE HAS A STORY BOOK WITH A DEAD DOG. SO SHE POINTS TO THE DEAD DOG AND ASKS IF IT'S BILLY!

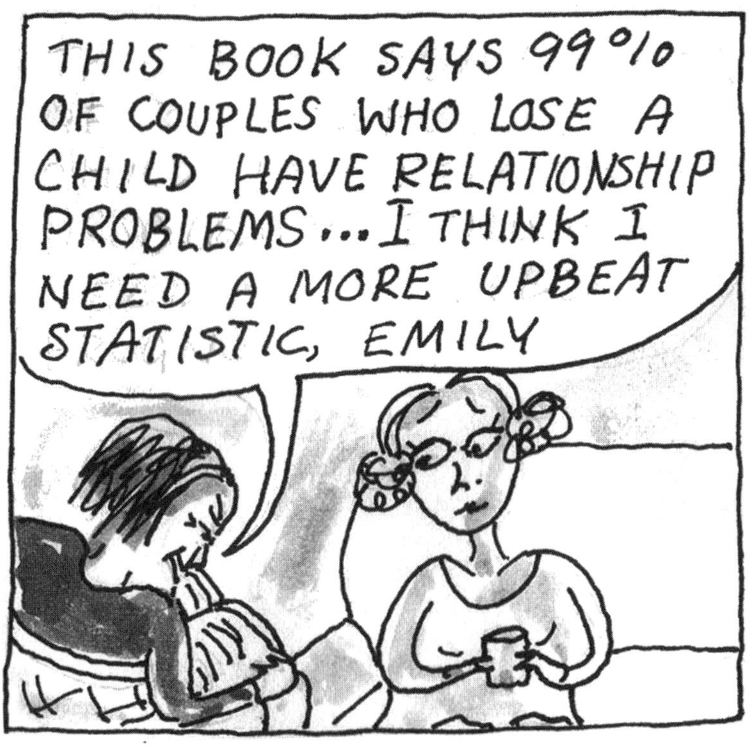
THIS BOOK SAYS 99% OF COUPLES WHO LOSE A CHILD HAVE RELATIONSHIP PROBLEMS... I THINK I NEED A MORE UPBEAT STATISTIC, EMILY

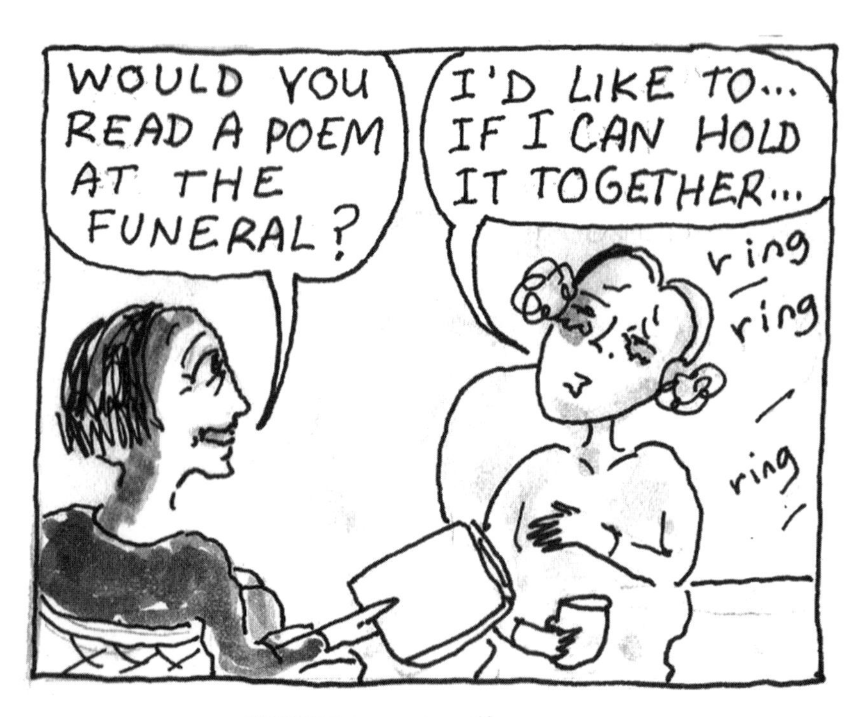
WOULD YOU READ A POEM AT THE FUNERAL?
I'D LIKE TO... IF I CAN HOLD IT TOGETHER...
ring
ring
ring

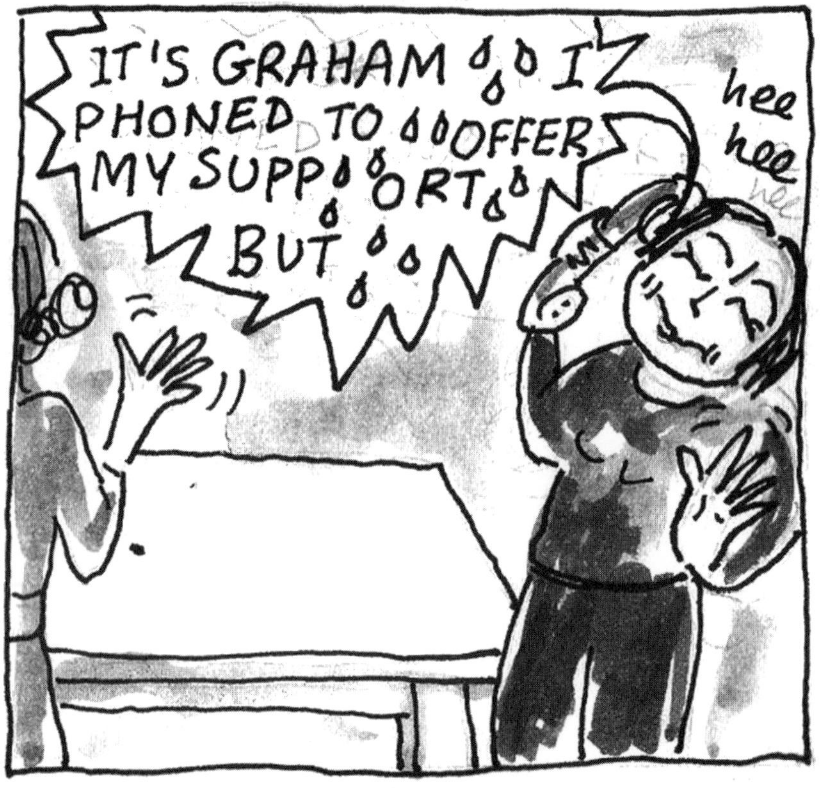
IT'S GRAHAM I PHONED TO OFFER MY SUPPORT BUT
hee
hee
hee

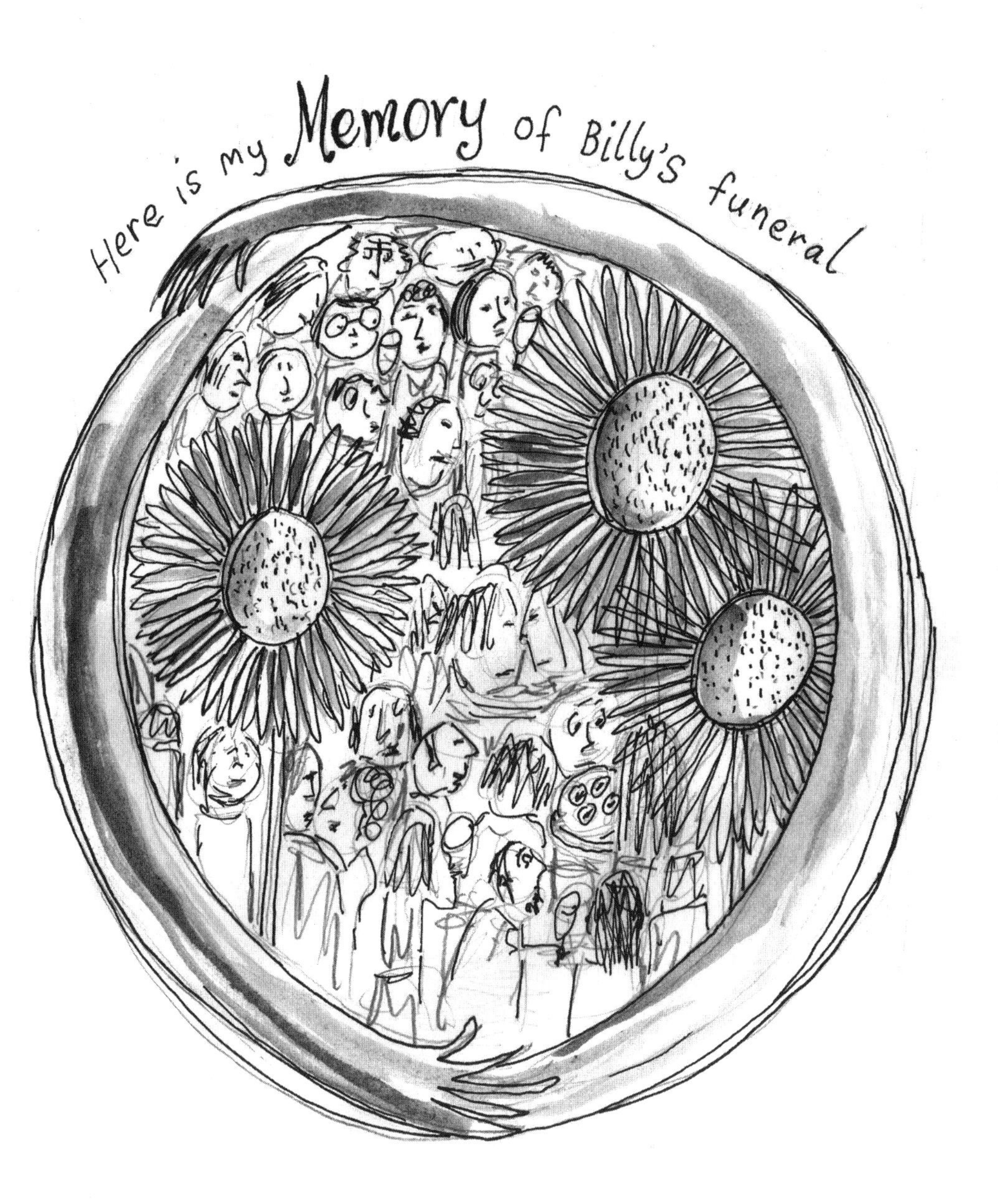
Here is my Memory of Billy's funeral

HERE ARE THE DETAILS I'D FORGOTTEN...

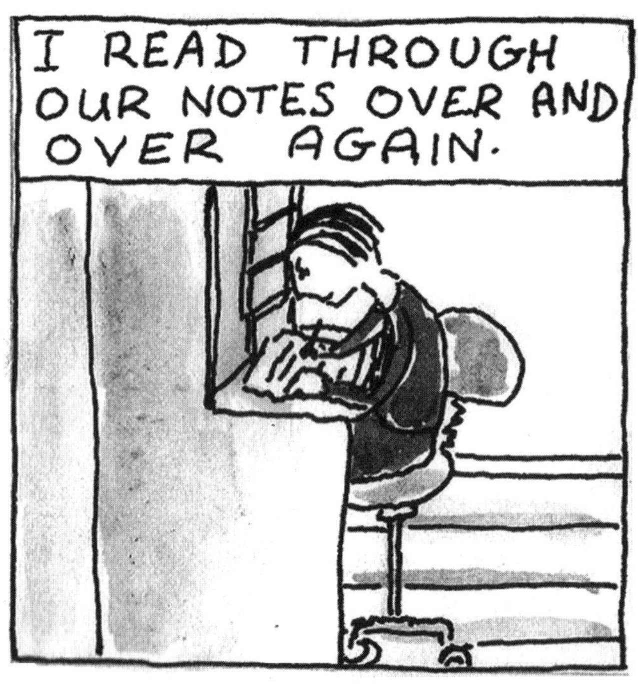
I READ THROUGH OUR NOTES OVER AND OVER AGAIN.

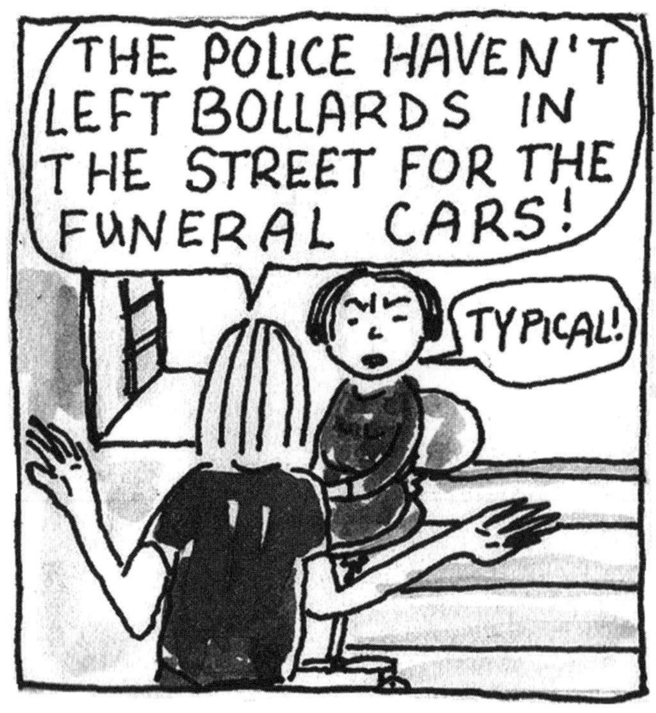
THE POLICE HAVEN'T LEFT BOLLARDS IN THE STREET FOR THE FUNERAL CARS!
TYPICAL!

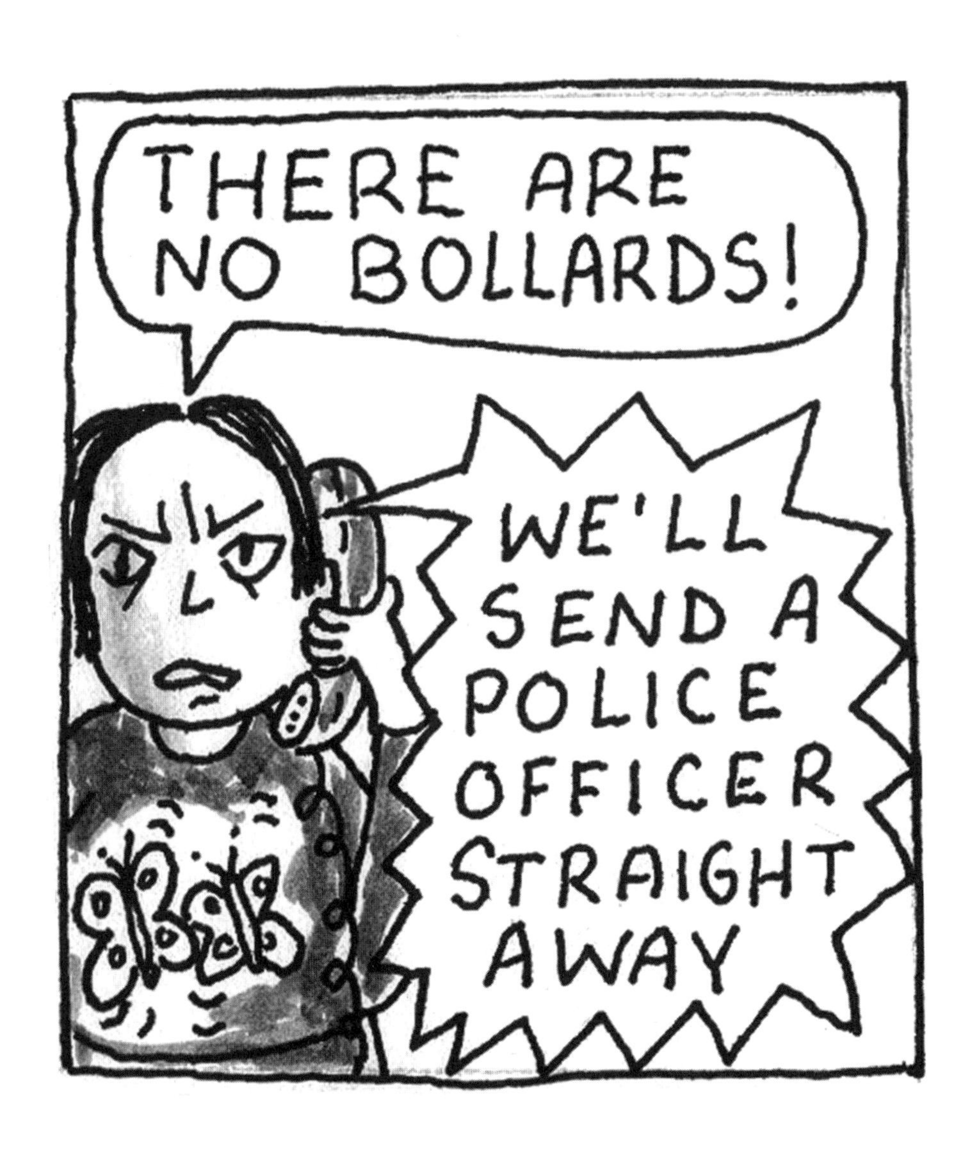
THERE ARE NO BOLLARDS!
WE'LL SEND A POLICE OFFICER STRAIGHT AWAY

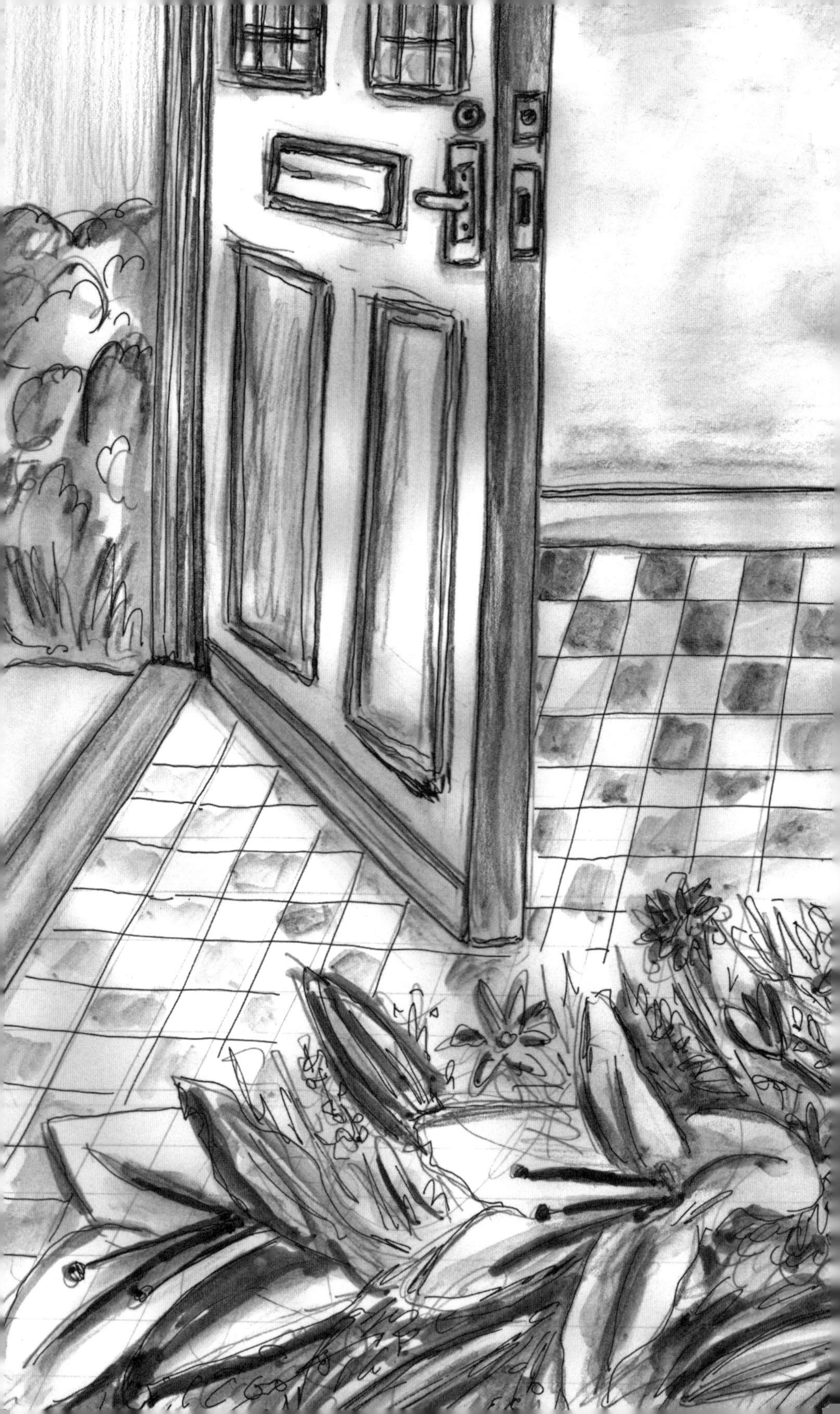

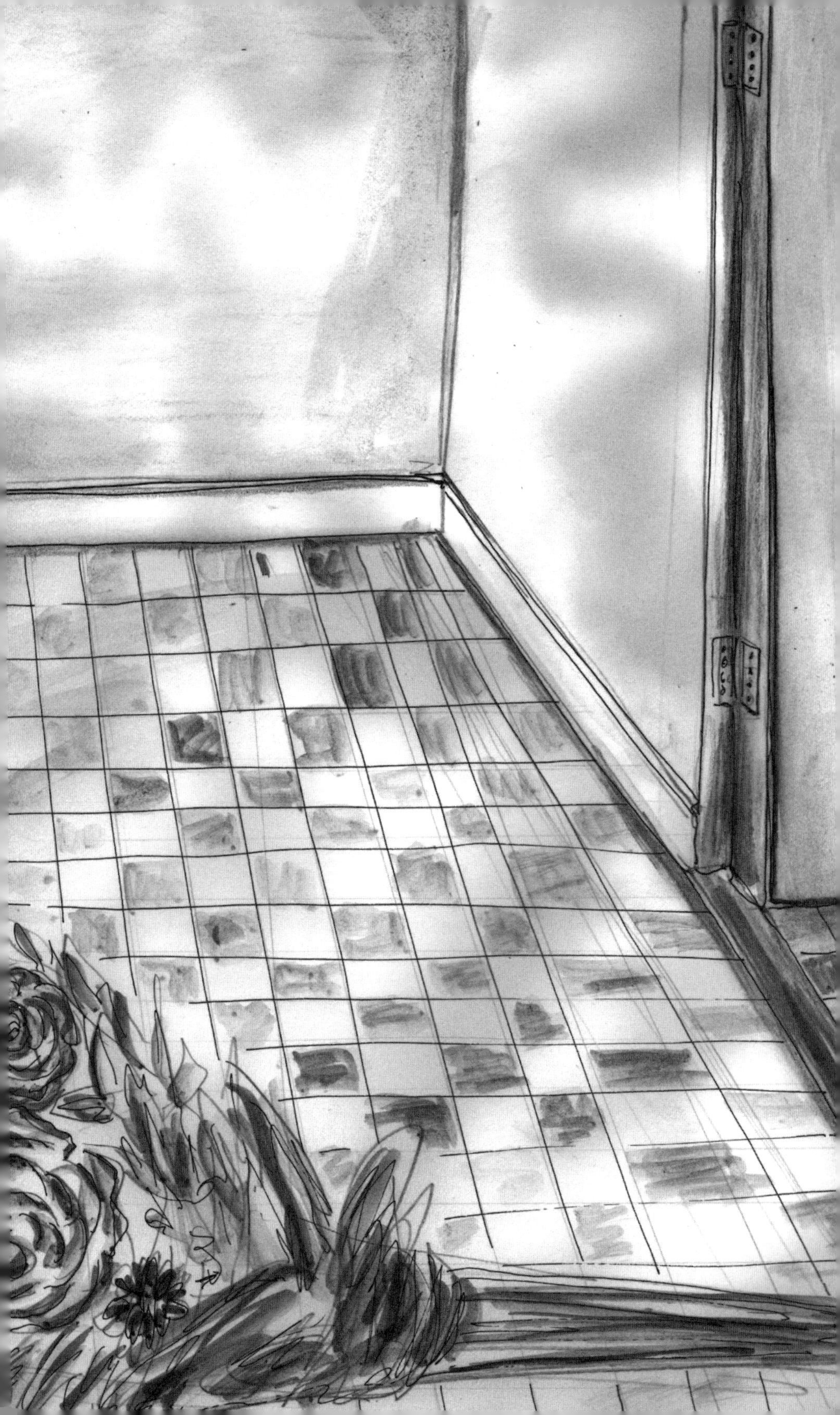

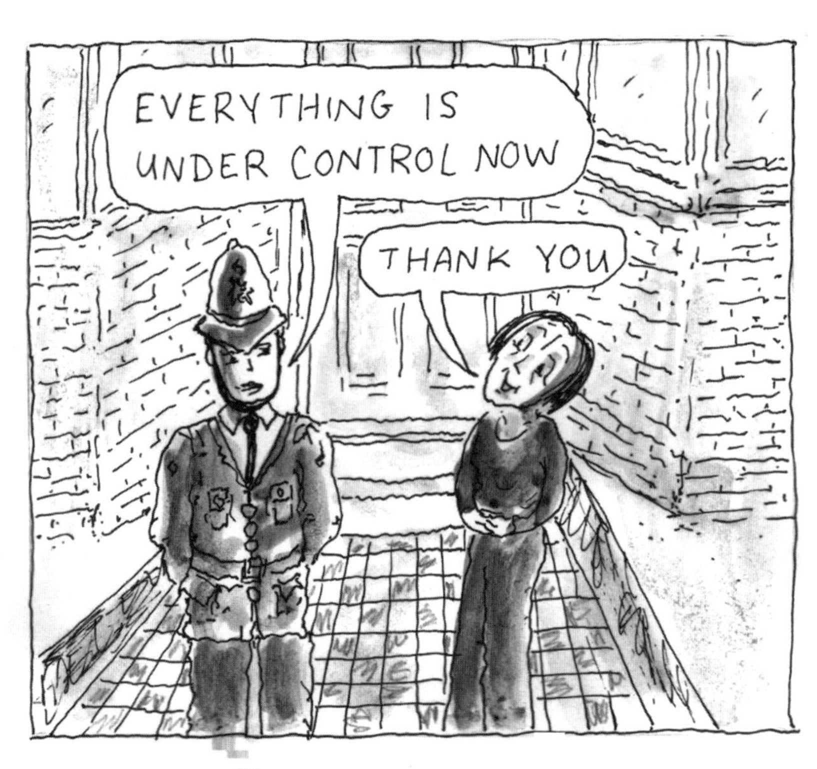
EVERYTHING IS UNDER CONTROL NOW
THANK YOU

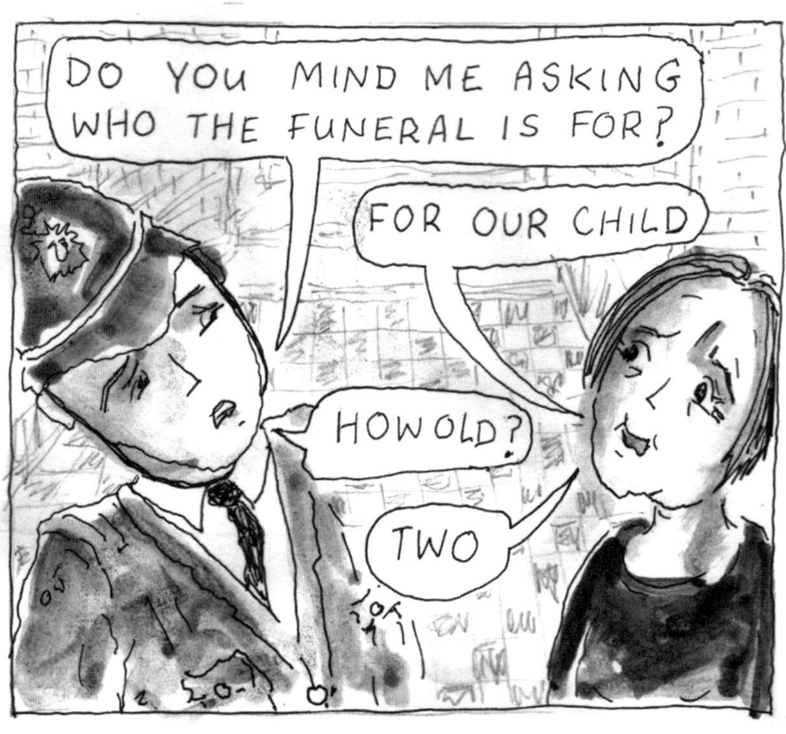
DO YOU MIND ME ASKING WHO THE FUNERAL IS FOR?
FOR OUR CHILD
HOW OLD?
TWO

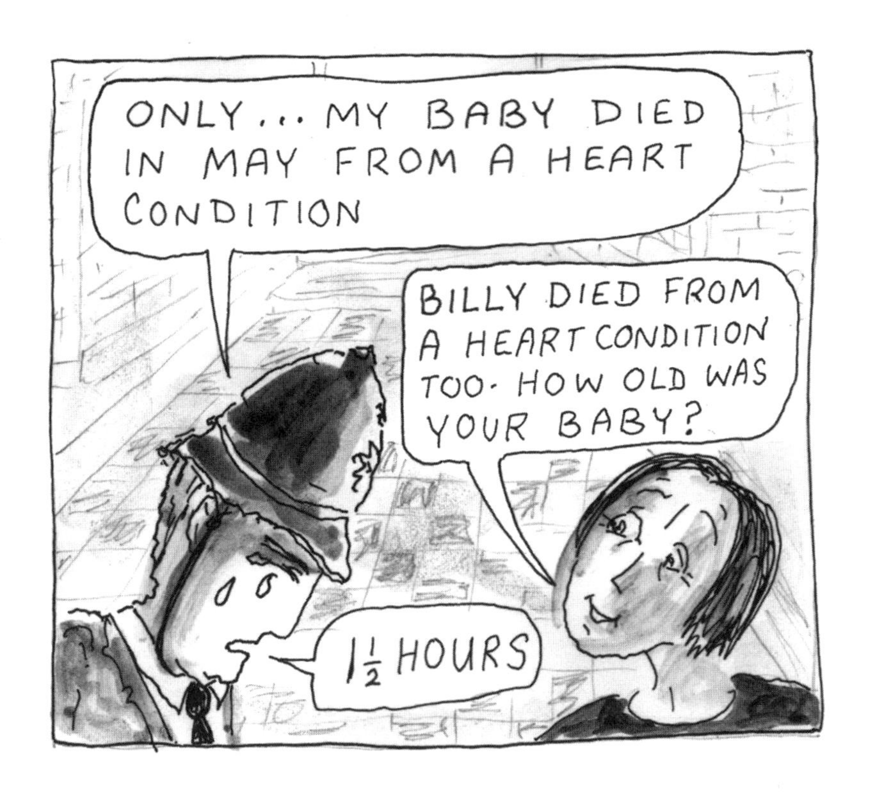
ONLY... MY BABY DIED IN MAY FROM A HEART CONDITION
BILLY DIED FROM A HEART CONDITION TOO. HOW OLD WAS YOUR BABY?
$1\frac{1}{2}$ HOURS

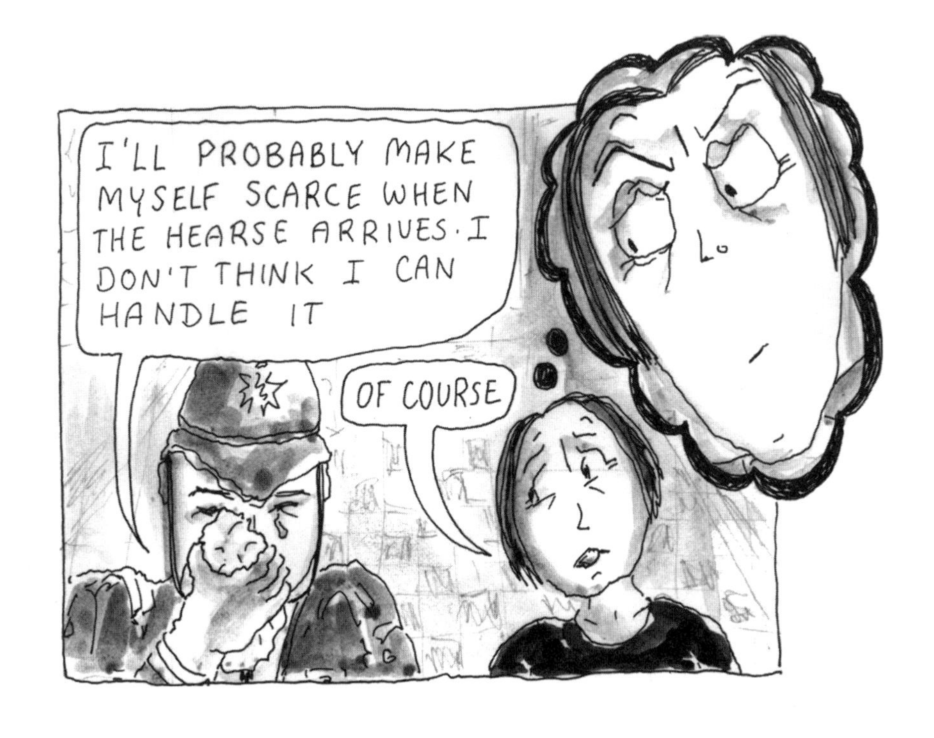
I'LL PROBABLY MAKE MYSELF SCARCE WHEN THE HEARSE ARRIVES. I DON'T THINK I CAN HANDLE IT
OF COURSE

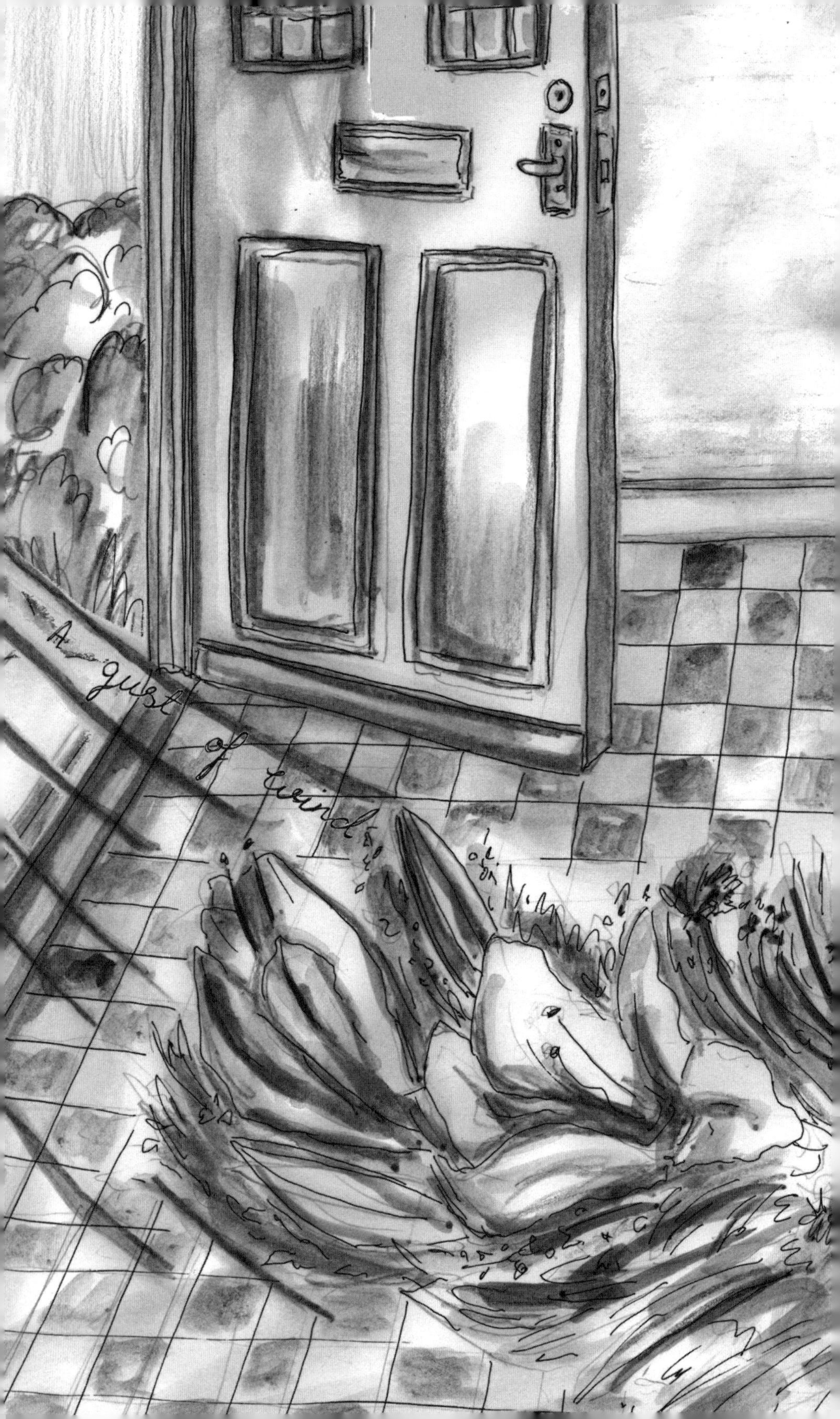
A gust of wind

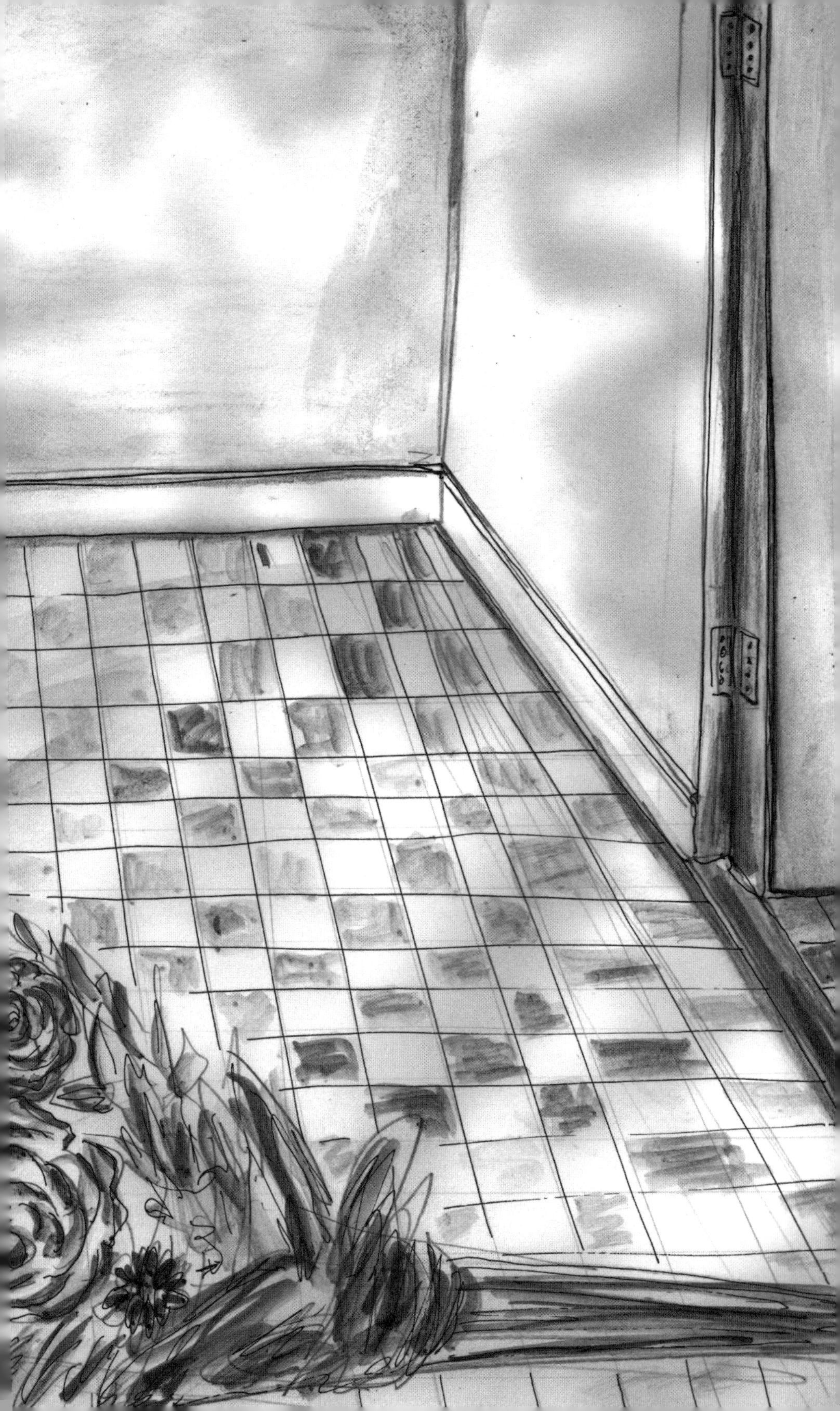

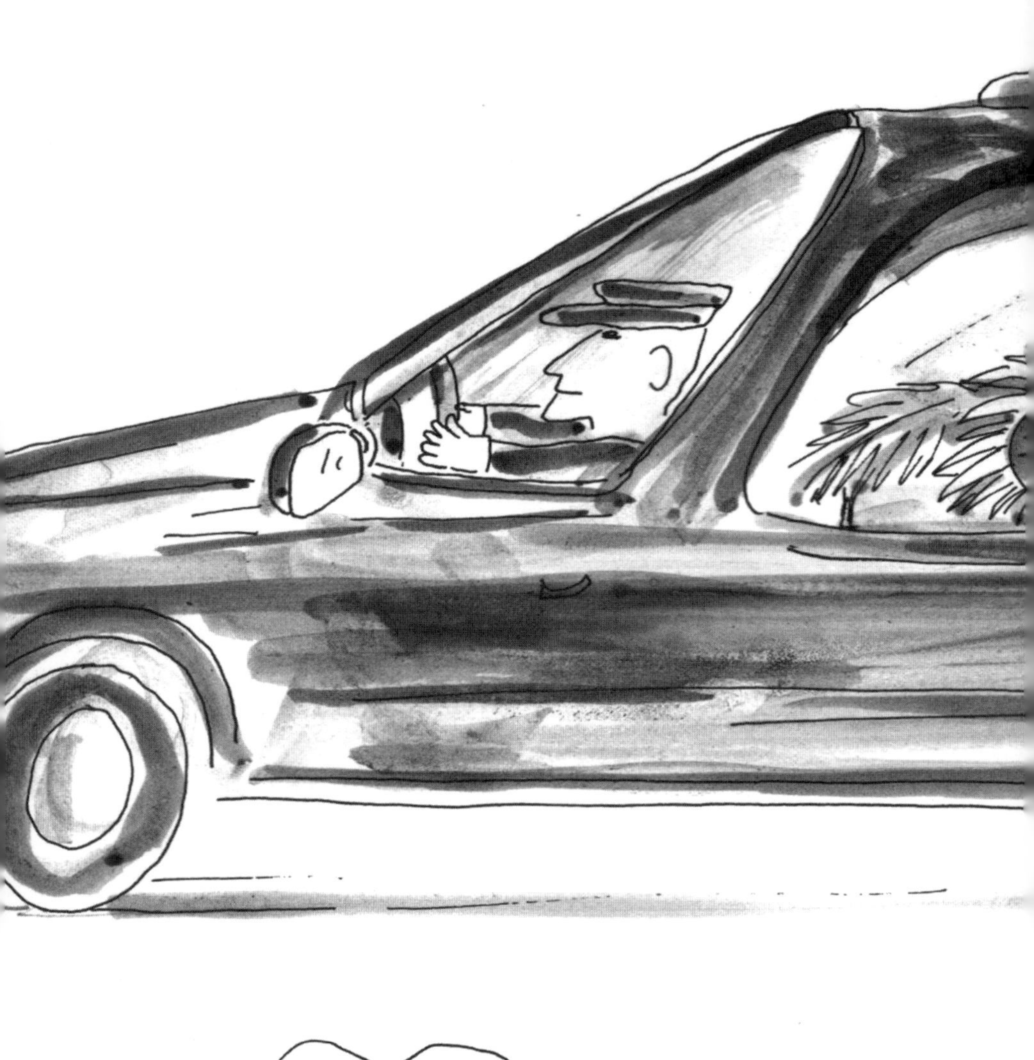

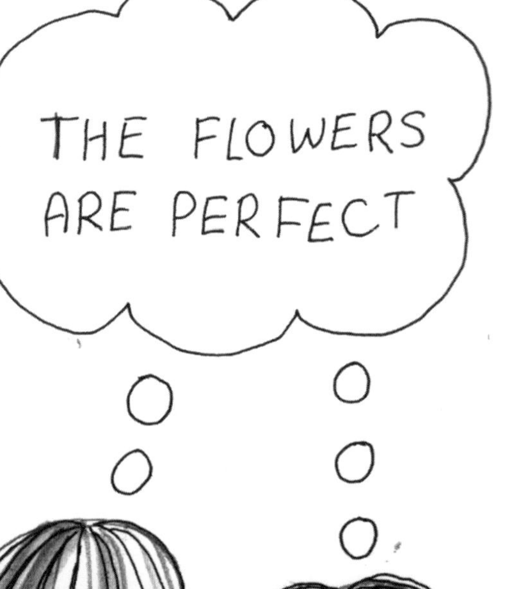
THE FLOWERS ARE PERFECT

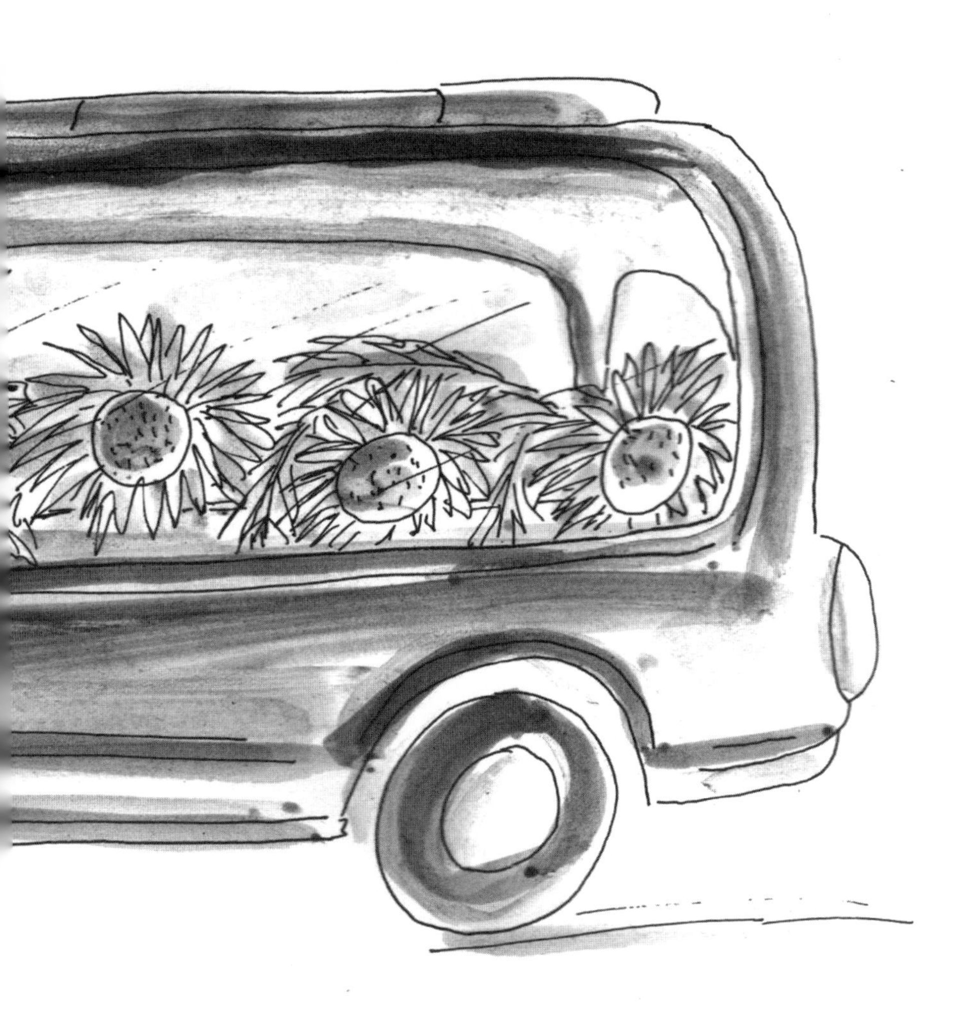

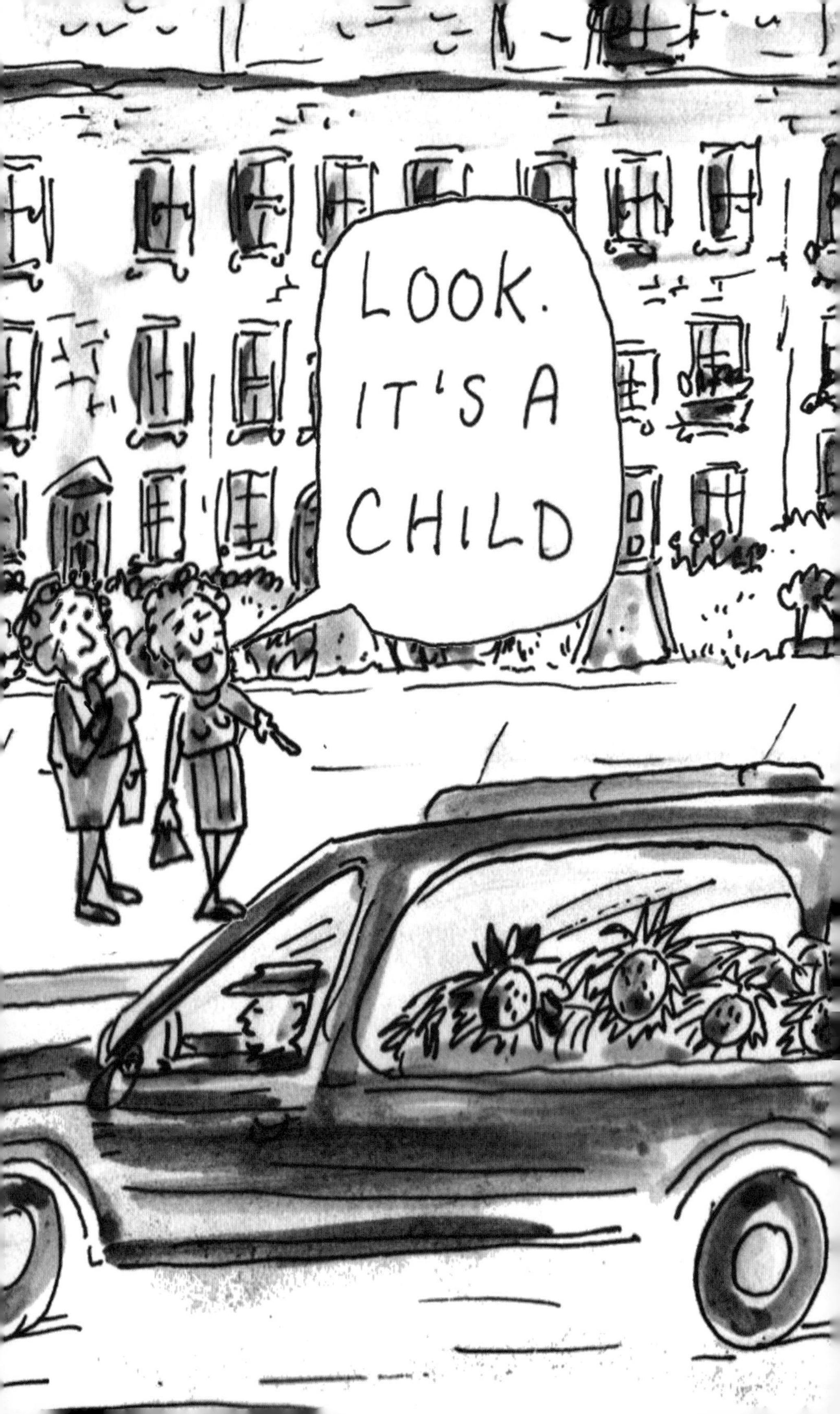
LOOK. IT'S A CHILD

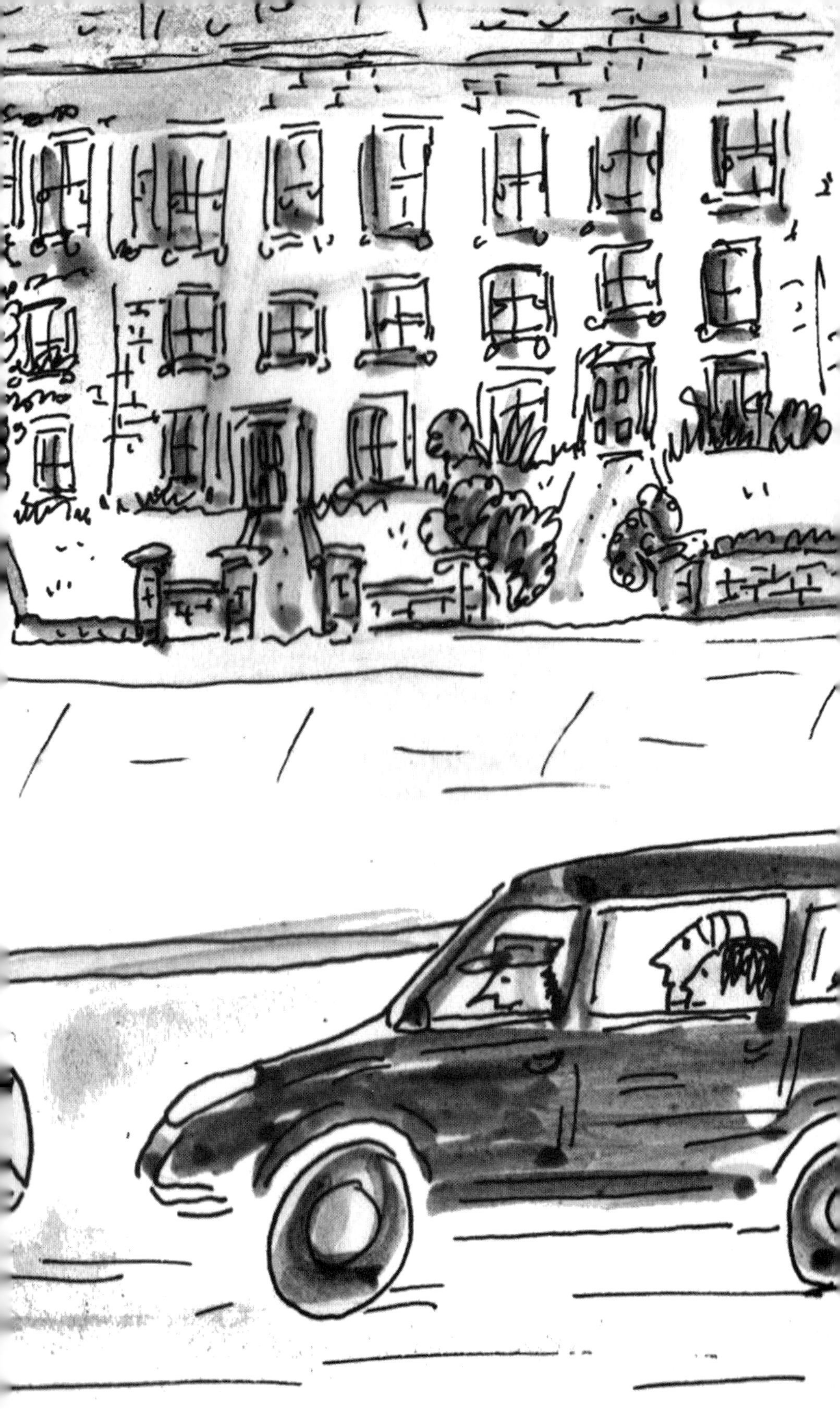

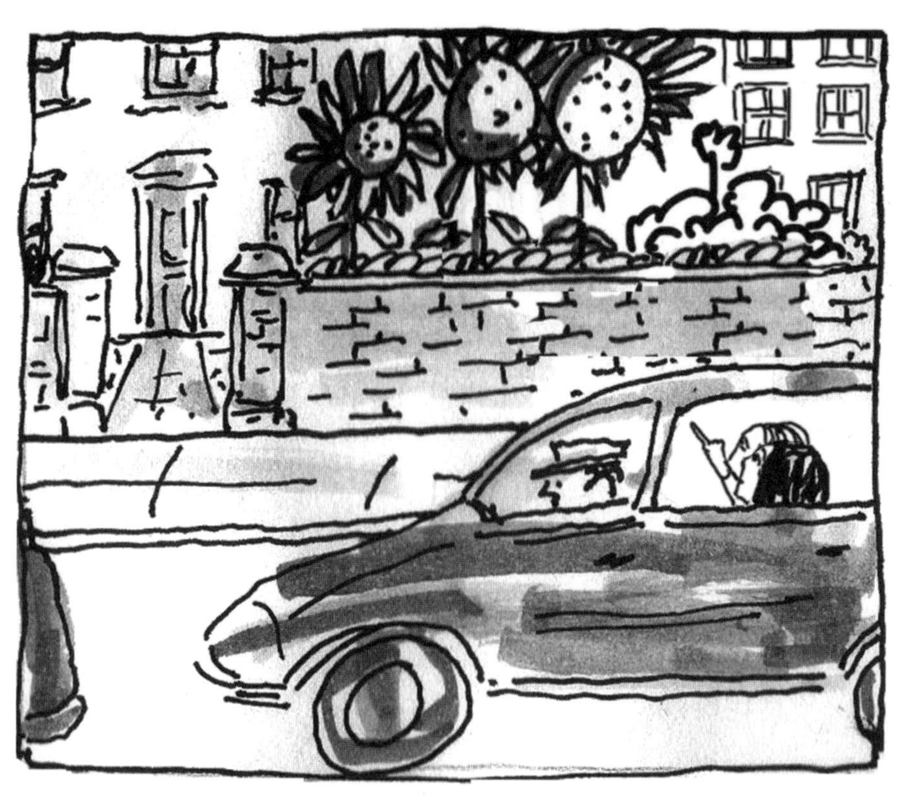

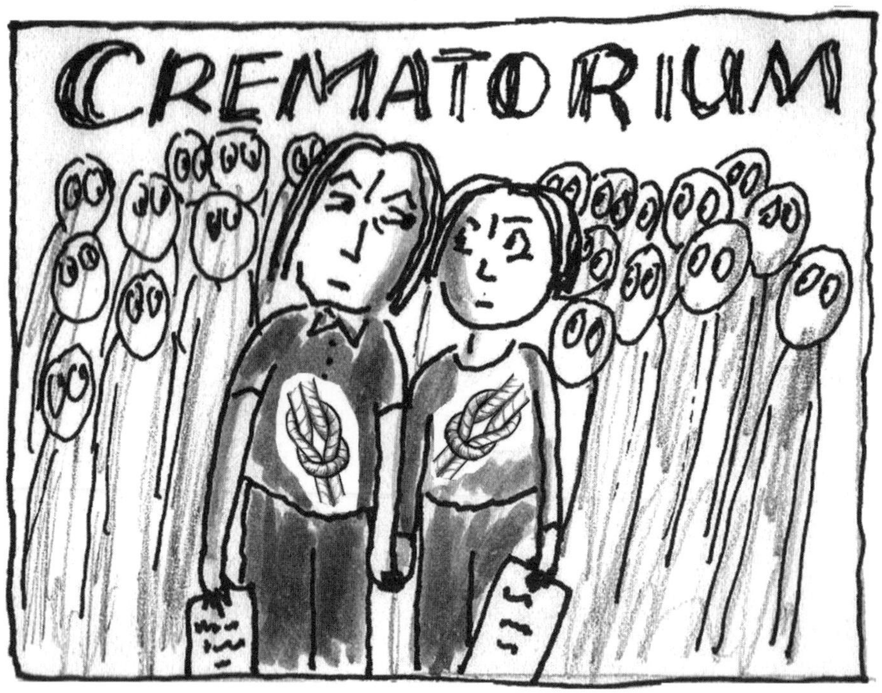
CREMATORIUM

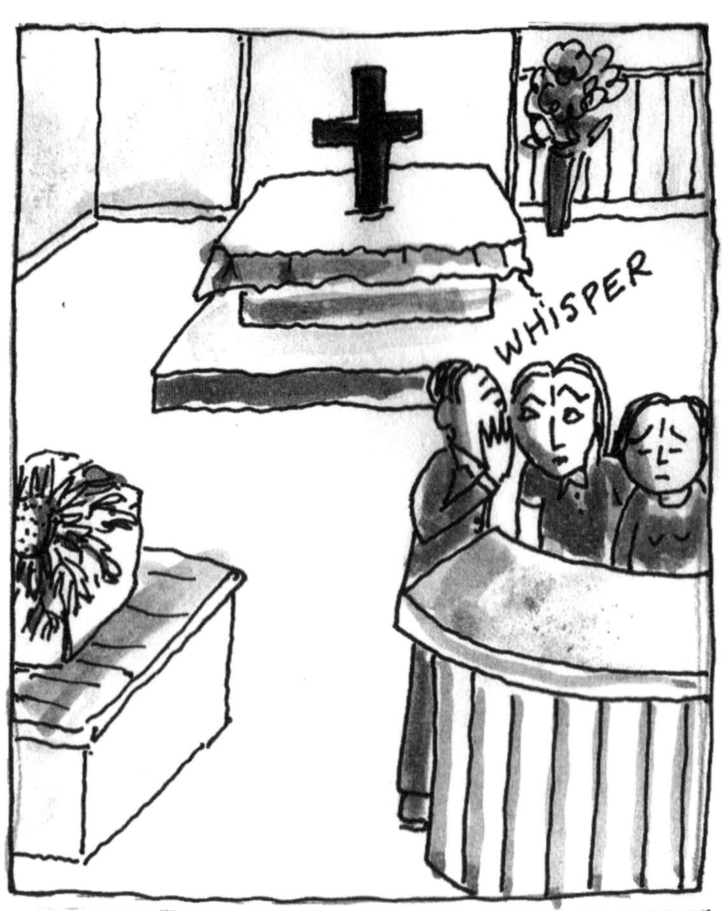
WHISPER

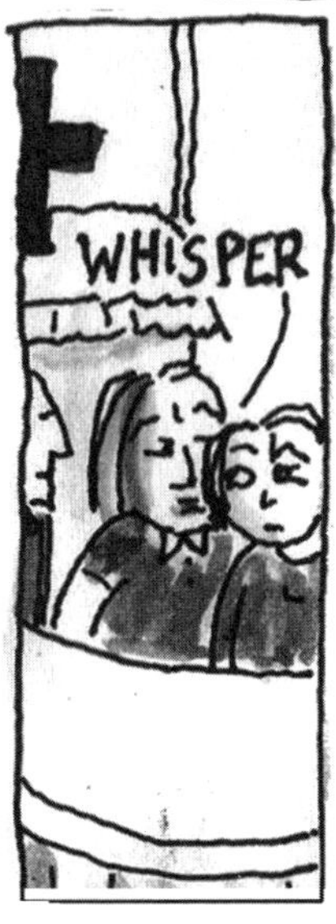
WHISPER

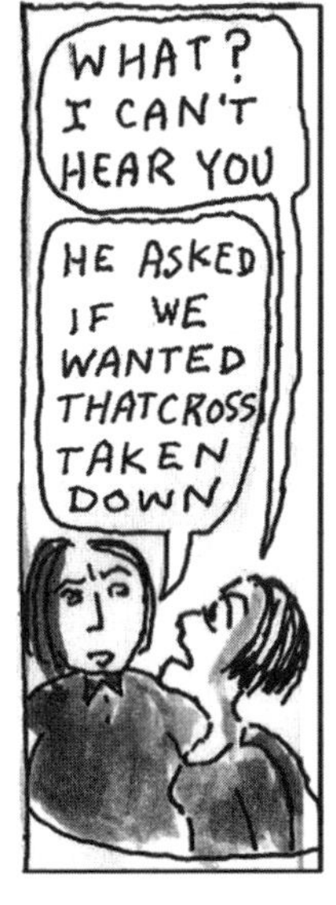
WHAT? I CAN'T HEAR YOU
HE ASKED IF WE WANTED THATCROSS TAKEN DOWN

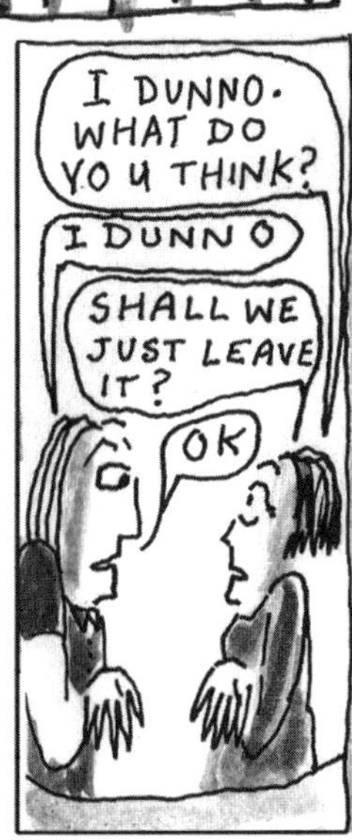
I DUNNO. WHAT DO YOU THINK?
I DUNNO
SHALL WE JUST LEAVE IT?
OK

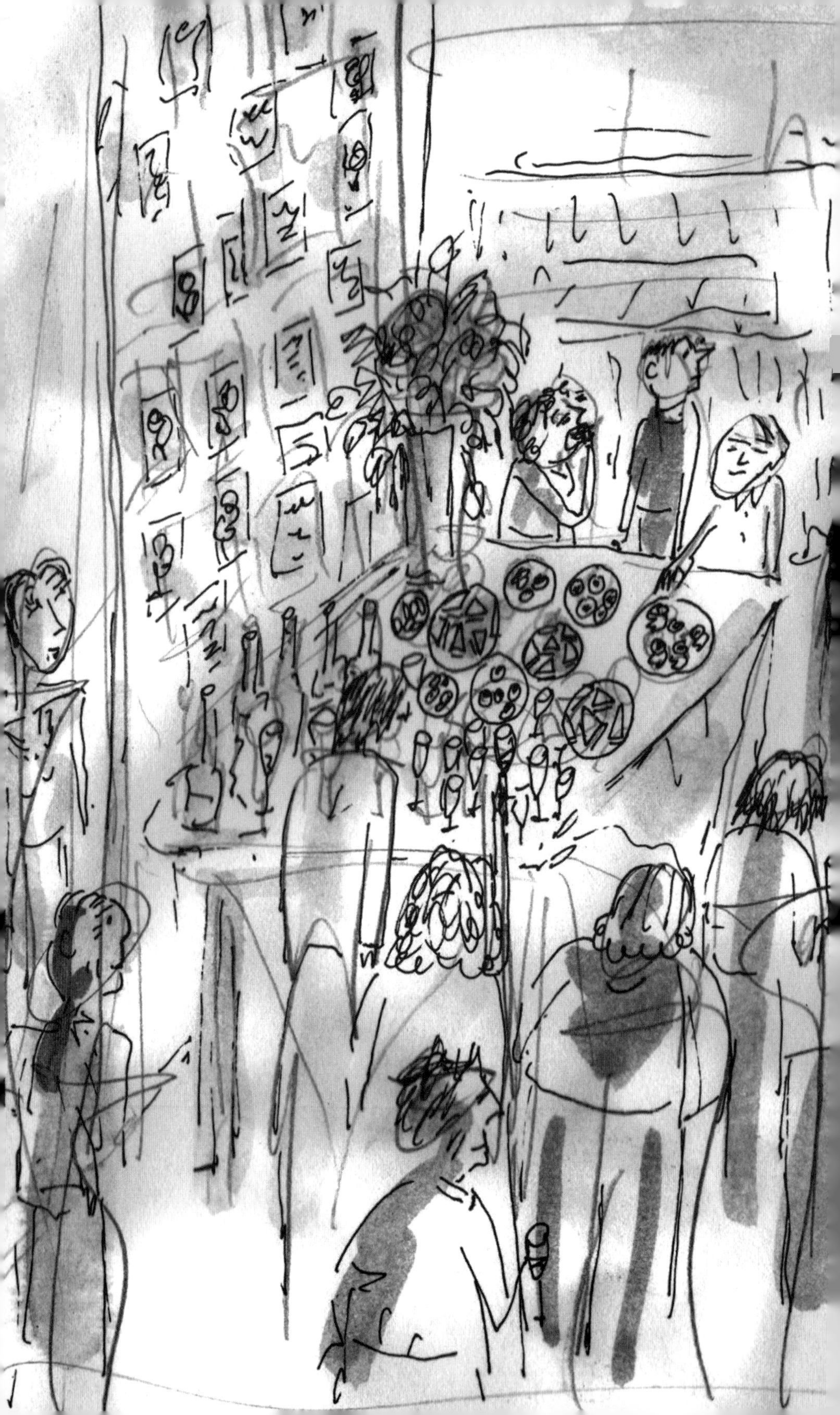

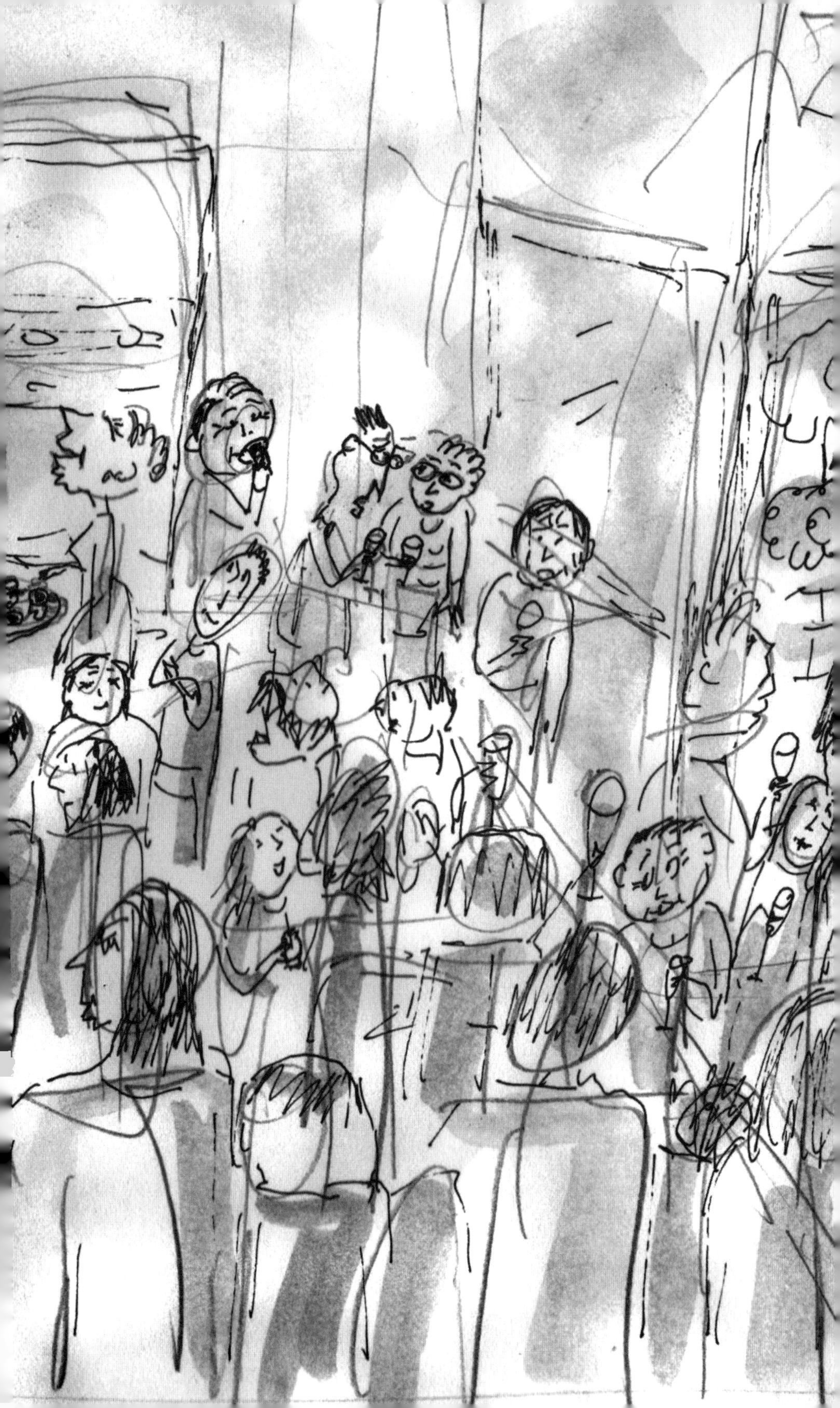

AFTERWARDS OUR NEXT-DOOR NEIGHBOUR KNOCKED AT THE DOOR.

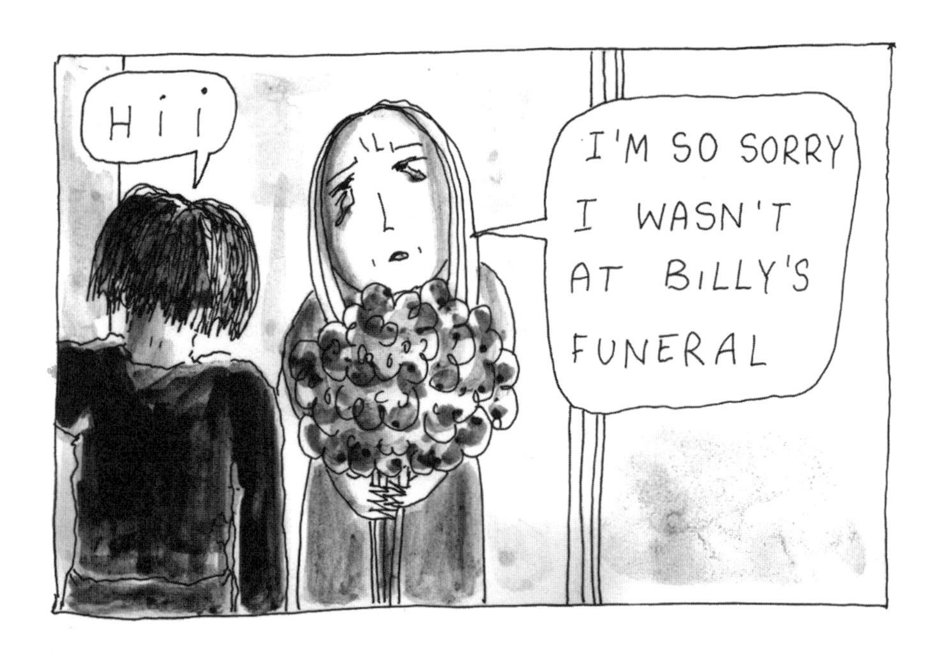
Hi i
I'M SO SORRY I WASN'T AT BILLY'S FUNERAL

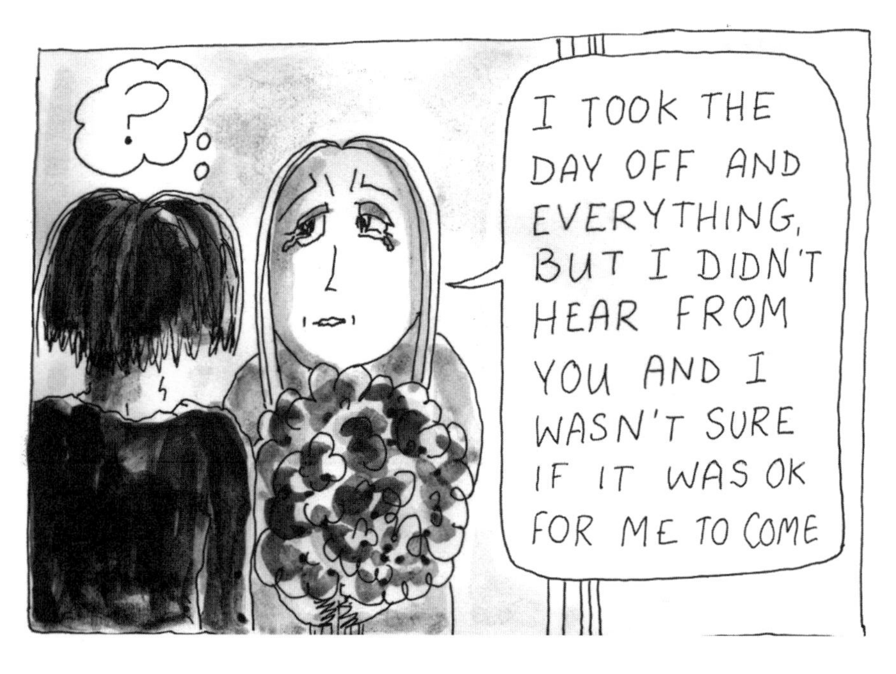
?
I TOOK THE DAY OFF AND EVERYTHING, BUT I DIDN'T HEAR FROM YOU AND I WASN'T SURE IF IT WAS OK FOR ME TO COME

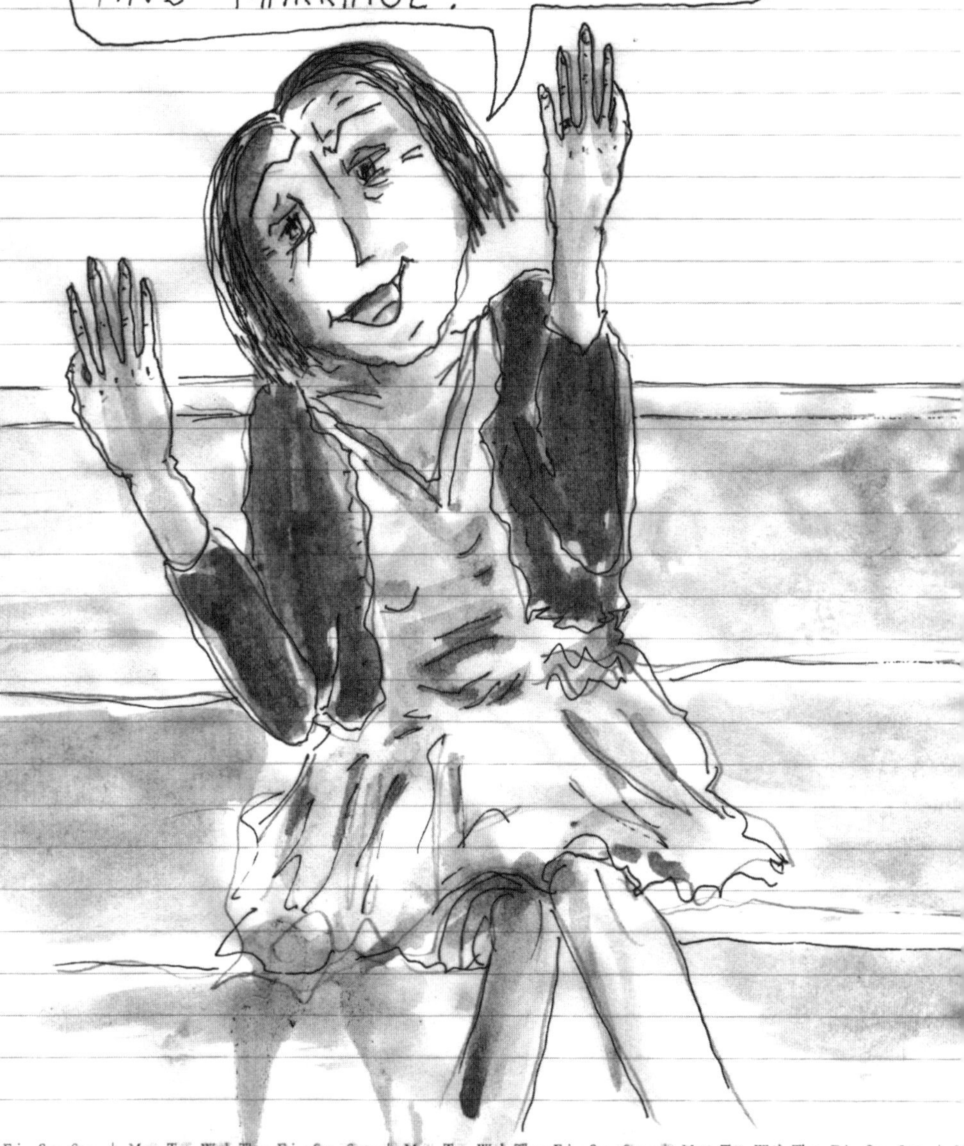
WHY IS FUNERAL ETIQUETTE SO UNCLEAR TO US WHEN DEATH IS AS COMMON AS BIRTHDAYS AND MARRIAGE?

Thu	Fri	Sat	Sun	Mon	Tue	Wed	Thu	Fri	Sat	Sun	Mon	Tue	Wed	Thu	Fri	Sat	Sun	Mon	Tue	Wed	Thu	Fri	Sat	Sun
4	5	6	7	8	9	10	11	12	13	14	15	16	17	18	19	20	21	22	23	24	25	26	27	28

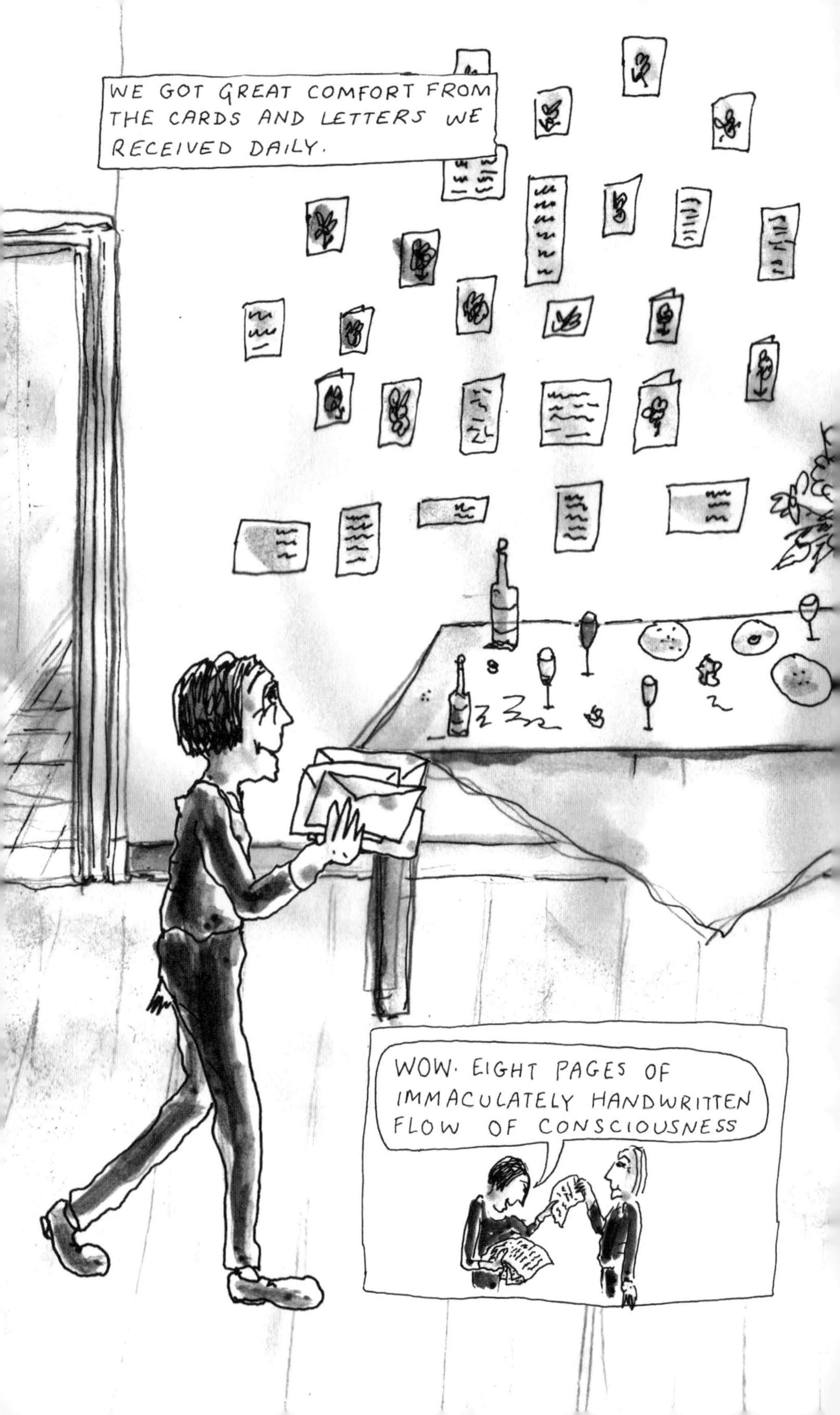
WE GOT GREAT COMFORT FROM THE CARDS AND LETTERS WE RECEIVED DAILY.
WOW. EIGHT PAGES OF IMMACULATELY HANDWRITTEN FLOW OF CONSCIOUSNESS

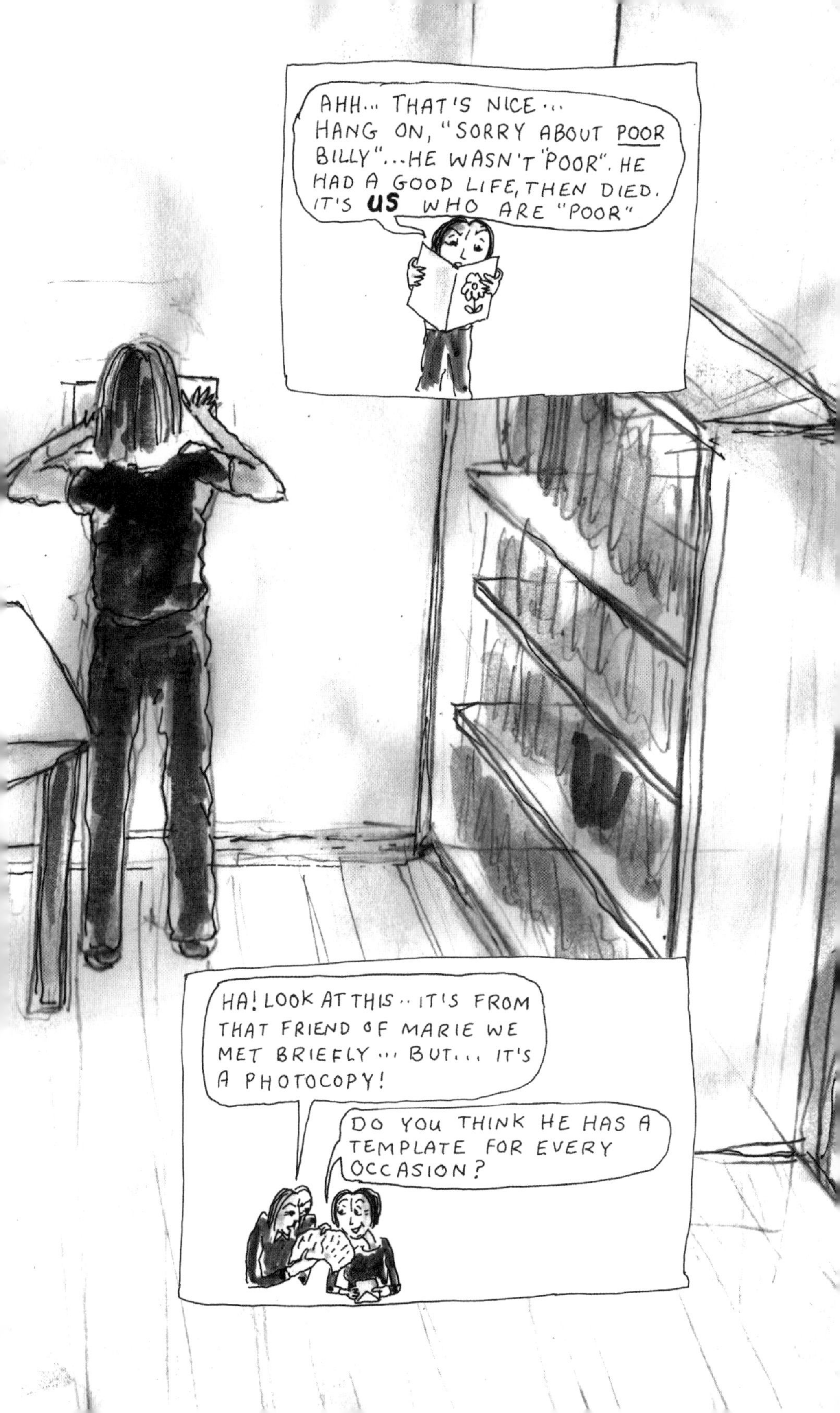
AHH... THAT'S NICE...
HANG ON, "SORRY ABOUT POOR BILLY"...HE WASN'T "POOR". HE HAD A GOOD LIFE, THEN DIED. IT'S US WHO ARE "POOR"
HA! LOOK AT THIS.. IT'S FROM THAT FRIEND OF MARIE WE MET BRIEFLY... BUT... IT'S A PHOTOCOPY!
DO YOU THINK HE HAS A TEMPLATE FOR EVERY OCCASION?

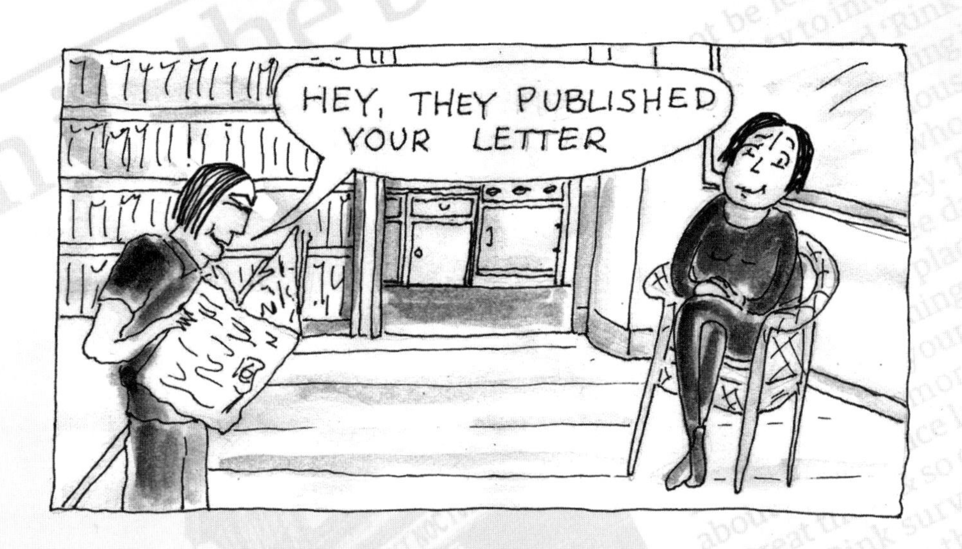
HEY, THEY PUBLISHED YOUR LETTER

Private Lives

Last week, a mother wrote of the despair she felt when her baby daughter died at just three days old. How can she begin to come to terms with her loss?

The comfort of strangers

OUR SON died the day before we read your letter. He was two and for six months he'd had an undiagnosed respiratory illness, maybe asthma.

Unlike you, we have had no religious input and in a way it is harder. The way we grieve is not set out and we have no prescription to follow. But it is your time to do whatever makes you cope. I tell you what we tell ourselves: your baby didn't suffer in her short, sweet life and all that was possible was done. If she had suffered and then died, you would have felt empty *and* guilty. But there is nothing to say for the emptiness inside you, except that time will make the pain less acute.

Nicola Streeten
Crouch End

WE HAD also been married for four years and my wife was in her mid-thirties when our first, much tried-for baby died at birth. We witnessed the whole gamut of responses from the incredibly supportive and helpful to the sad, silly and stupid. The latter included supposedly close friends who never contacted us at the

SOME WEEKS LATER THE WORLD AROUND US RETURNED TO ITS EVERYDAY PREOCCUPATIONS ... AND WE TRIED TO AS WELL...

I SAW WOMEN ON THEIR WAY TO WORK

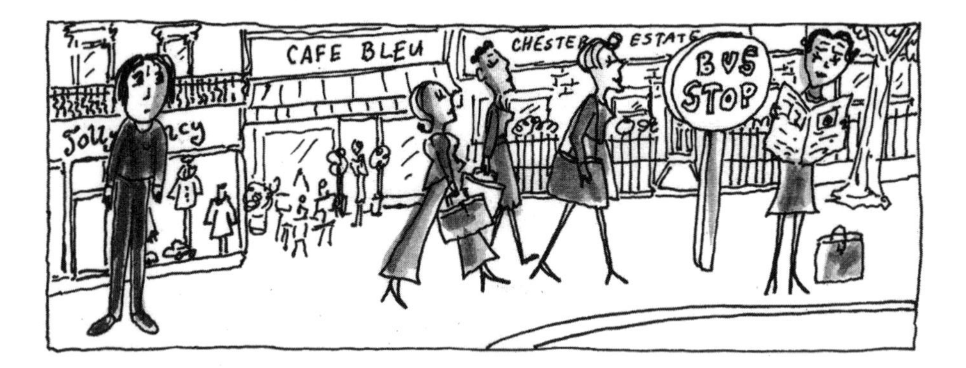

AND WOMEN OFF TO THE PARK WITH CHILDREN

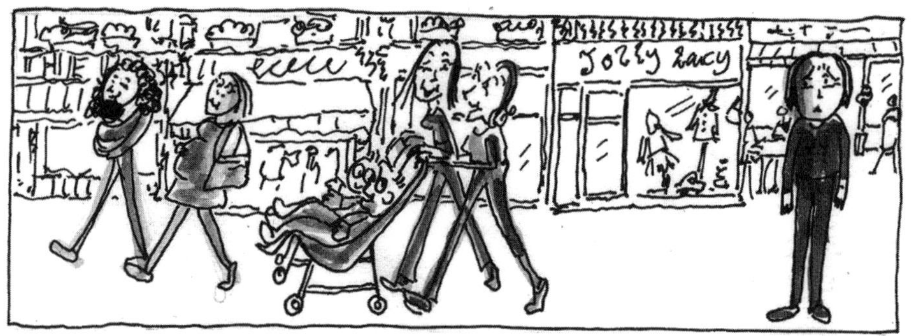

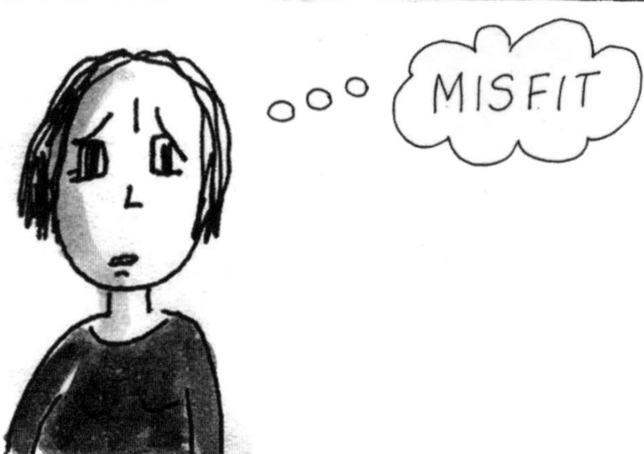

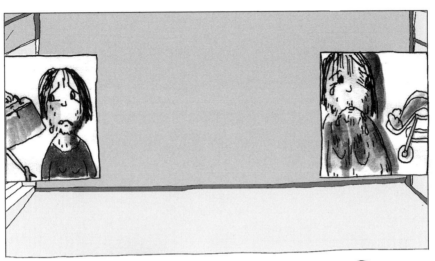

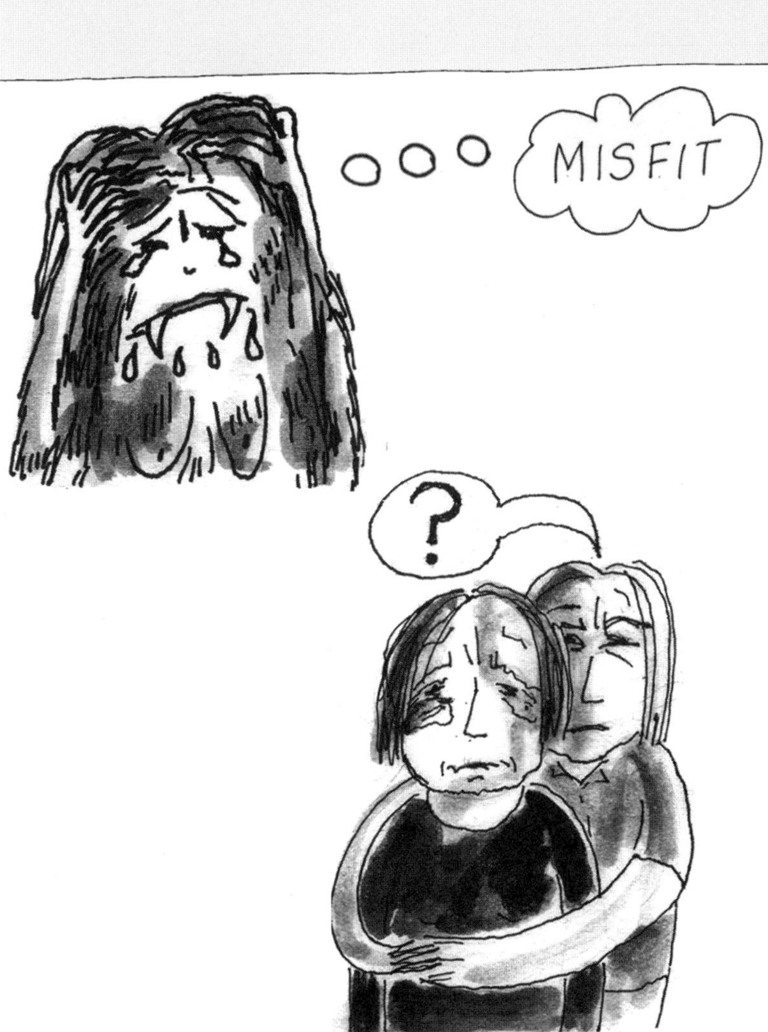
MISFIT
?

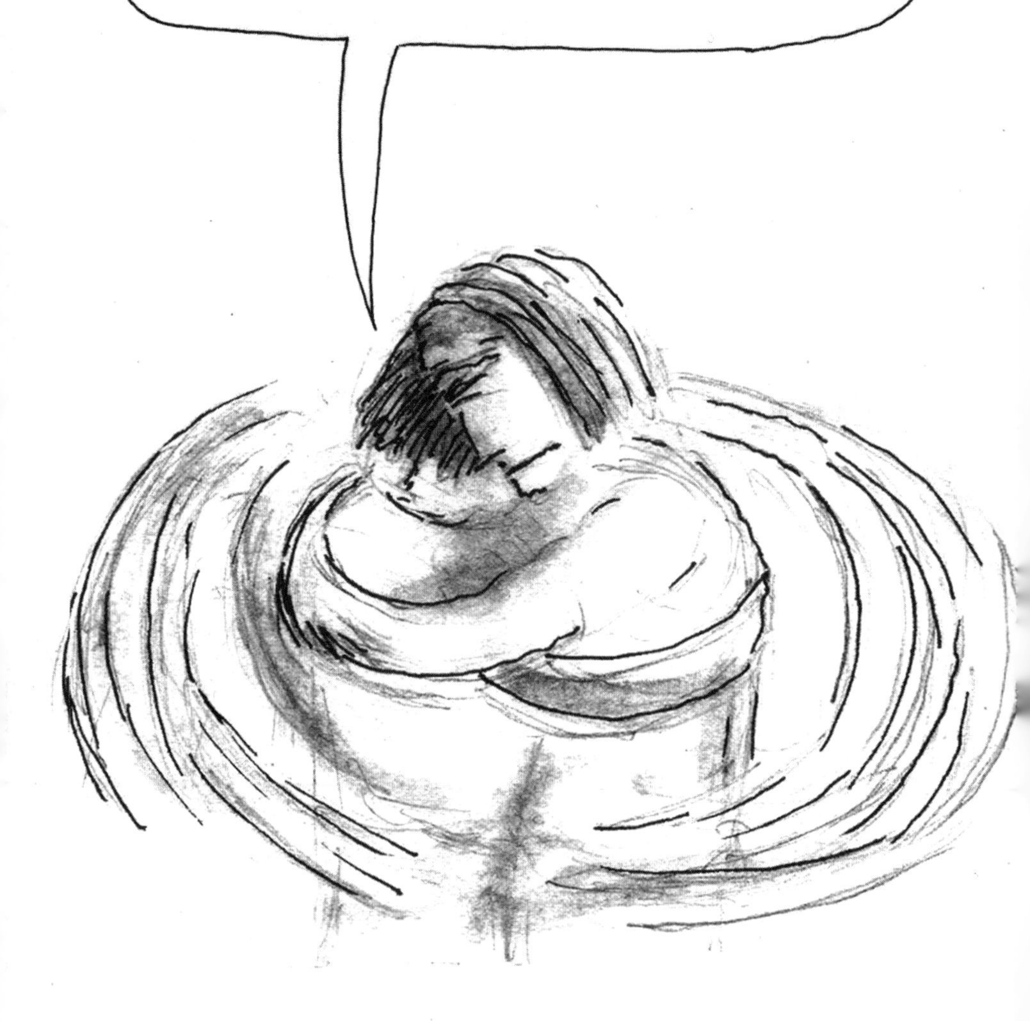
I'M NOT A MOTHER, BUT I'M NOT NOT A MOTHER. I DON'T HAVE A SCRIPT TO FOLLOW ANY MORE

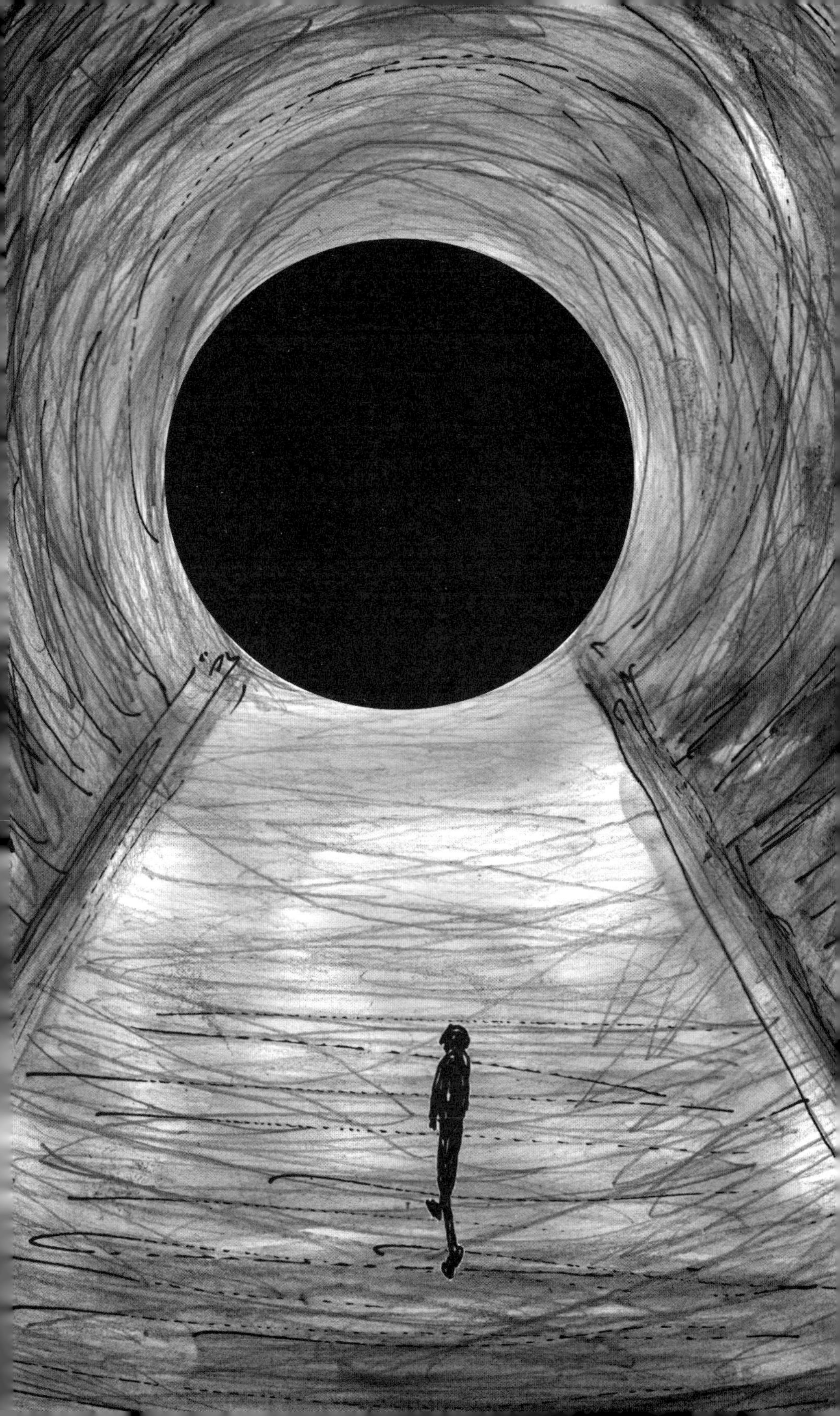

I DECIDED I NEEDED TO DRAMATICALLY ALTER MY APPEARANCE TO REFLECT MY CHANGED IDENTITY... SO I BOOKED IN WITH JEANA.

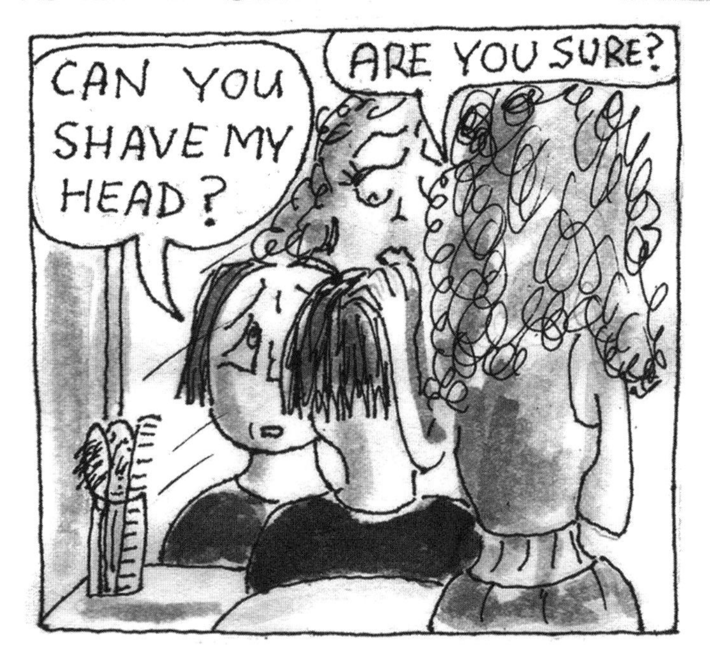
CAN YOU SHAVE MY HEAD?
ARE YOU SURE?

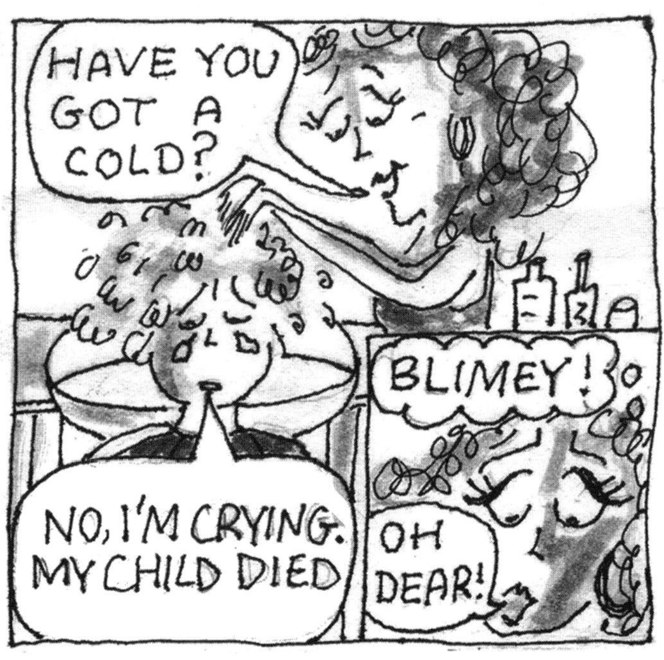
HAVE YOU GOT A COLD?
NO, I'M CRYING. MY CHILD DIED
BLIMEY!
OH DEAR!

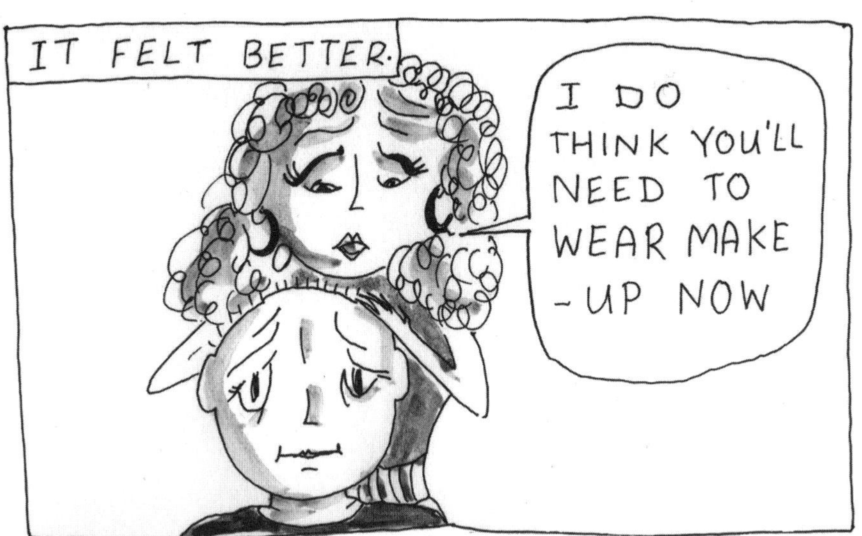
IT FELT BETTER.
I DO THINK YOU'LL NEED TO WEAR MAKE-UP NOW

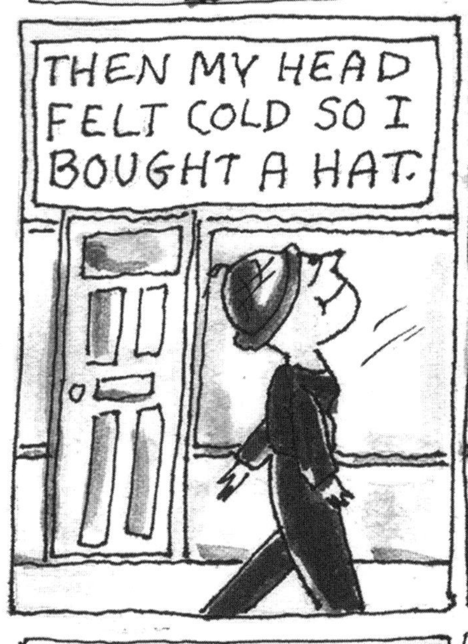
THEN MY HEAD FELT COLD SO I BOUGHT A HAT.

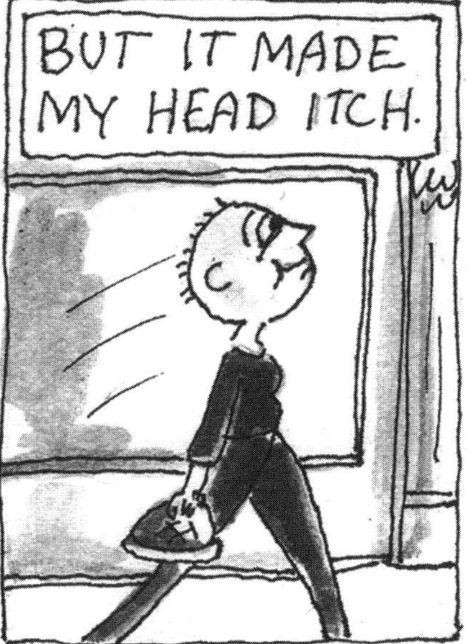
BUT IT MADE MY HEAD ITCH.

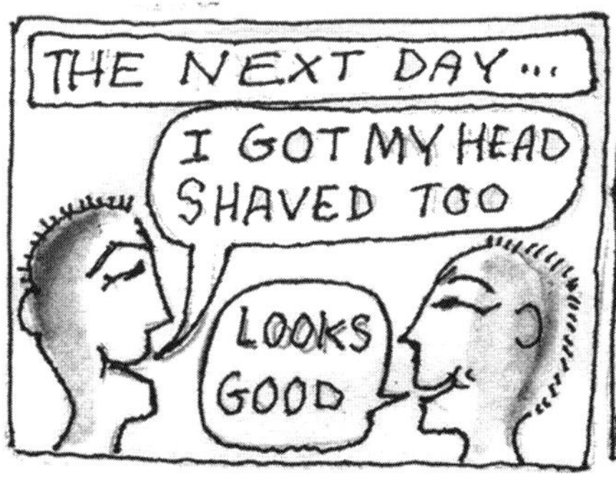
THE NEXT DAY...
I GOT MY HEAD SHAVED TOO
LOOKS GOOD

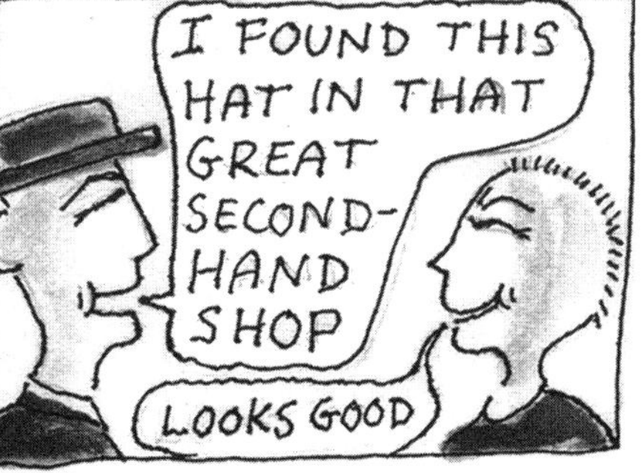
I FOUND THIS HAT IN THAT GREAT SECOND-HAND SHOP
LOOKS GOOD

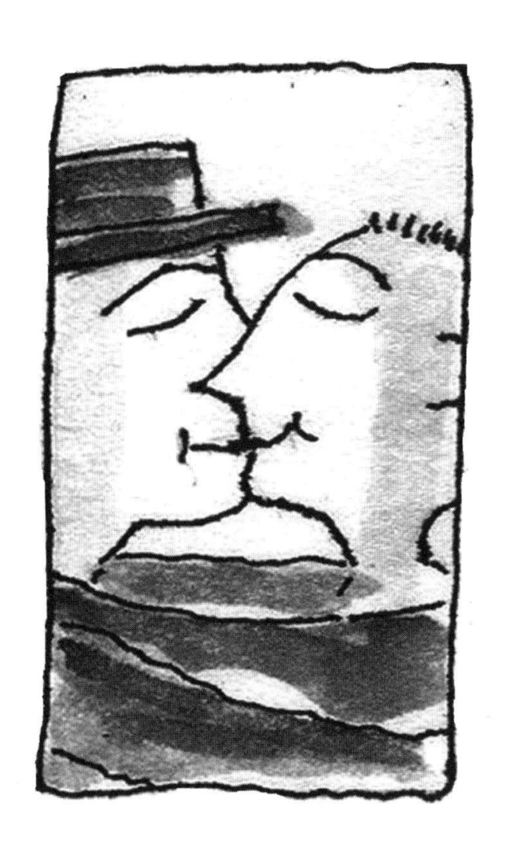

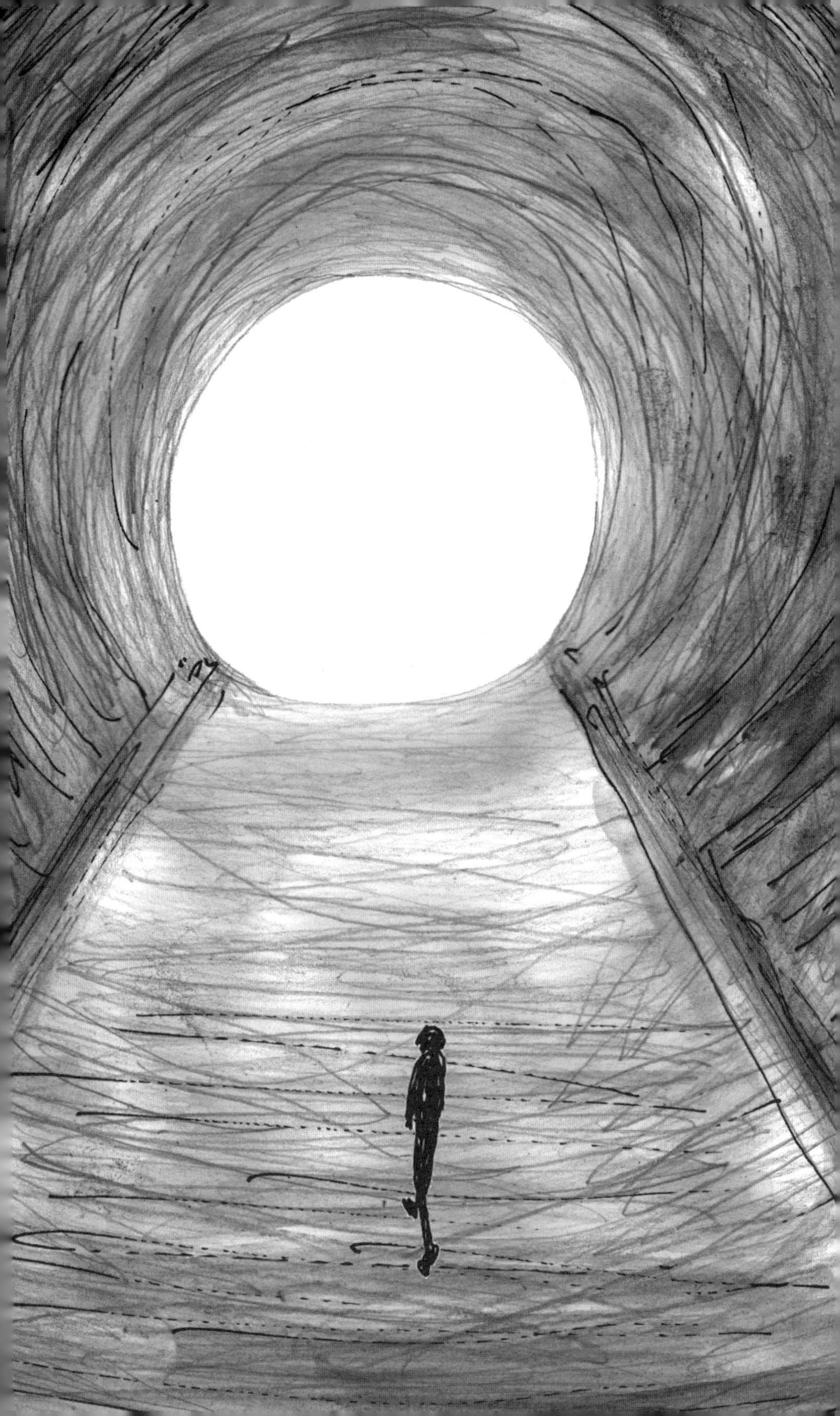

PART TWO

TIME ... I KNEW IT WAS THE HEALER, BUT IN THOSE EARLY MONTHS IT WAS MY TORMENTOR... SLOW ... JEERING ... TIME ... COMBINED WITH A SEARING SENSUAL DEPRIVATION ...

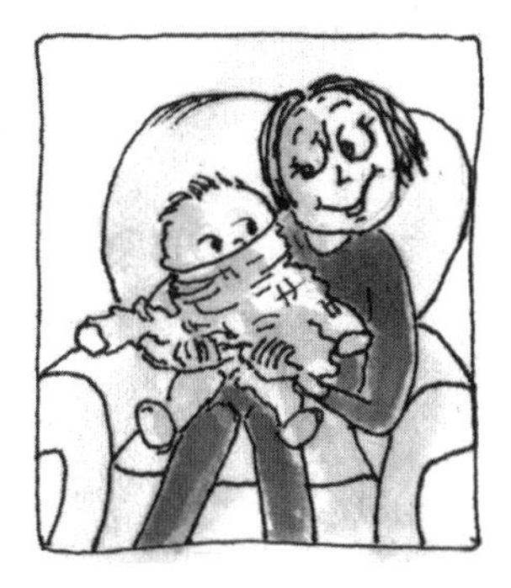
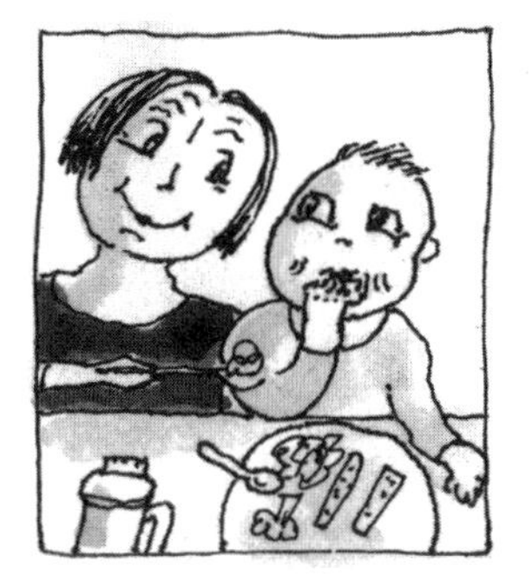
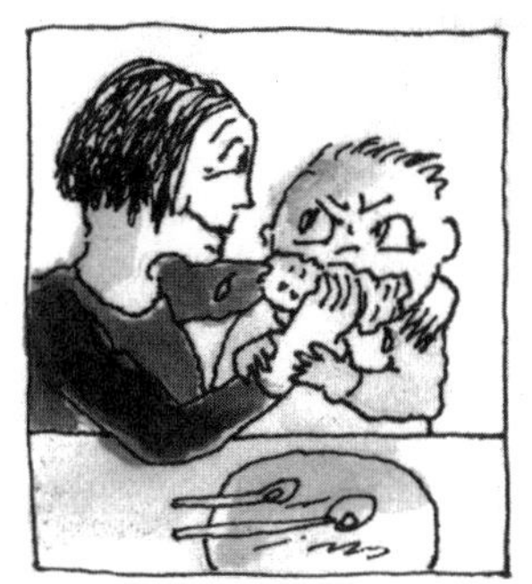

THERE'S SO MUCH TOUCH INVOLVED IN LOOKING AFTER A YOUNG CHILD...

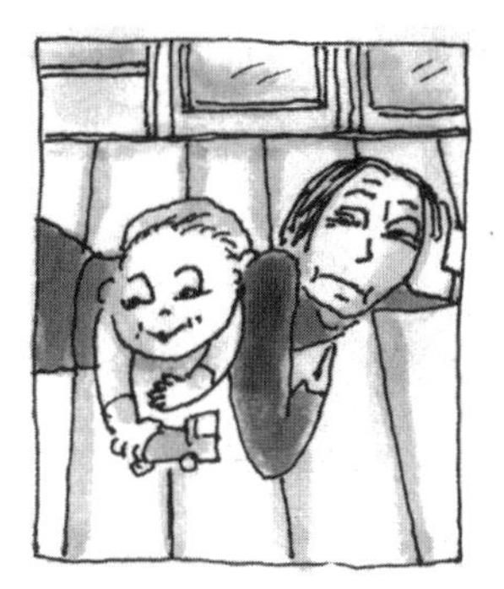
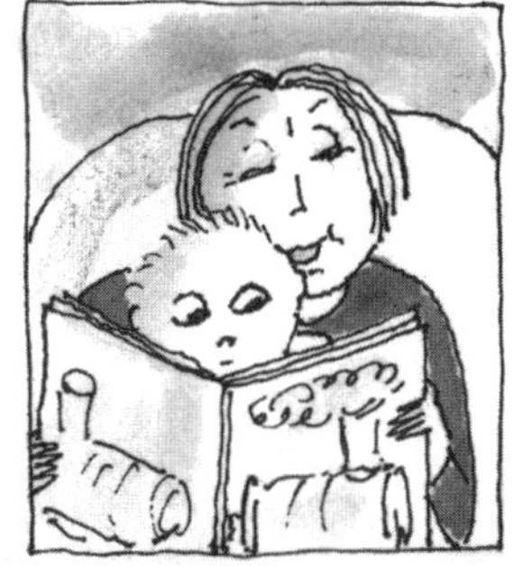
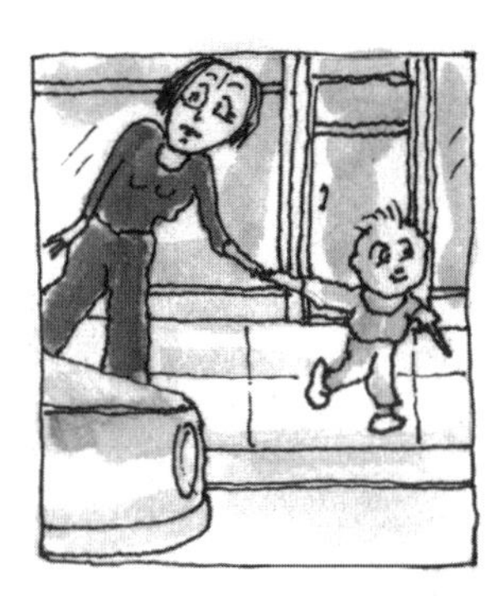

AND YOU HAVE TO LOOK, HEAR AND TASTE FOR THEM TOO.

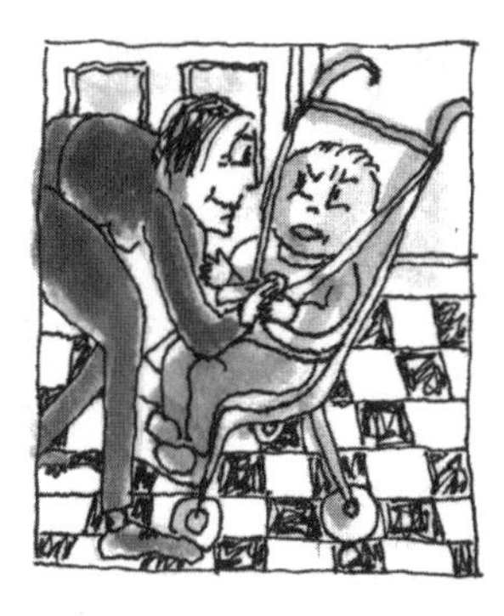
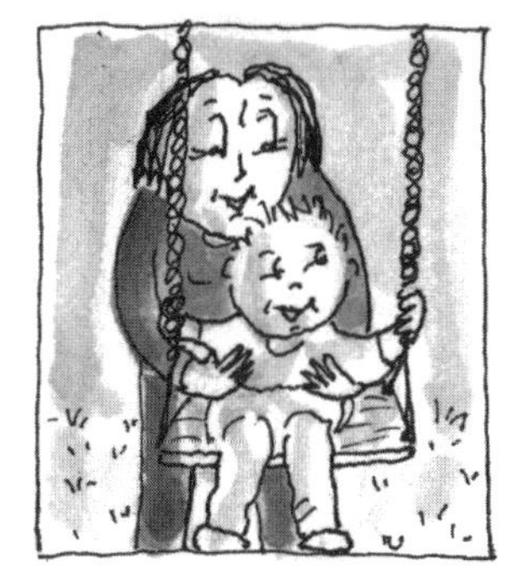
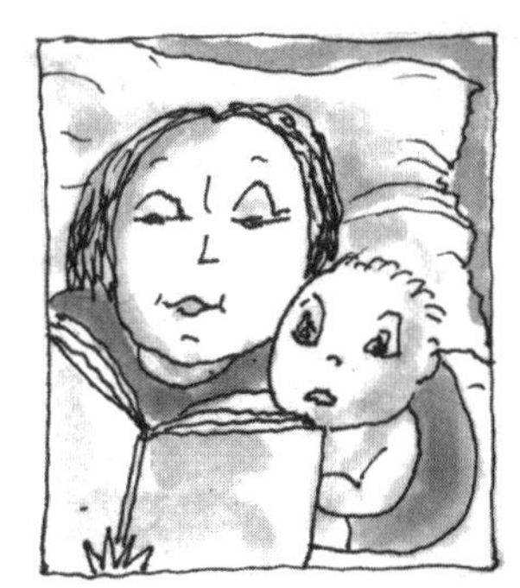

MY ARMS WERE EMPTY,
MY SENSES NUMBED.

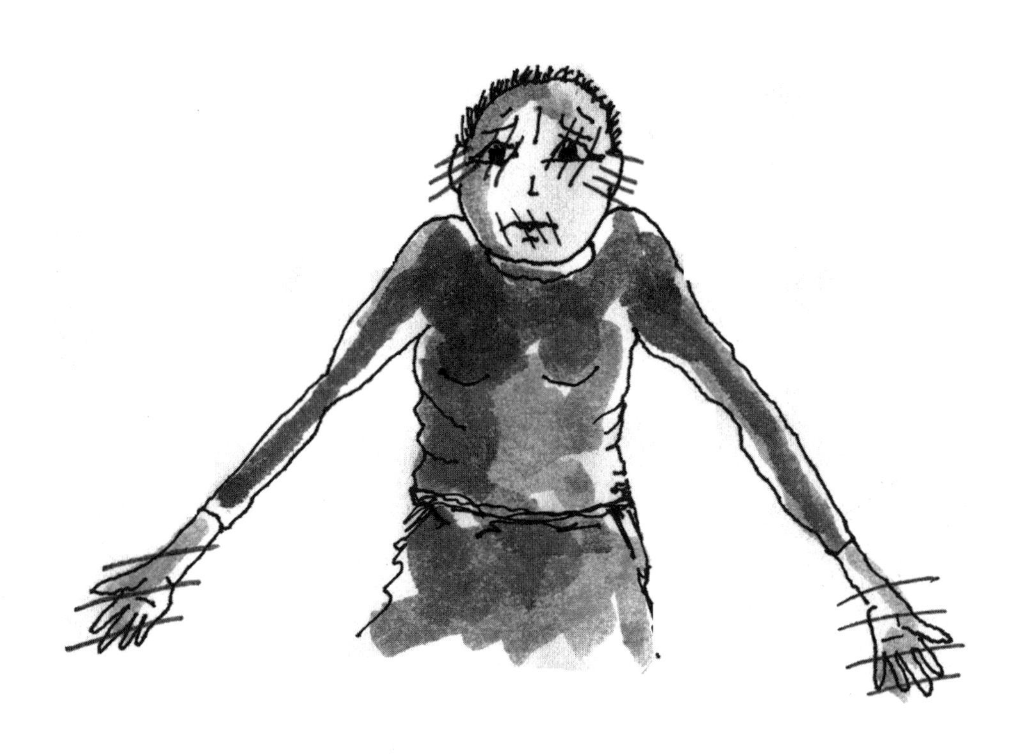

AND **TIME** WAS A
VESSEL FOR THIS ACHING
—VOID—

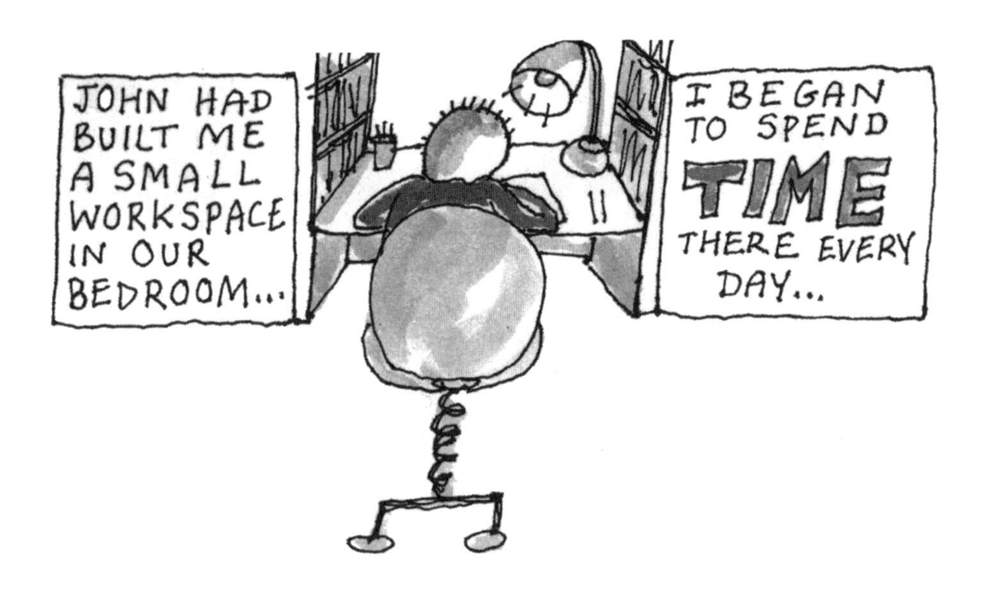
JOHN HAD BUILT ME A SMALL WORKSPACE IN OUR BEDROOM...
I BEGAN TO SPEND TIME THERE EVERY DAY...

DRAWING FILLED THIS VACUUM
... ENTIRELY ... WHOLLY...

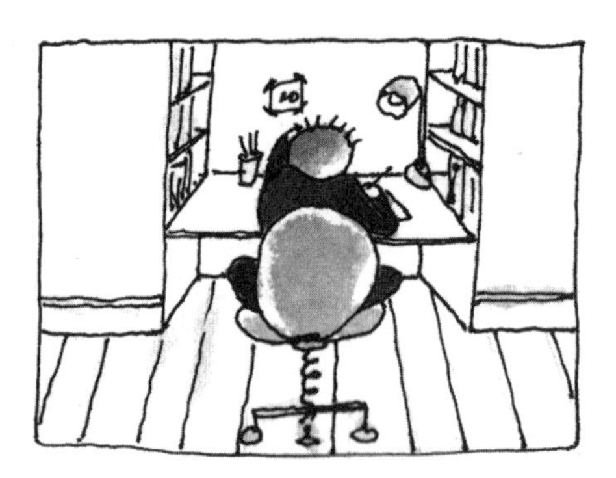

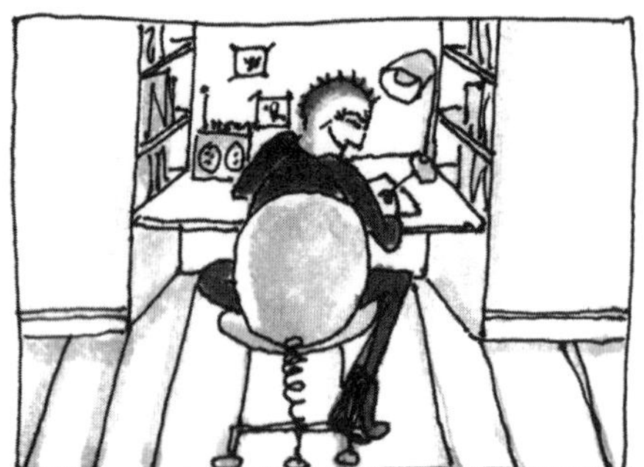

AND I DREW WHAT HAD CONSUMED MY LIFE.

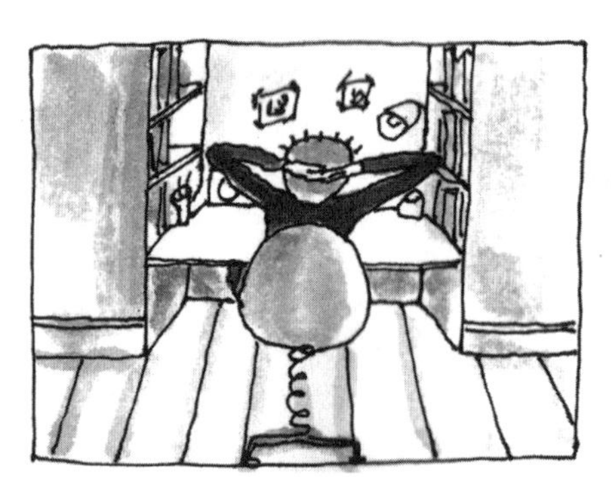

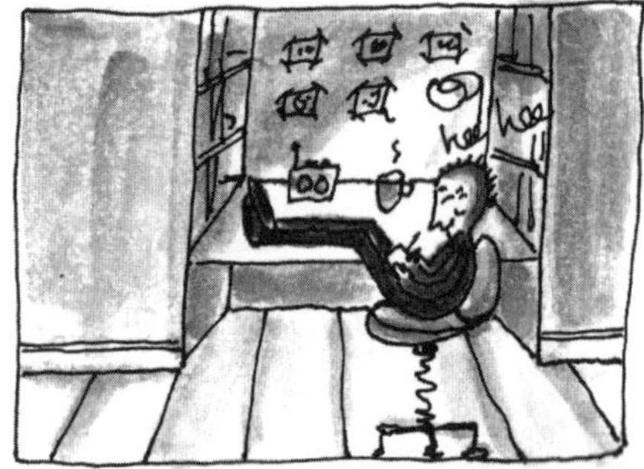

I DREW MY EXPERIENCE OF PARENTING.

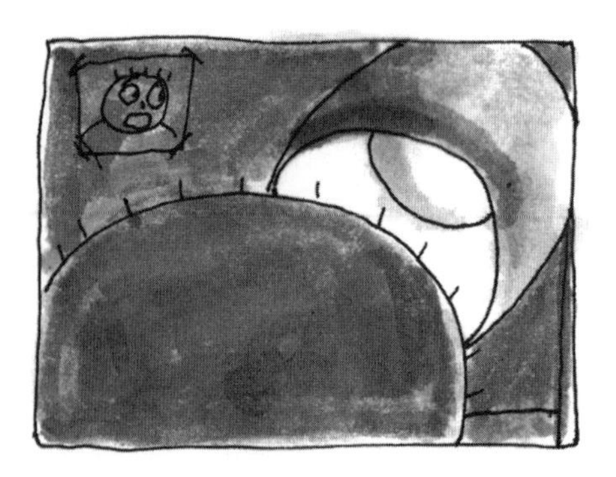

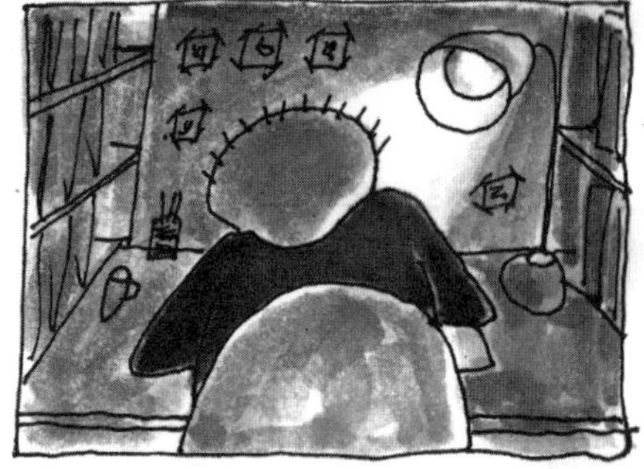

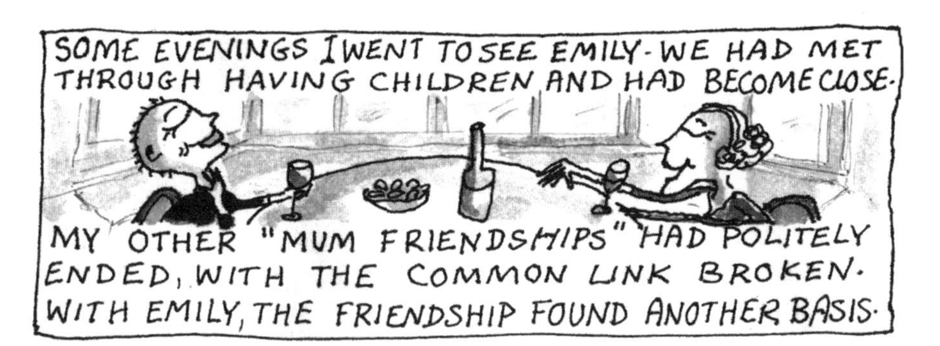

SOME EVENINGS I WENT TO SEE EMILY - WE HAD MET THROUGH HAVING CHILDREN AND HAD BECOME CLOSE.
MY OTHER "MUM FRIENDSHIPS" HAD POLITELY ENDED, WITH THE COMMON LINK BROKEN. WITH EMILY, THE FRIENDSHIP FOUND ANOTHER BASIS.

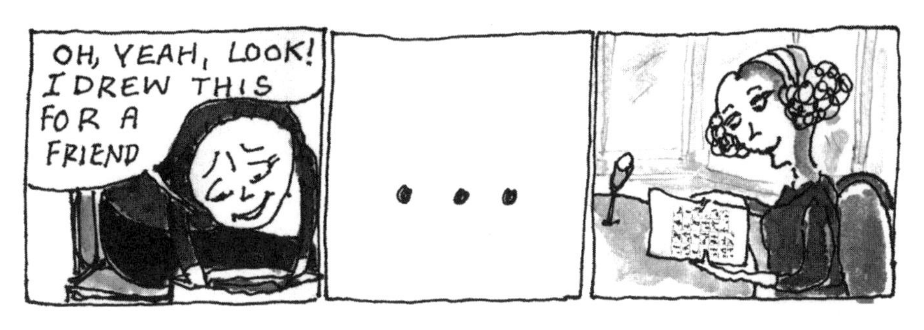

OH, YEAH, LOOK! I DREW THIS FOR A FRIEND
. . .

IF YOU CHANGED THE FORMAT IT WOULD MAKE A GOOD GREETING CARD. SHALL I SHOW MY PARTNER?*

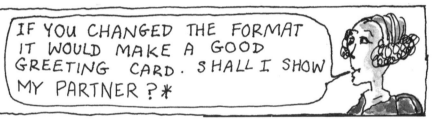

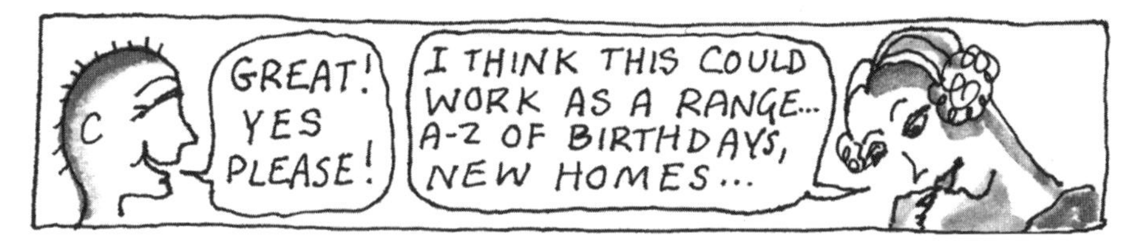

GREAT! YES PLEASE!
I THINK THIS COULD WORK AS A RANGE... A-Z OF BIRTHDAYS, NEW HOMES...

HER PARTNER THOUGHT THEY WOULDN'T SELL, BUT AGREED TO COMMISSION SIX TITLES BECAUSE EMILY LIKED THE IDEA.

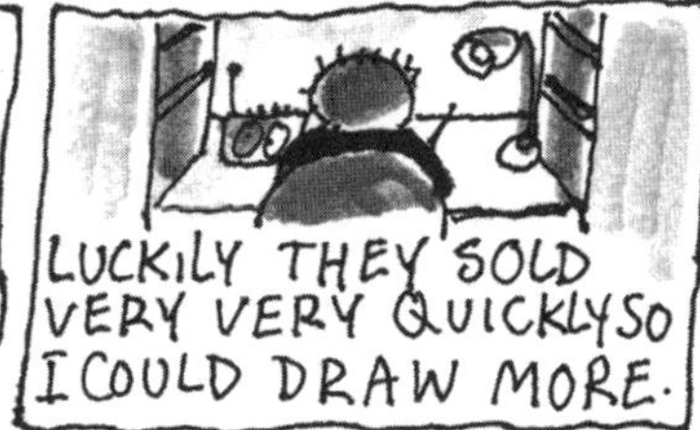

LUCKILY THEY SOLD VERY VERY QUICKLY SO I COULD DRAW MORE.

* A GREETING CARD PUBLISHER

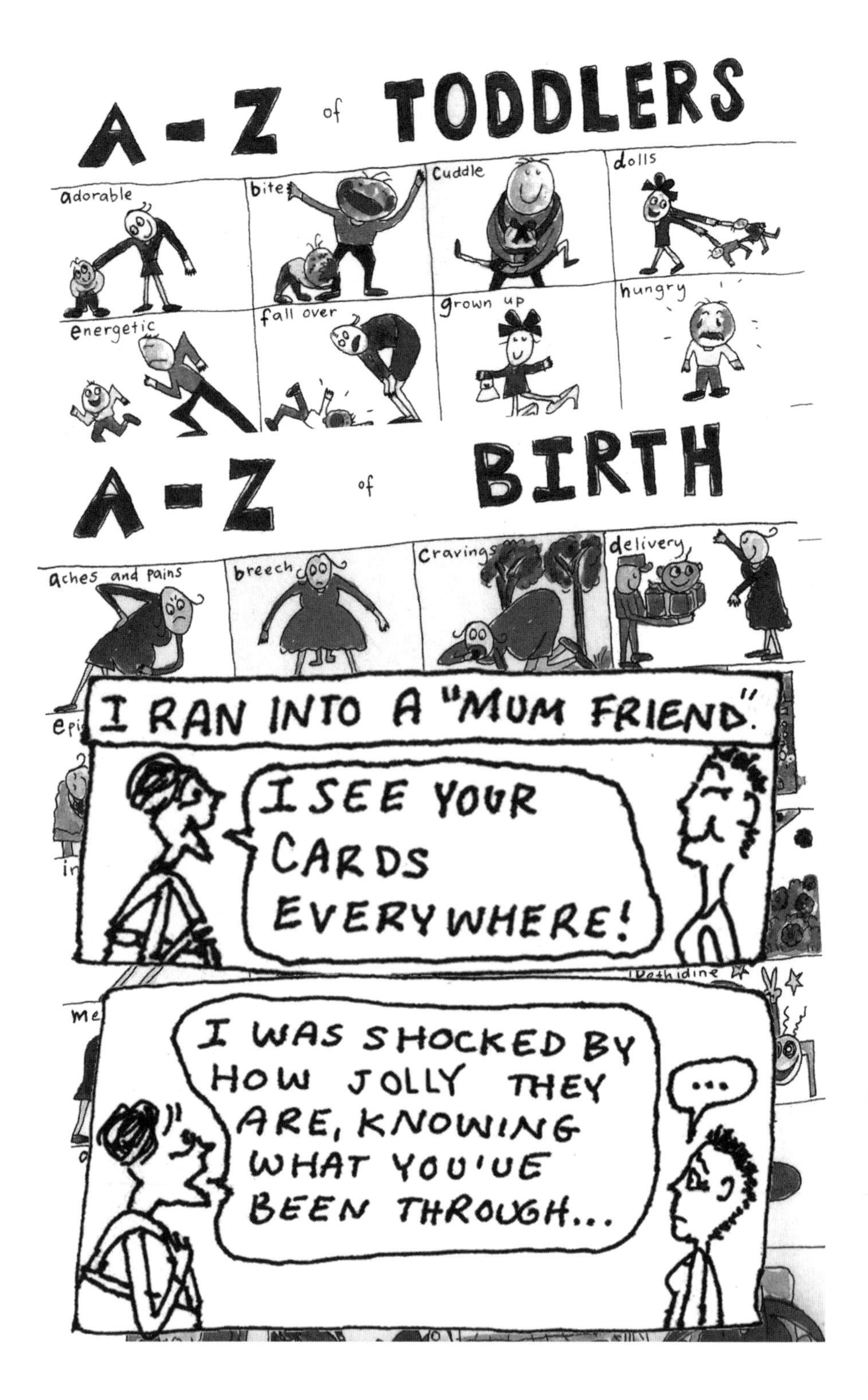
A-Z of TODDLERS
adorable
bite
cuddle
dolls
energetic
fall over
grown up
hungry
A-Z of BIRTH
aches and pains
breech
cravings
delivery
I RAN INTO A "MUM FRIEND".
I SEE YOUR CARDS EVERYWHERE!
I WAS SHOCKED BY HOW JOLLY THEY ARE, KNOWING WHAT YOU'VE BEEN THROUGH...
...

DRAWING ALLEVIATED MY NEED TO TALK ABOUT DEATH, BUT I STILL THOUGHT ABOUT IT CONSTANTLY. I GREW DEATH ANTENNAE.

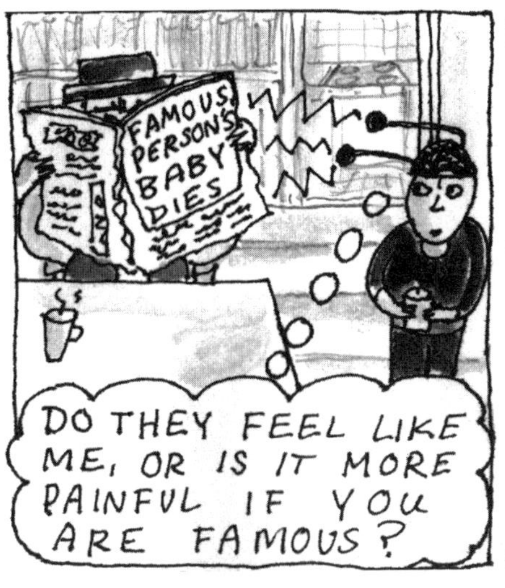

FAMOUS PERSON'S BABY DIES
DO THEY FEEL LIKE ME, OR IS IT MORE PAINFUL IF YOU ARE FAMOUS?

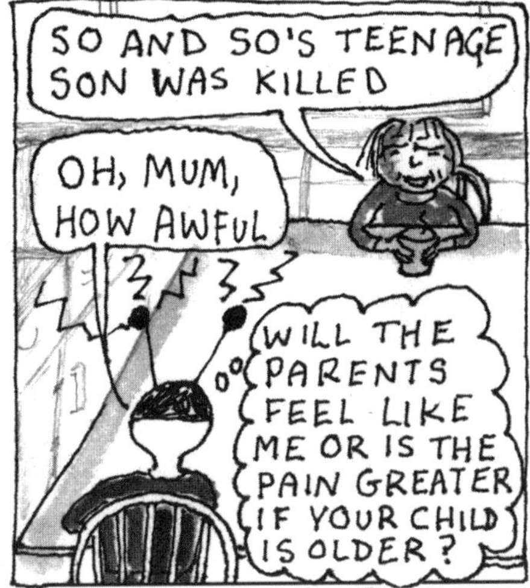

SO AND SO'S TEENAGE SON WAS KILLED
OH, MUM, HOW AWFUL
WILL THE PARENTS FEEL LIKE ME OR IS THE PAIN GREATER IF YOUR CHILD IS OLDER?

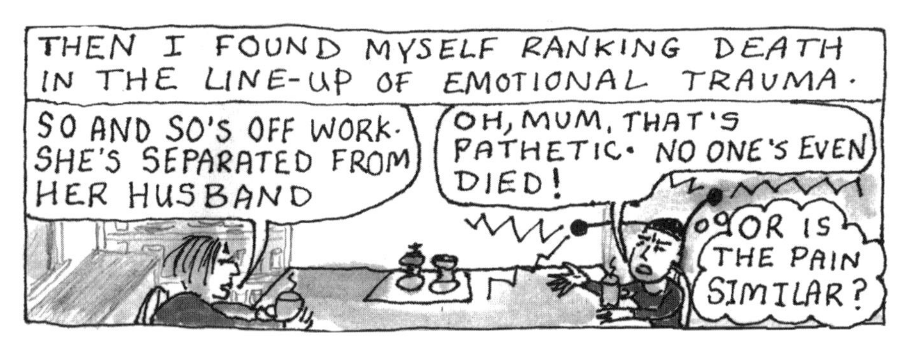

THEN I FOUND MYSELF RANKING DEATH IN THE LINE-UP OF EMOTIONAL TRAUMA.
SO AND SO'S OFF WORK. SHE'S SEPARATED FROM HER HUSBAND
OH, MUM, THAT'S PATHETIC. NO ONE'S EVEN DIED!
OR IS THE PAIN SIMILAR?

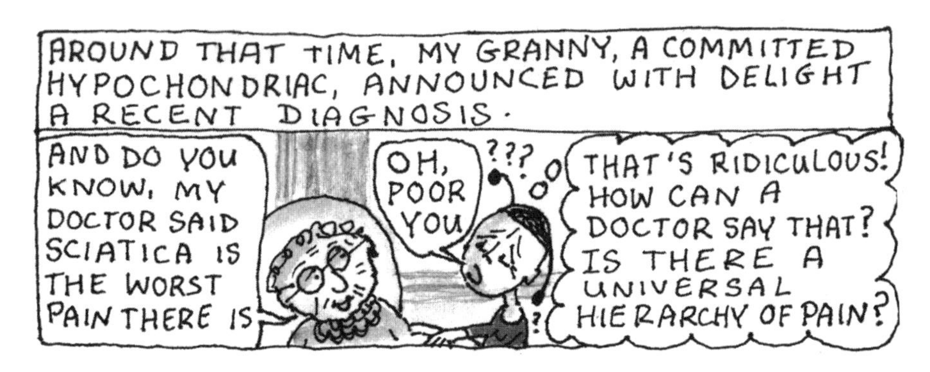

AROUND THAT TIME, MY GRANNY, A COMMITTED HYPOCHONDRIAC, ANNOUNCED WITH DELIGHT A RECENT DIAGNOSIS.
AND DO YOU KNOW, MY DOCTOR SAID SCIATICA IS THE WORST PAIN THERE IS
OH, POOR YOU
???
THAT'S RIDICULOUS! HOW CAN A DOCTOR SAY THAT? IS THERE A UNIVERSAL HIERARCHY OF PAIN?

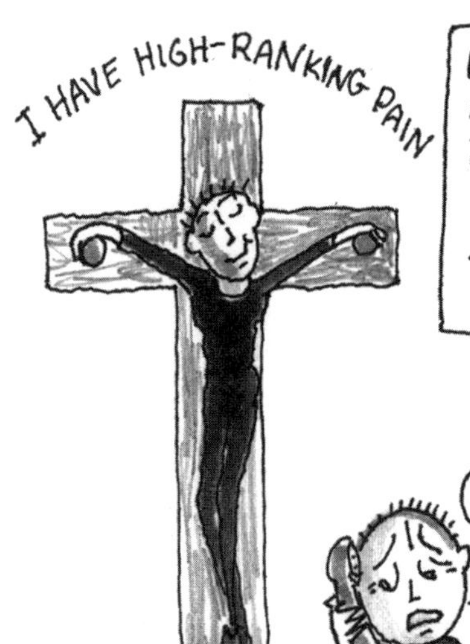
I HAVE HIGH-RANKING PAIN

ANYWAY... I APPOINTED MYSELF AS SOMETHING OF A DEATH EXPERT. SO WHEN MY FRIEND'S FATHER DIED I WAS TAKEN ABACK BY MY RESPONSE...

OH. I'M SORRY

SIMPLE ACKNOWLEDGEMENT CAN'T CAUSE OFFENCE ...OR IS IT TOO LITTLE?

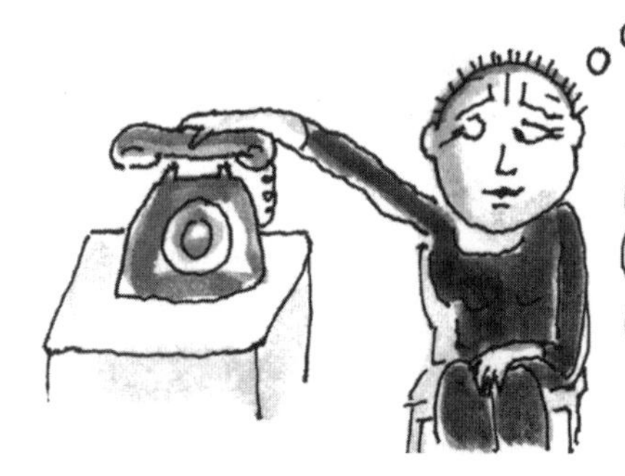

SHOULD I SEND FLOWERS? ARE LILIES NAFF? DO I WRITE A LETTER? DO I NEED AN INVITATION TO THE FUNERAL?

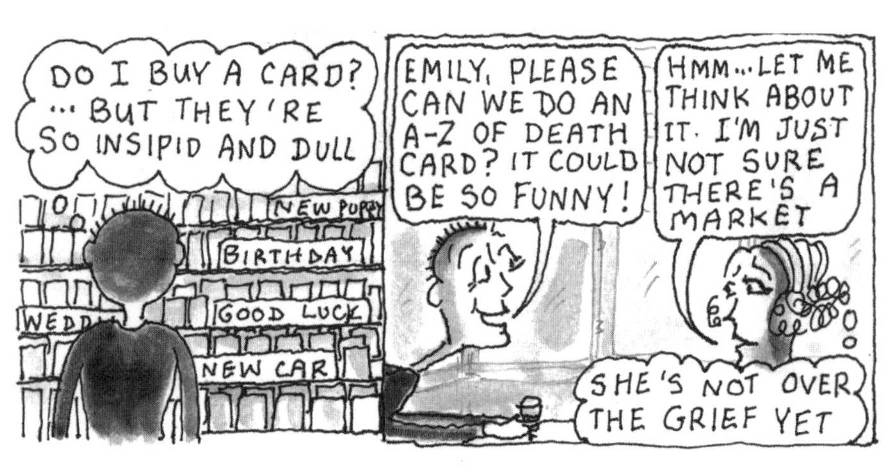
DO I BUY A CARD? ... BUT THEY'RE SO INSIPID AND DULL
NEW PUPPY
BIRTHDAY
GOOD LUCK
WEDD
NEW CAR
EMILY, PLEASE CAN WE DO AN A-Z OF DEATH CARD? IT COULD BE SO FUNNY!
HMM... LET ME THINK ABOUT IT. I'M JUST NOT SURE THERE'S A MARKET
SHE'S NOT OVER THE GRIEF YET

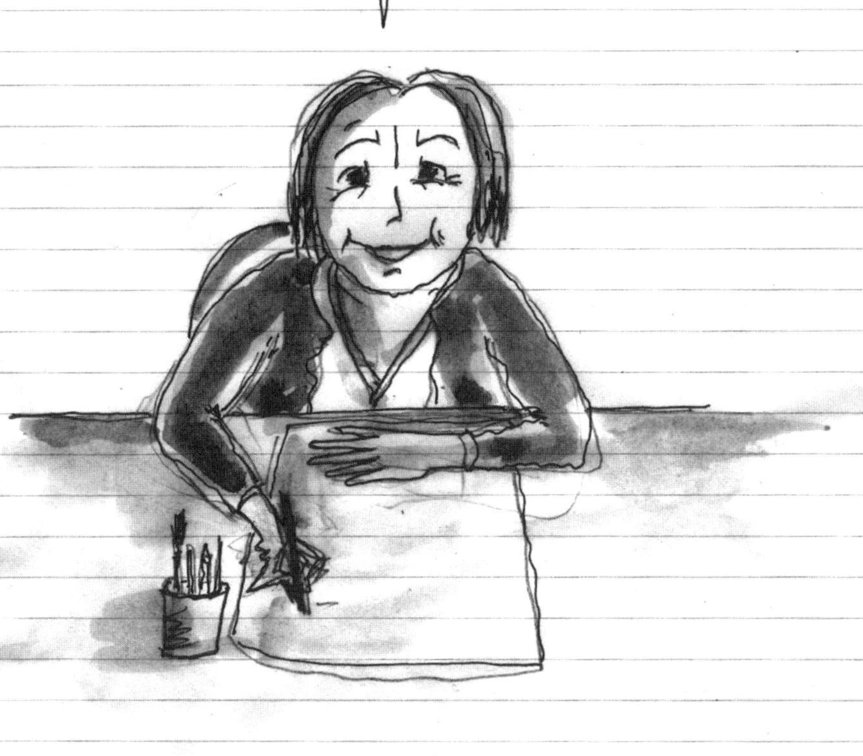
FOR JOHN, CREATIVE
ACTIVITY WAS ALSO A BALM

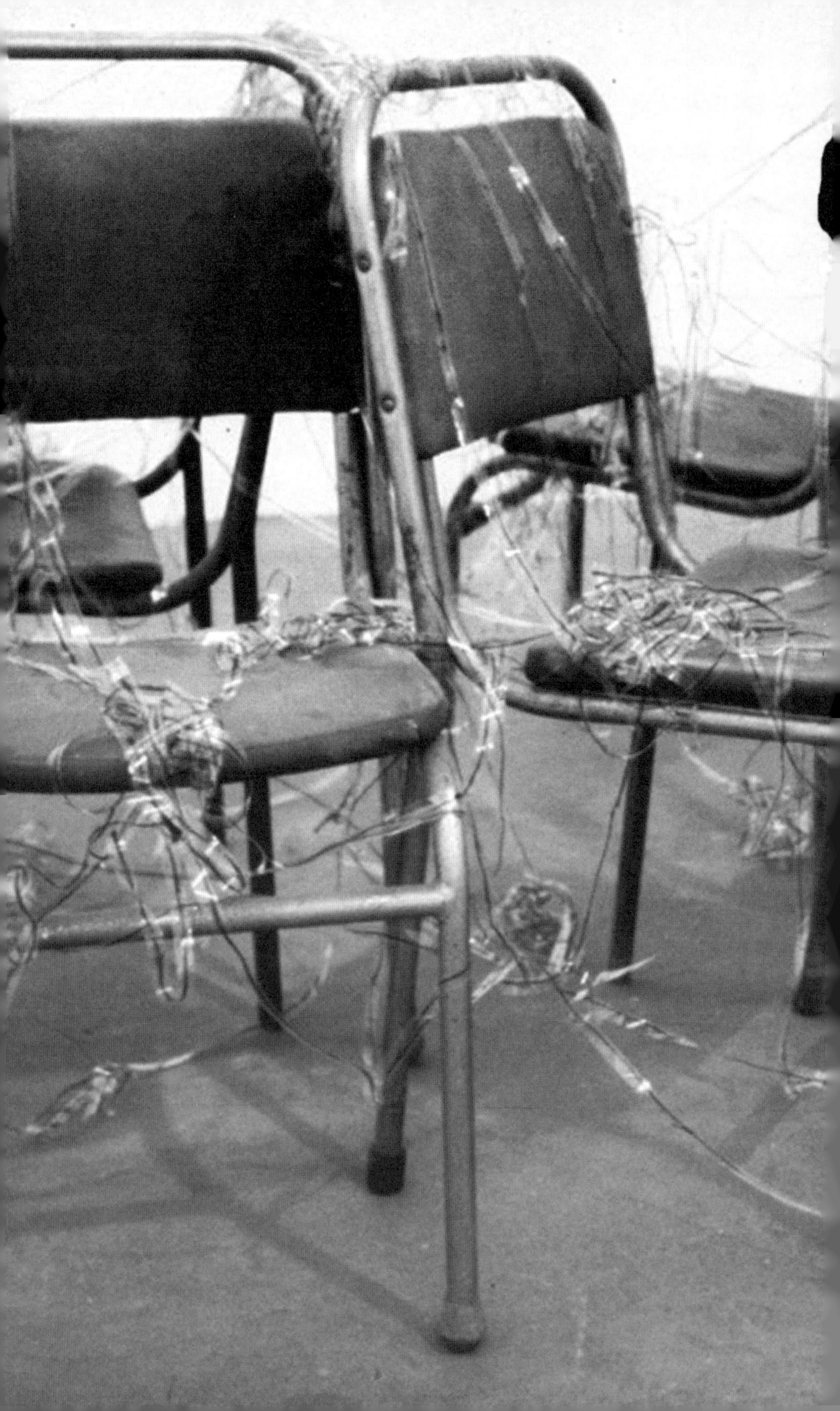

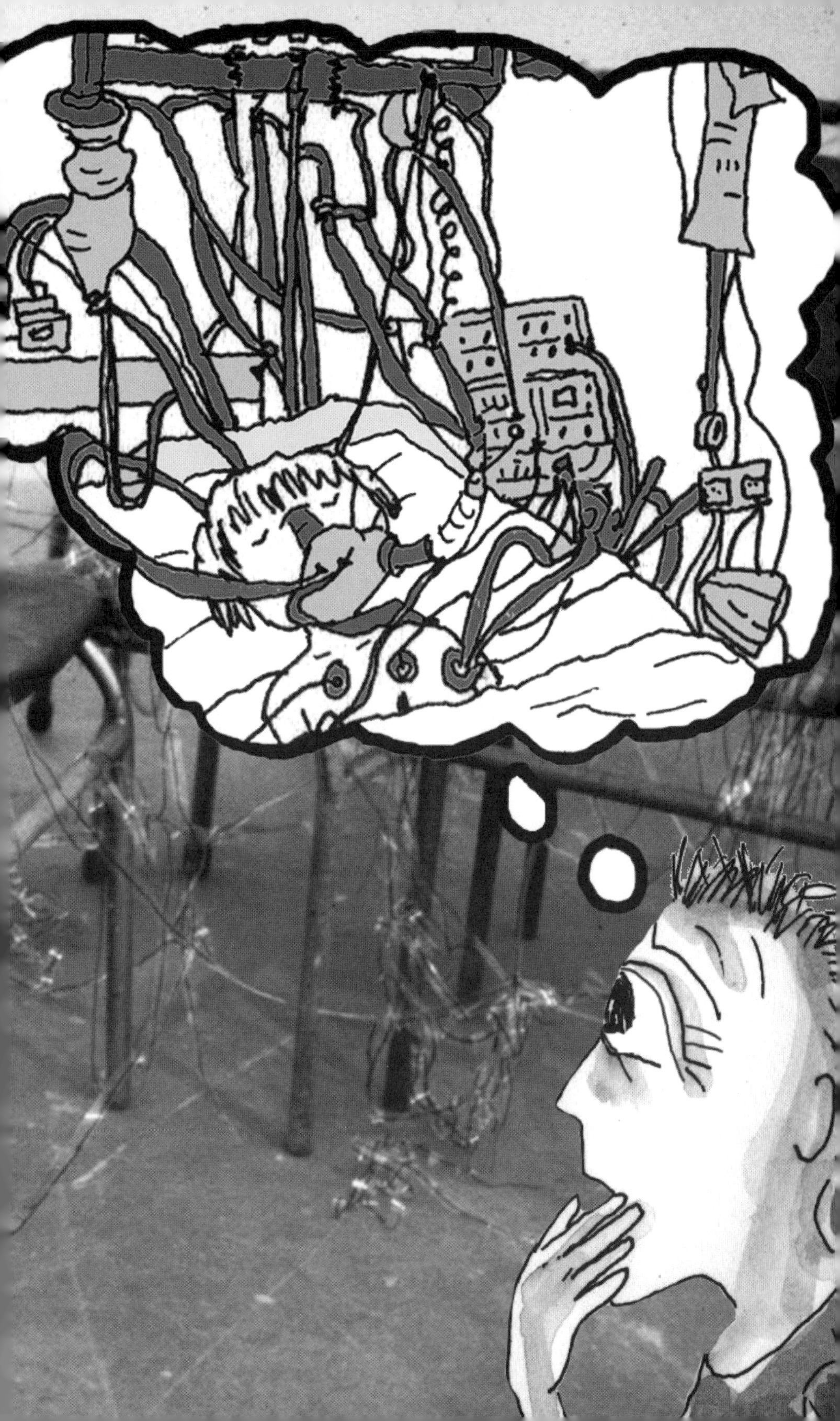

HIS RETURN TO PART-TIME ART TEACHING IN ADULT EDUCATION WAS LESS HELPFUL...

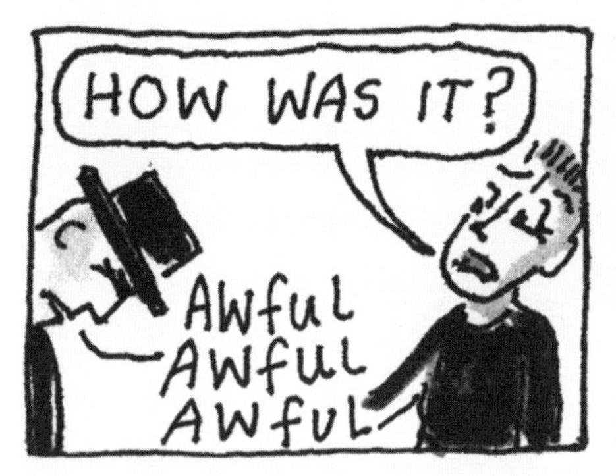

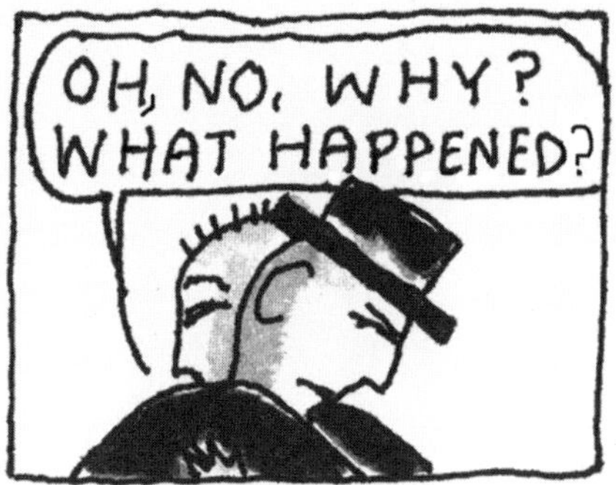

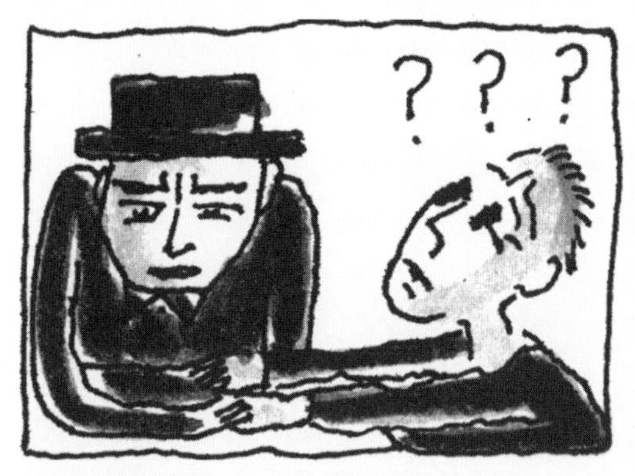

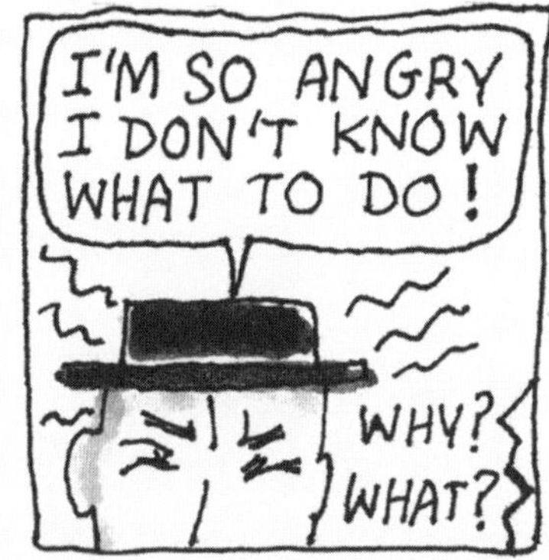

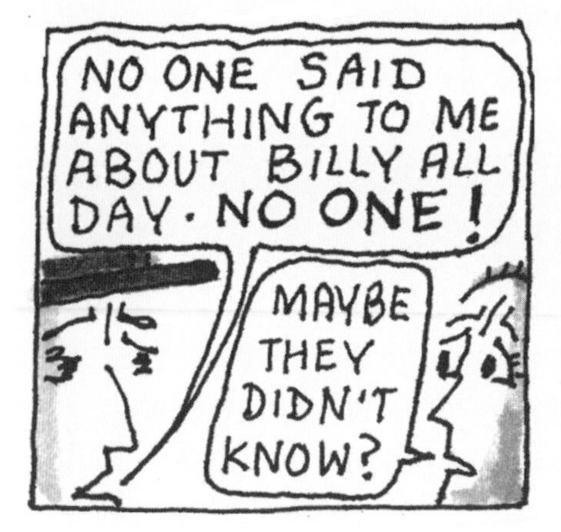

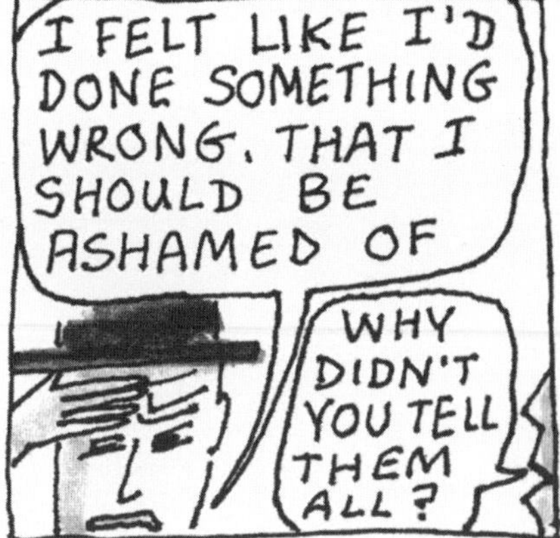

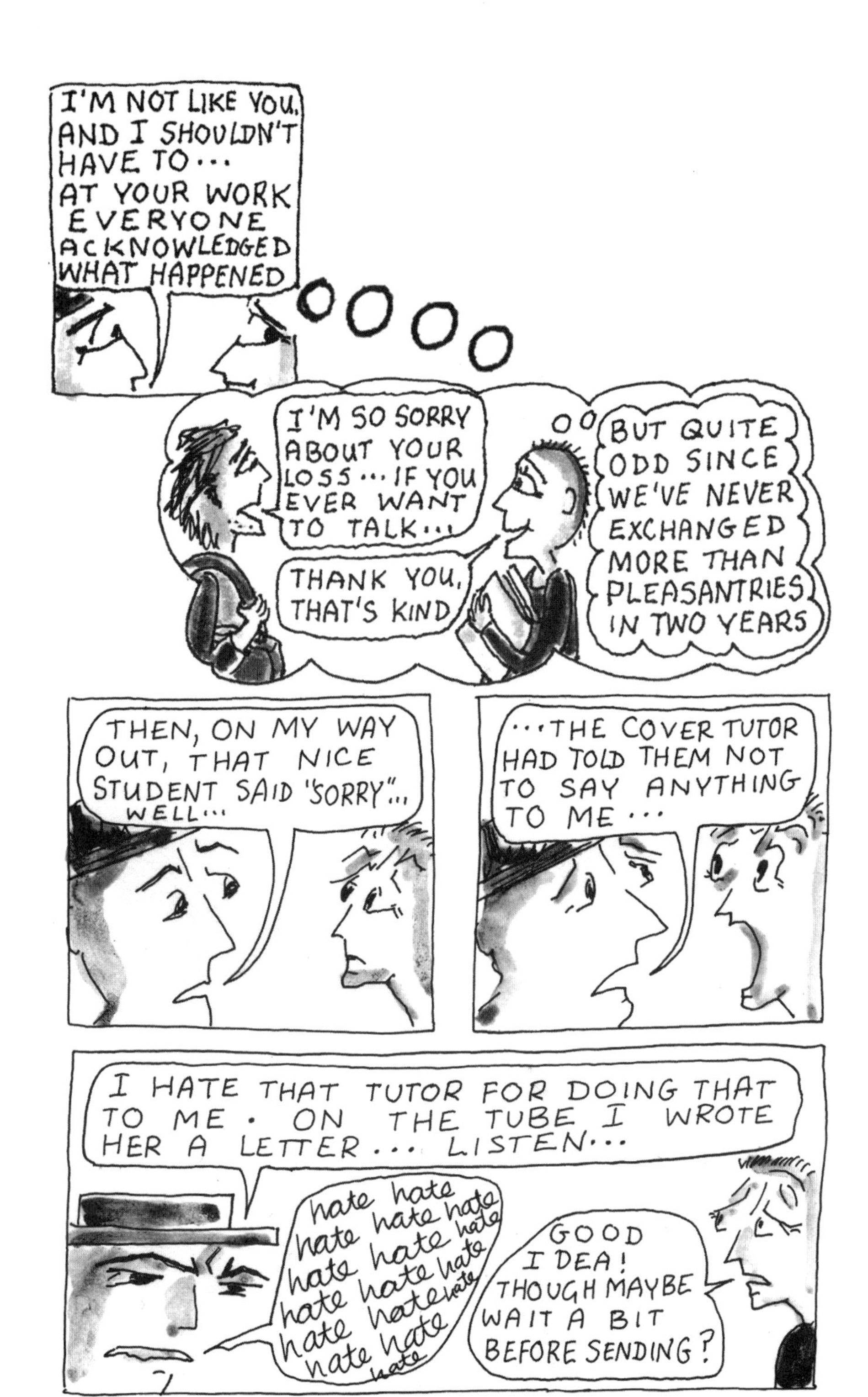
I'M NOT LIKE YOU, AND I SHOULDN'T HAVE TO... AT YOUR WORK EVERYONE ACKNOWLEDGED WHAT HAPPENED
I'M SO SORRY ABOUT YOUR LOSS... IF YOU EVER WANT TO TALK...
THANK YOU, THAT'S KIND
BUT QUITE ODD SINCE WE'VE NEVER EXCHANGED MORE THAN PLEASANTRIES IN TWO YEARS
THEN, ON MY WAY OUT, THAT NICE STUDENT SAID "SORRY"... WELL...
...THE COVER TUTOR HAD TOLD THEM NOT TO SAY ANYTHING TO ME...
I HATE THAT TUTOR FOR DOING THAT TO ME. ON THE TUBE I WROTE HER A LETTER... LISTEN...
hate hate hate hate hate hate hate hate hate hate hate hate hate hate hate hate hate hate hate hate hate
GOOD IDEA! THOUGH MAYBE WAIT A BIT BEFORE SENDING?

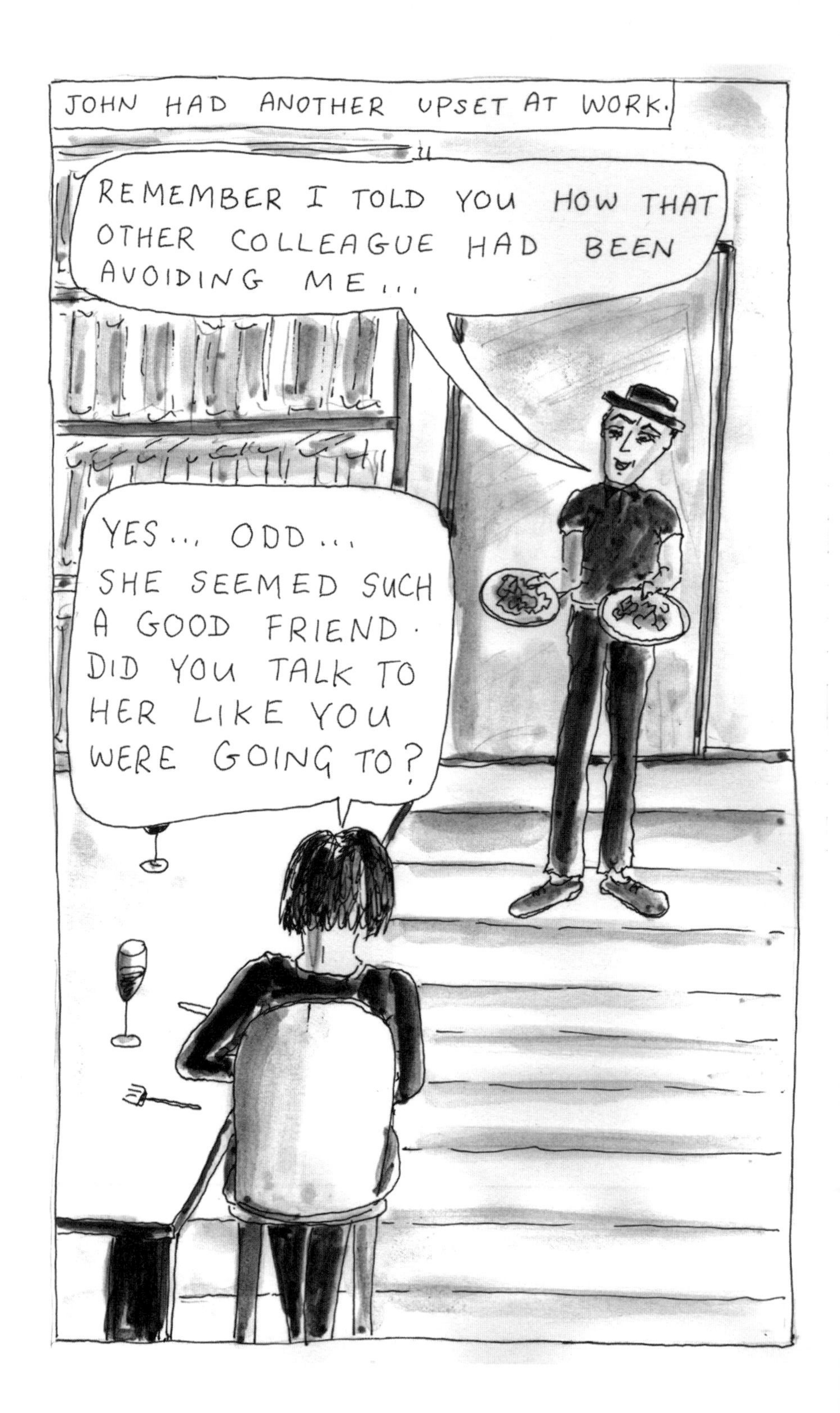
JOHN HAD ANOTHER UPSET AT WORK.
REMEMBER I TOLD YOU HOW THAT OTHER COLLEAGUE HAD BEEN AVOIDING ME...
YES... ODD... SHE SEEMED SUCH A GOOD FRIEND. DID YOU TALK TO HER LIKE YOU WERE GOING TO?

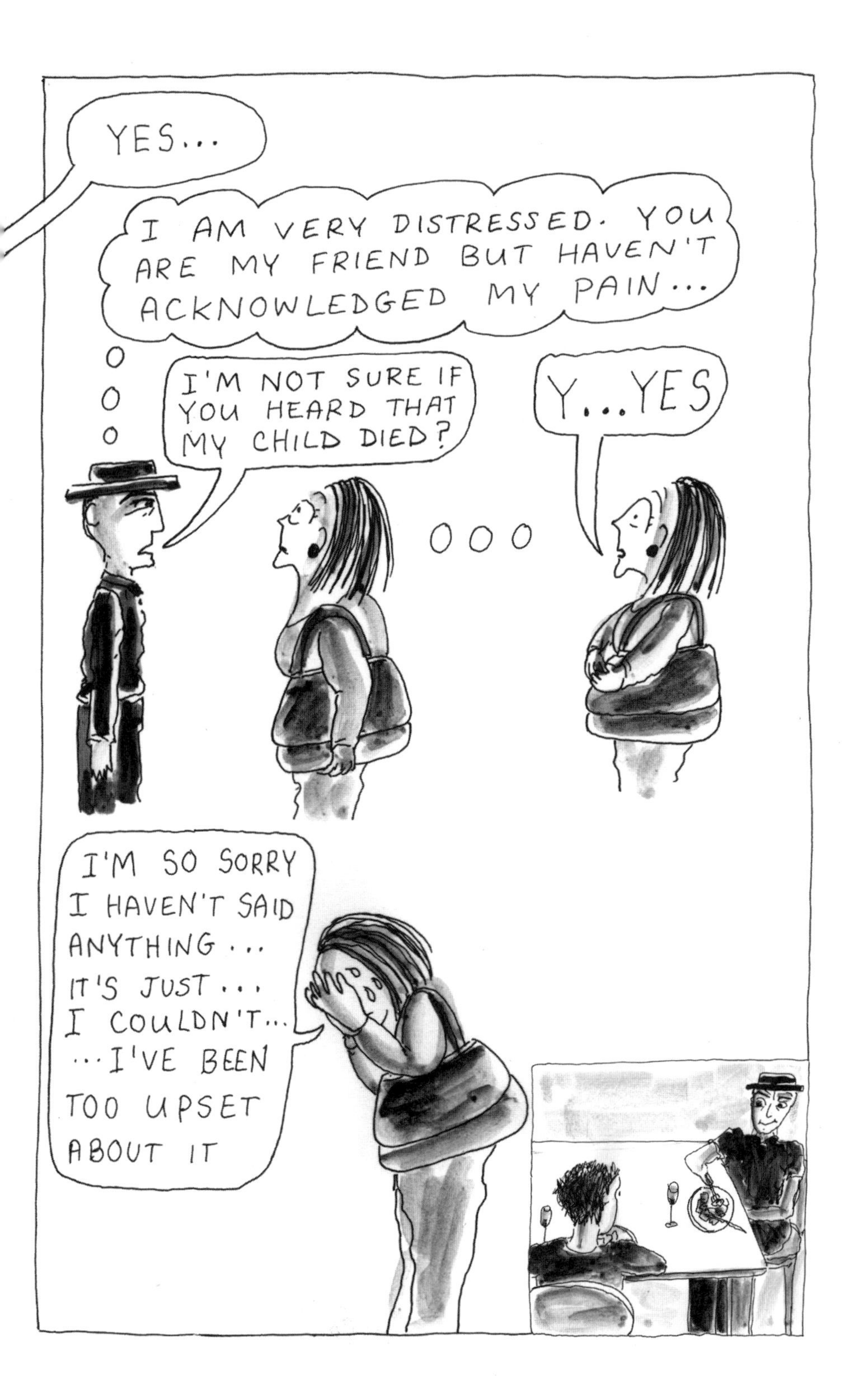
YES...
I AM VERY DISTRESSED. YOU ARE MY FRIEND BUT HAVEN'T ACKNOWLEDGED MY PAIN...
I'M NOT SURE IF YOU HEARD THAT MY CHILD DIED?
Y...YES
I'M SO SORRY I HAVEN'T SAID ANYTHING... IT'S JUST... I COULDN'T... ...I'VE BEEN TOO UPSET ABOUT IT

CURIOUS ABOUT THE SUBJECT OF BEREAVEMENT, I CAME UPON A THEORY OF THE STAGES OF GRIEF.

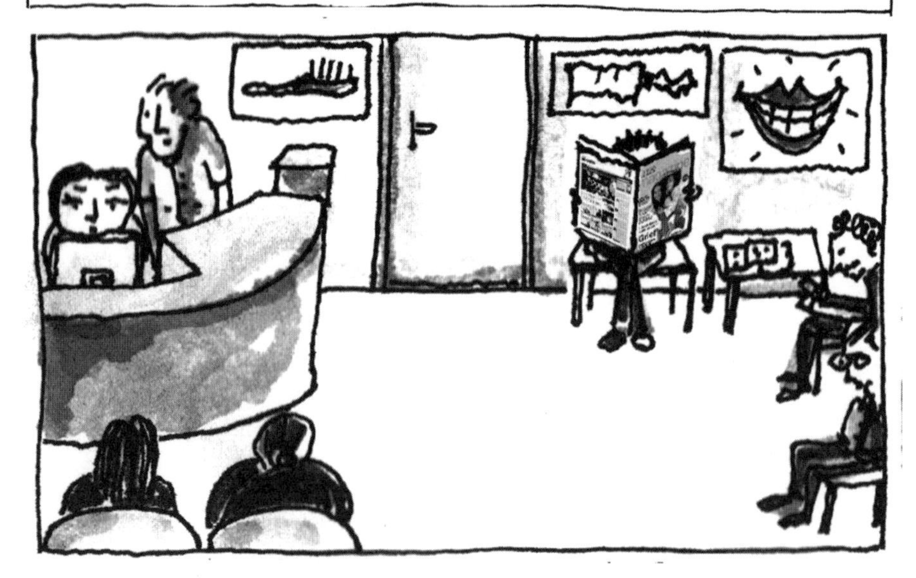

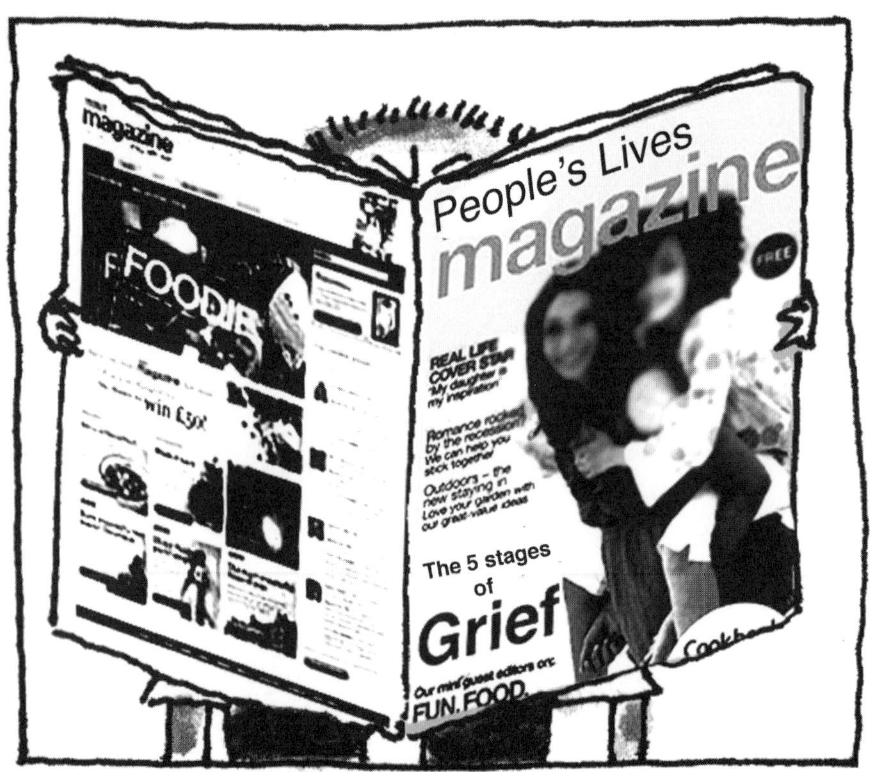

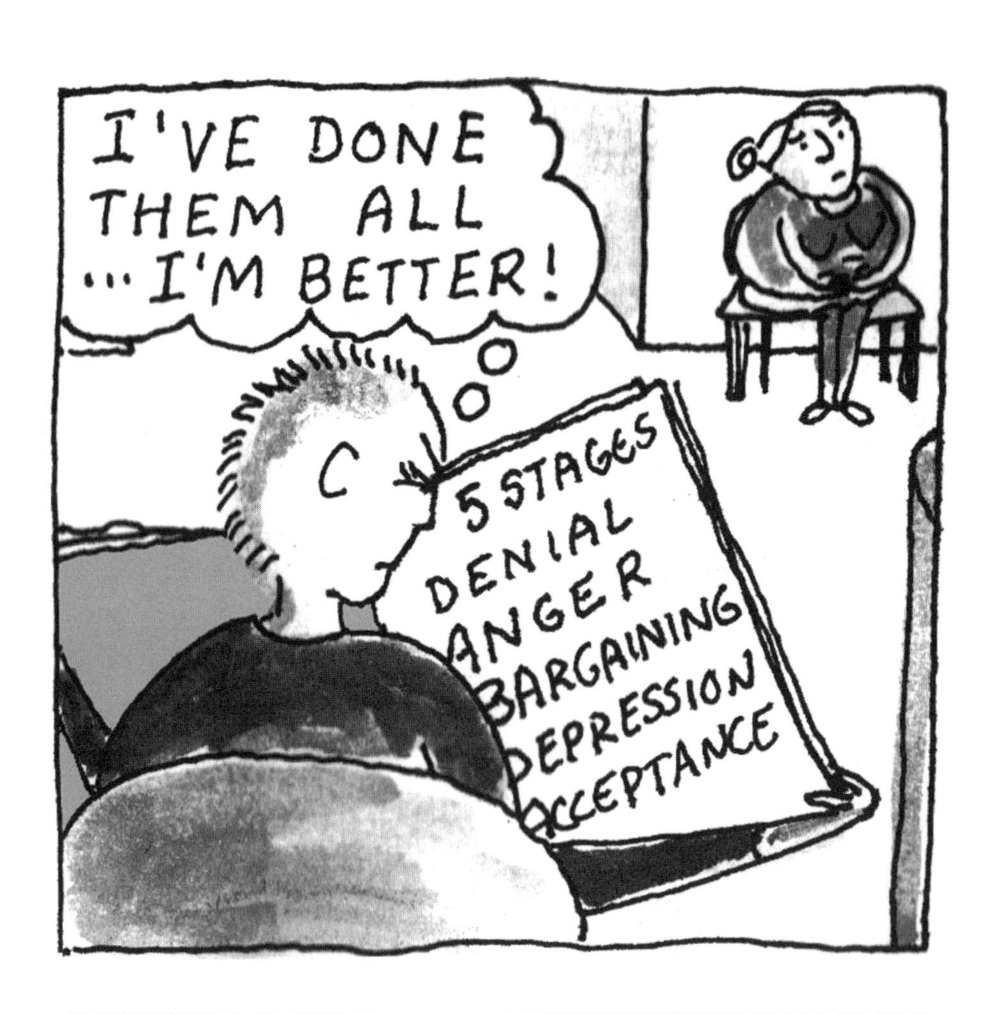
I'VE DONE THEM ALL ...I'M BETTER!
5 STAGES
DENIAL
ANGER
BARGAINING
DEPRESSION
ACCEPTANCE

I UNDERSTOOD THE THEORY RATHER SIMPLISTICALLY. IN HINDSIGHT, THE LIVING OF THESE STAGES WAS LESS TIDY.

AS MONTHS WENT BY, JOHN AND I FOUND WALKING AND TALKING BECAME IMPORTANT.

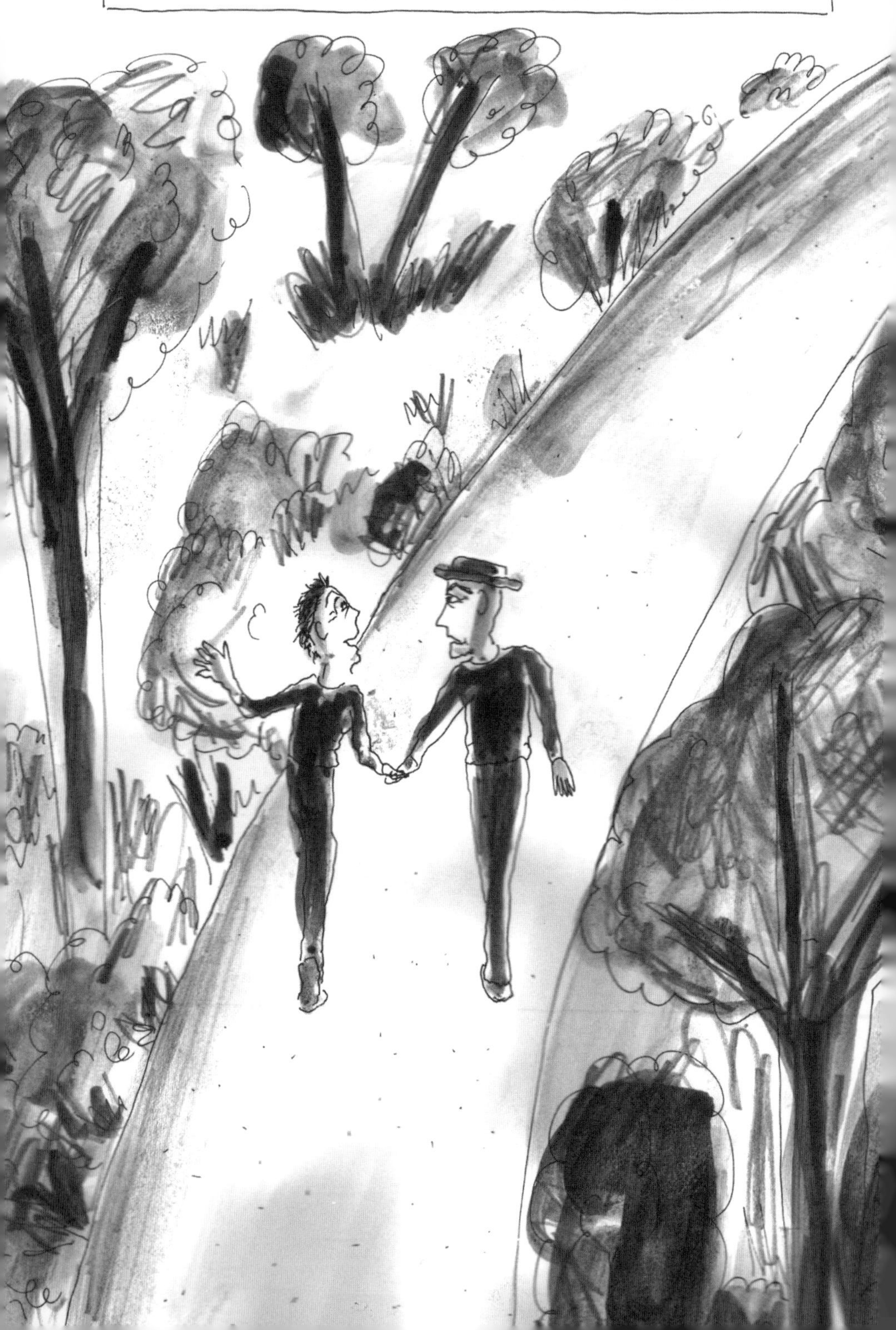

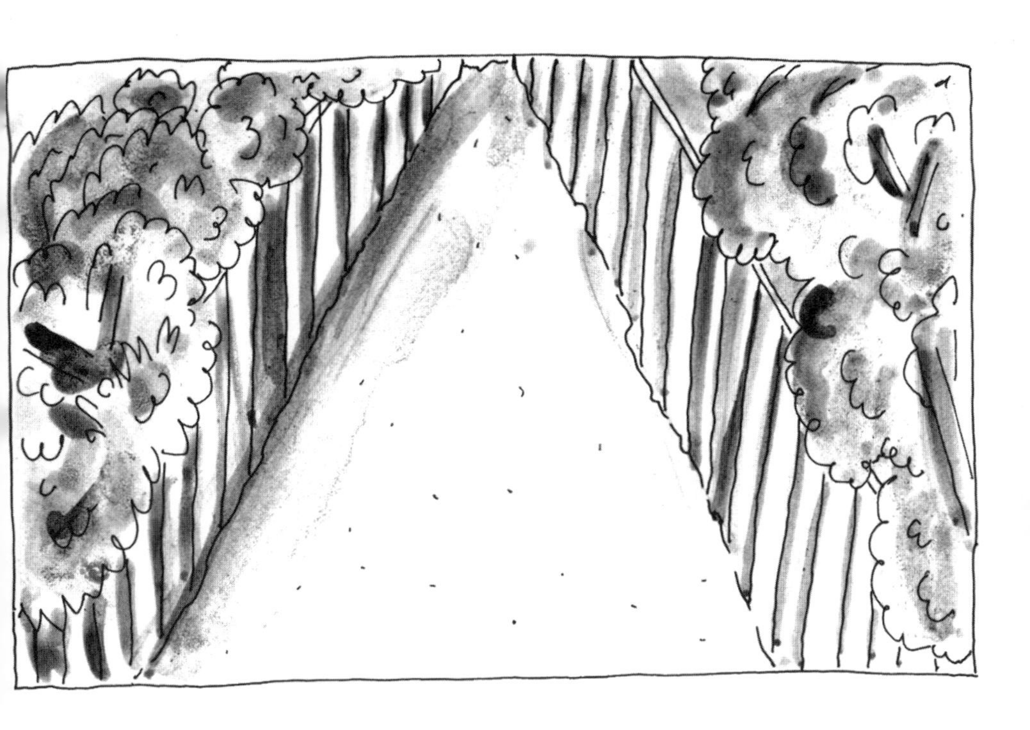

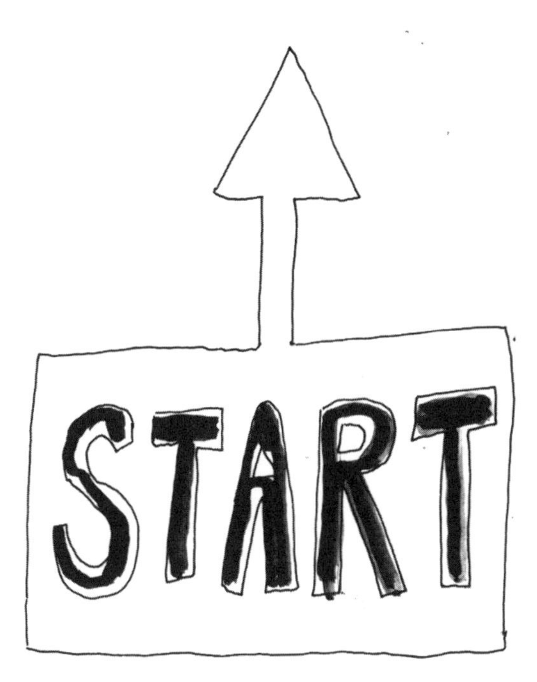
START

SOMETIMES...

WHY DO YOU DO THAT EVERY TIME

FINE. LET'S SPLIT UP THEN! I'LL LEAVE!

STOP IT! THAT'S SO STUPID

SO NOW I'M STUPID

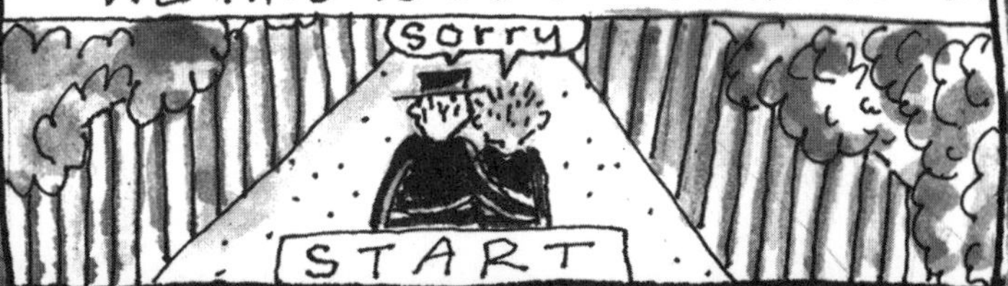

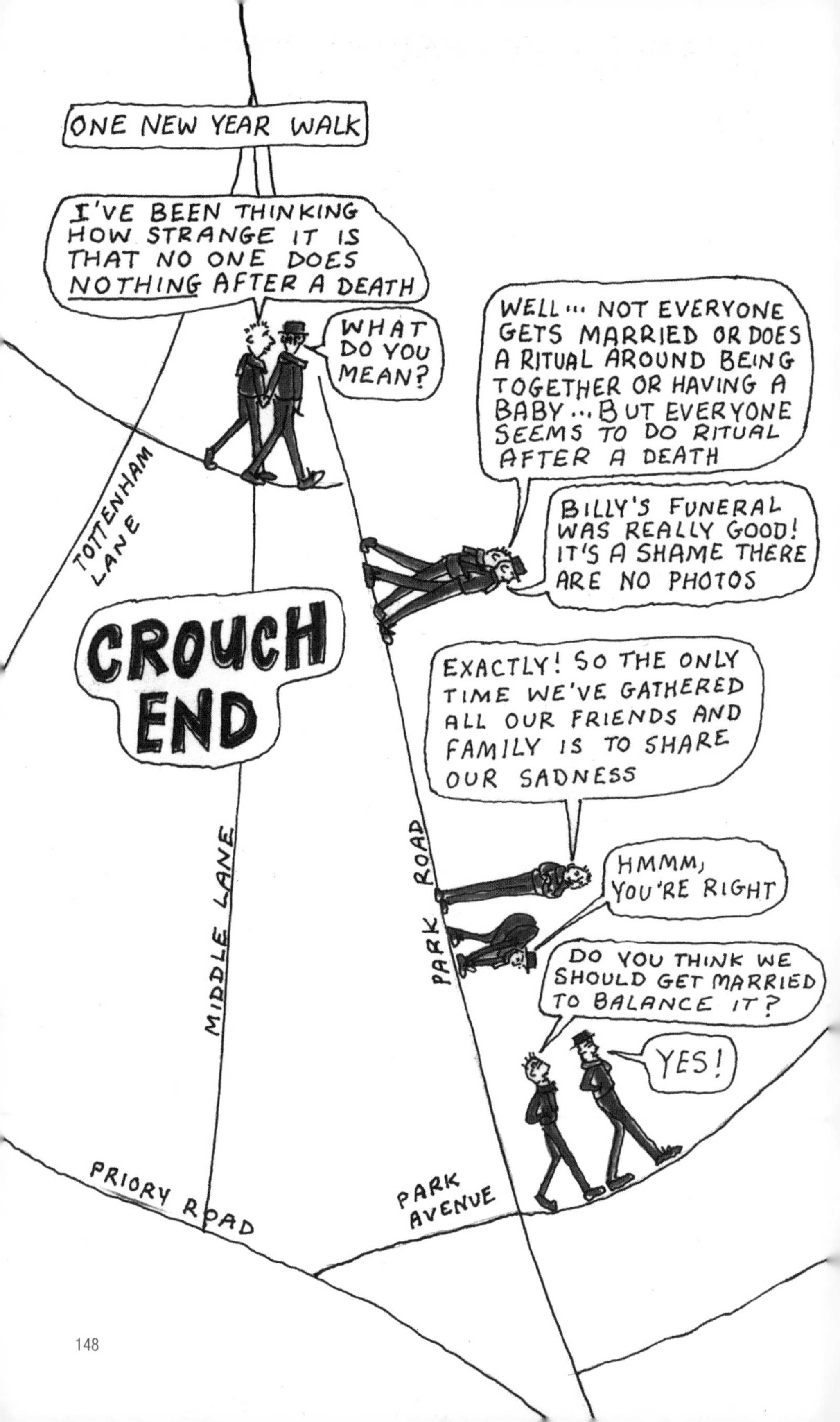
ONE NEW YEAR WALK
I'VE BEEN THINKING HOW STRANGE IT IS THAT NO ONE DOES NOTHING AFTER A DEATH
WHAT DO YOU MEAN?
WELL... NOT EVERYONE GETS MARRIED OR DOES A RITUAL AROUND BEING TOGETHER OR HAVING A BABY... BUT EVERYONE SEEMS TO DO RITUAL AFTER A DEATH
BILLY'S FUNERAL WAS REALLY GOOD! IT'S A SHAME THERE ARE NO PHOTOS
EXACTLY! SO THE ONLY TIME WE'VE GATHERED ALL OUR FRIENDS AND FAMILY IS TO SHARE OUR SADNESS
HMMM, YOU'RE RIGHT
DO YOU THINK WE SHOULD GET MARRIED TO BALANCE IT?
YES!
TOTTENHAM LANE
CROUCH END
MIDDLE LANE
PARK ROAD
PRIORY ROAD
PARK AVENUE

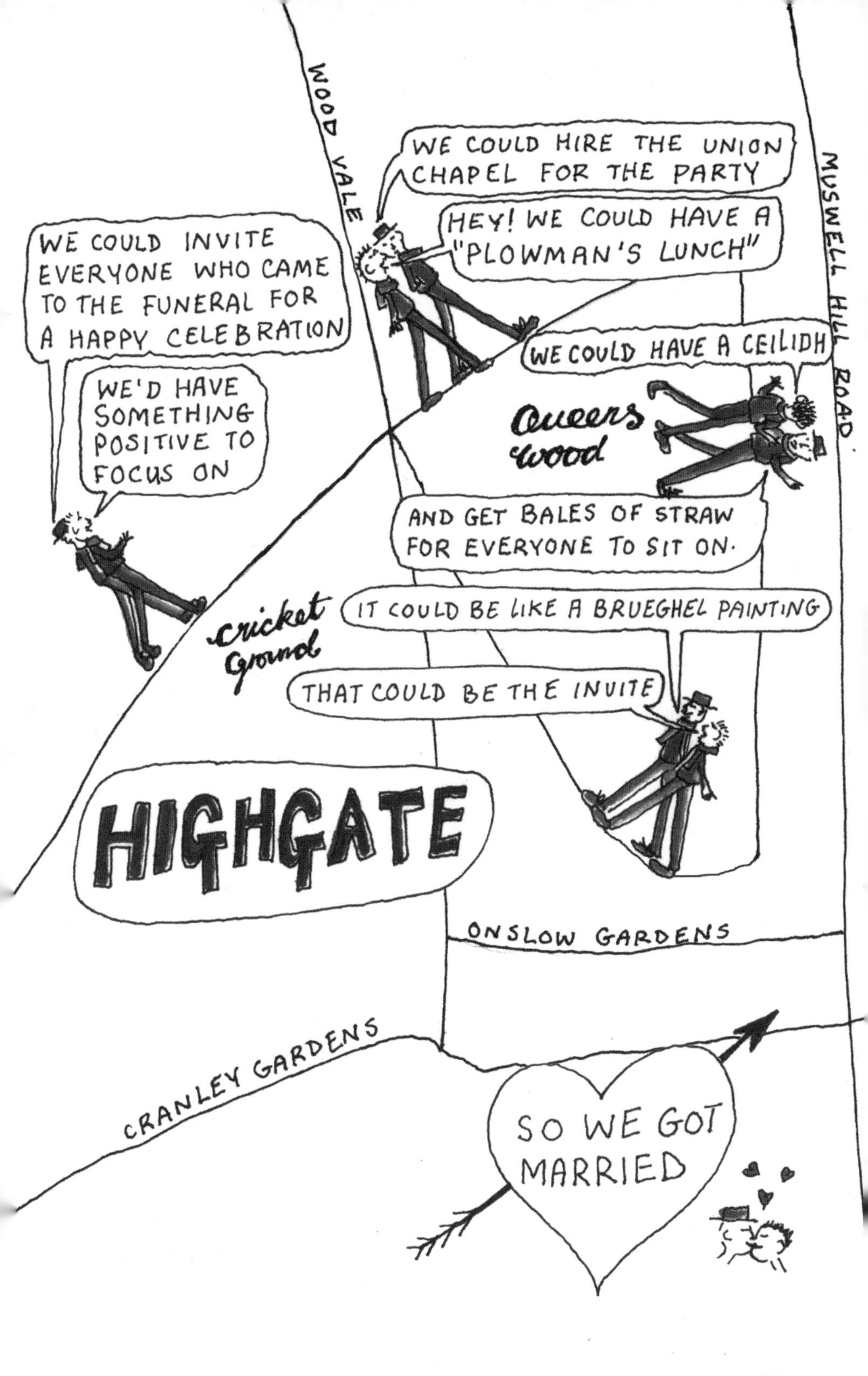
WOOD VALE
MUSWELL HILL ROAD
WE COULD INVITE EVERYONE WHO CAME TO THE FUNERAL FOR A HAPPY CELEBRATION
WE'D HAVE SOMETHING POSITIVE TO FOCUS ON
WE COULD HIRE THE UNION CHAPEL FOR THE PARTY
HEY! WE COULD HAVE A "PLOWMAN'S LUNCH"
WE COULD HAVE A CEILIDH
Queens wood
AND GET BALES OF STRAW FOR EVERYONE TO SIT ON.
cricket ground
IT COULD BE LIKE A BRUEGHEL PAINTING
THAT COULD BE THE INVITE
HIGHGATE
ONSLOW GARDENS
CRANLEY GARDENS
SO WE GOT MARRIED

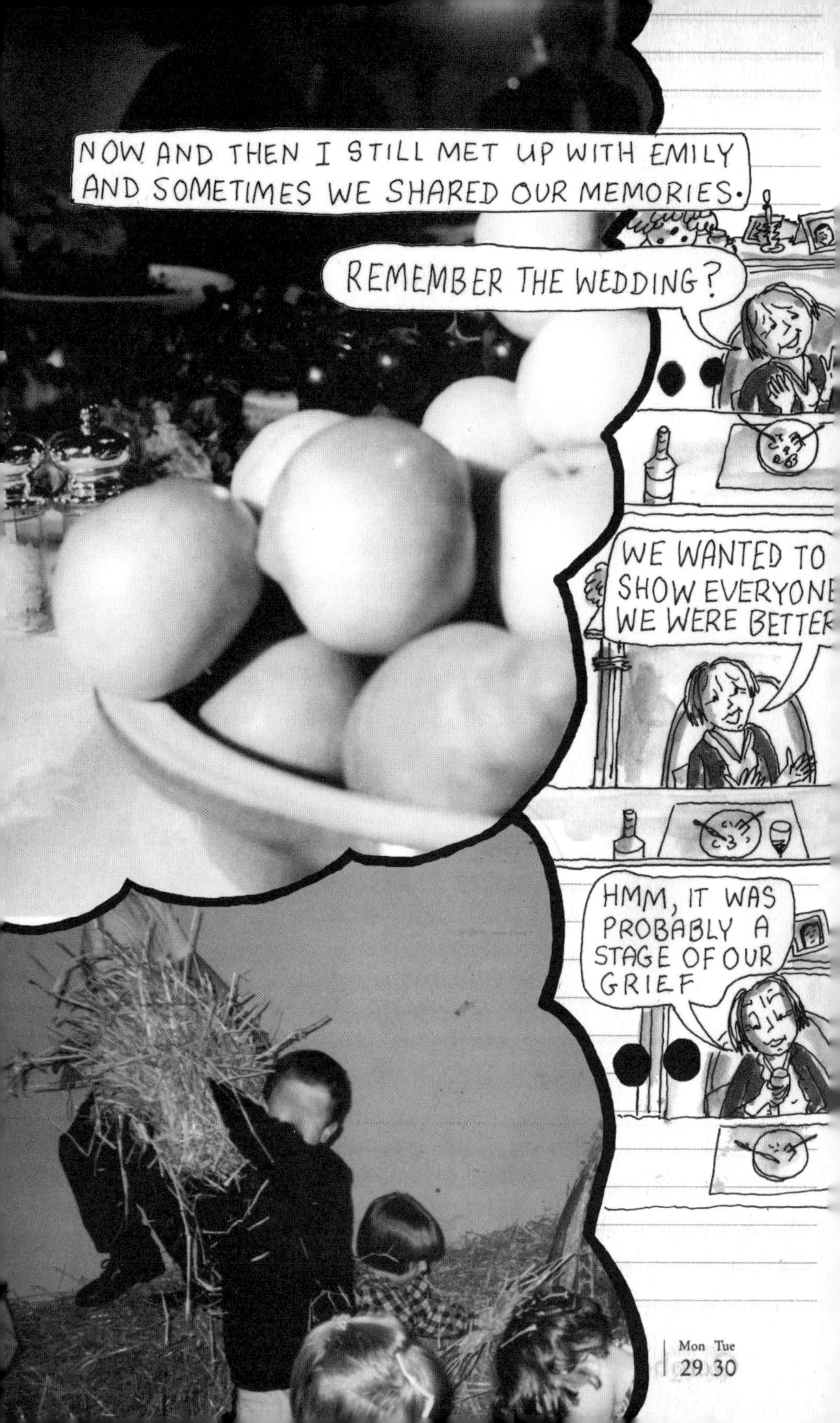
NOW AND THEN I STILL MET UP WITH EMILY AND SOMETIMES WE SHARED OUR MEMORIES.
REMEMBER THE WEDDING?
WE WANTED TO SHOW EVERYONE WE WERE BETTER
HMM, IT WAS PROBABLY A STAGE OF OUR GRIEF
Mon Tue
29 30

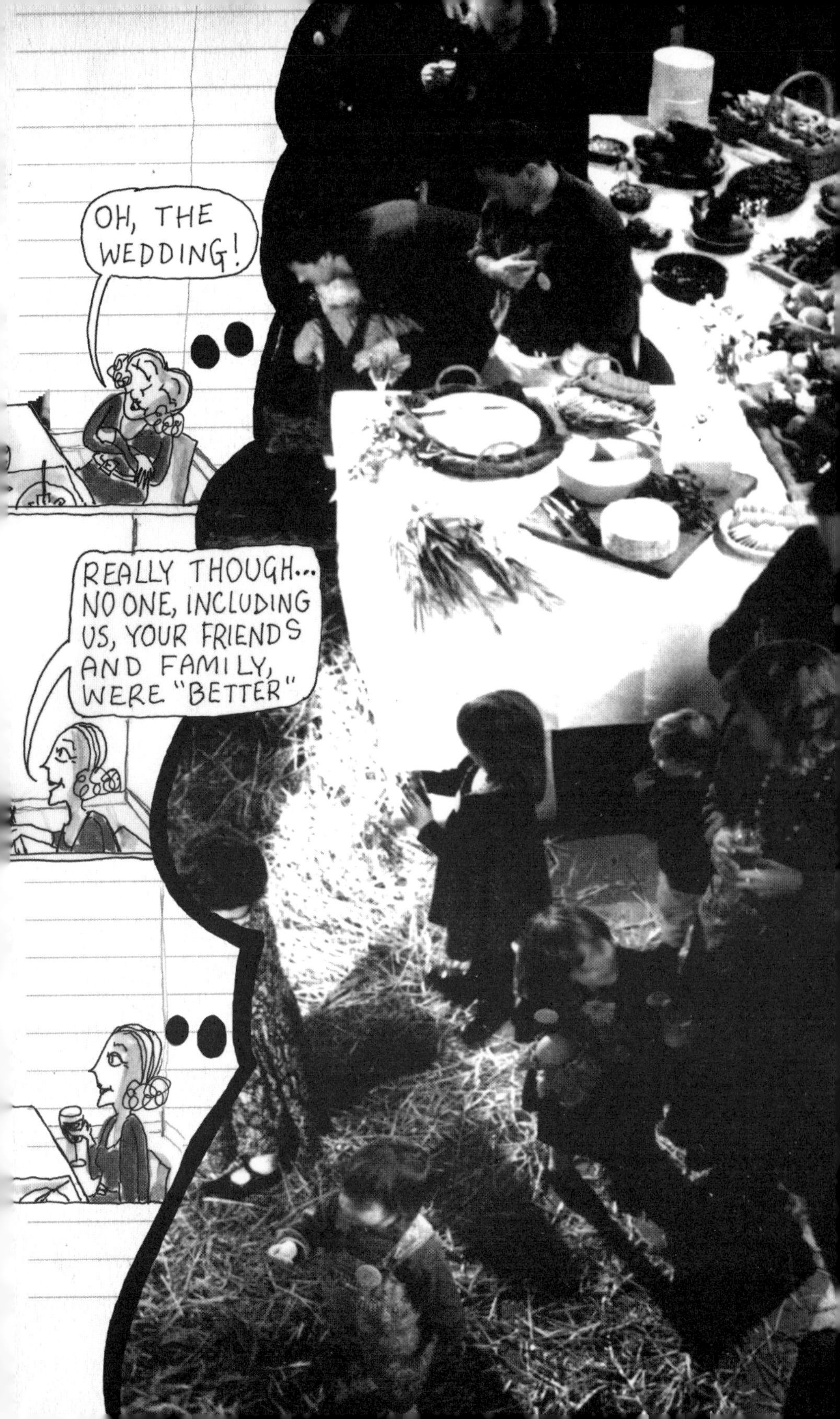
OH, THE WEDDING!
REALLY THOUGH... NO ONE, INCLUDING US, YOUR FRIENDS AND FAMILY, WERE "BETTER"

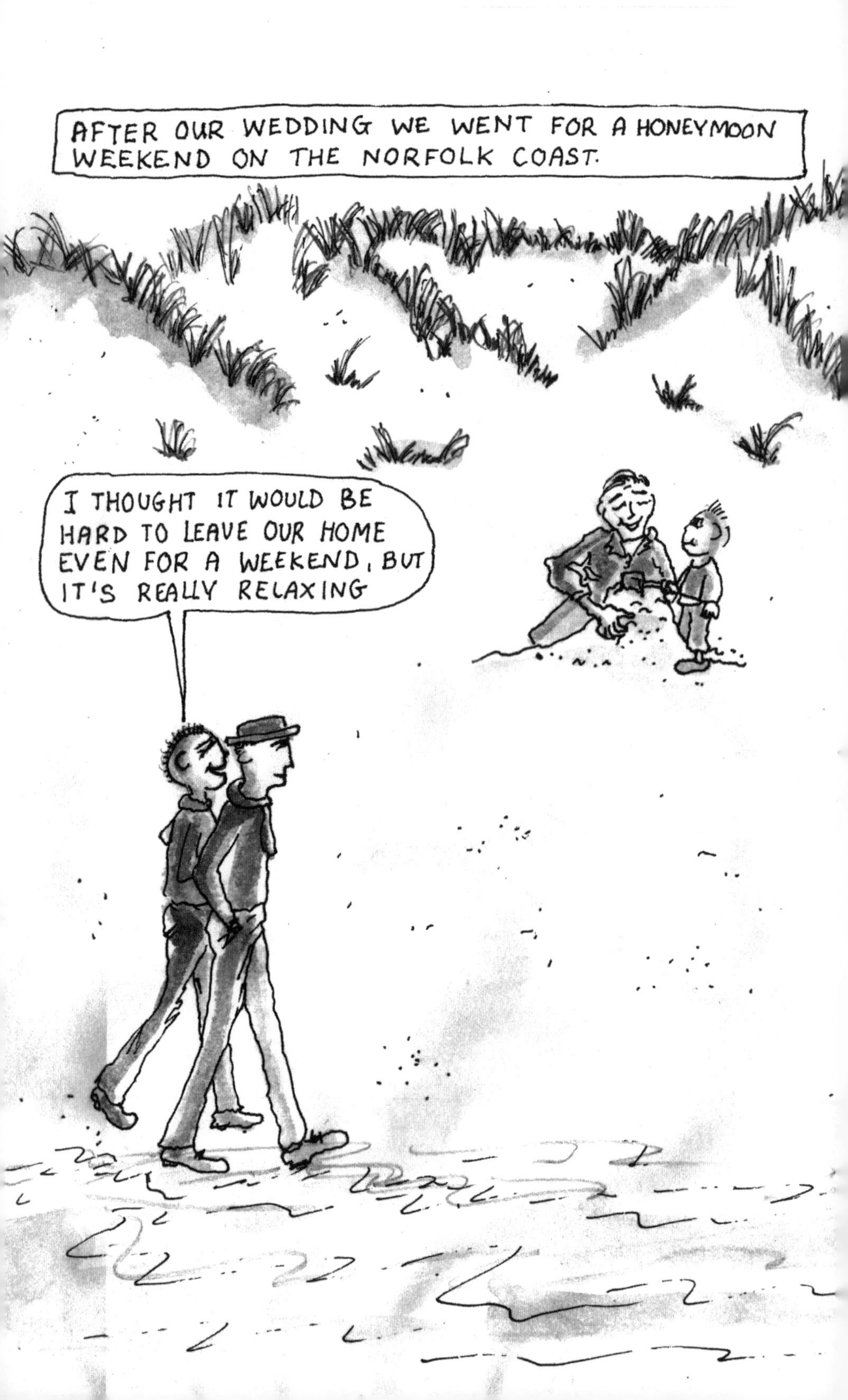
AFTER OUR WEDDING WE WENT FOR A HONEYMOON WEEKEND ON THE NORFOLK COAST.
I THOUGHT IT WOULD BE HARD TO LEAVE OUR HOME EVEN FOR A WEEKEND, BUT IT'S REALLY RELAXING

DID YOU SEE THAT MAN PLAYING WITH HIS LITTLE BOY... WHO LOOKED LIKE ... I WANT TO PLAY WITH BILLY

MARSEILLE, FRANCE. JOHN WAS INVITED TO EXHIBIT HIS ARTWORK. I WENT WITH HIM TO HELP INSTALL THE PIECE.

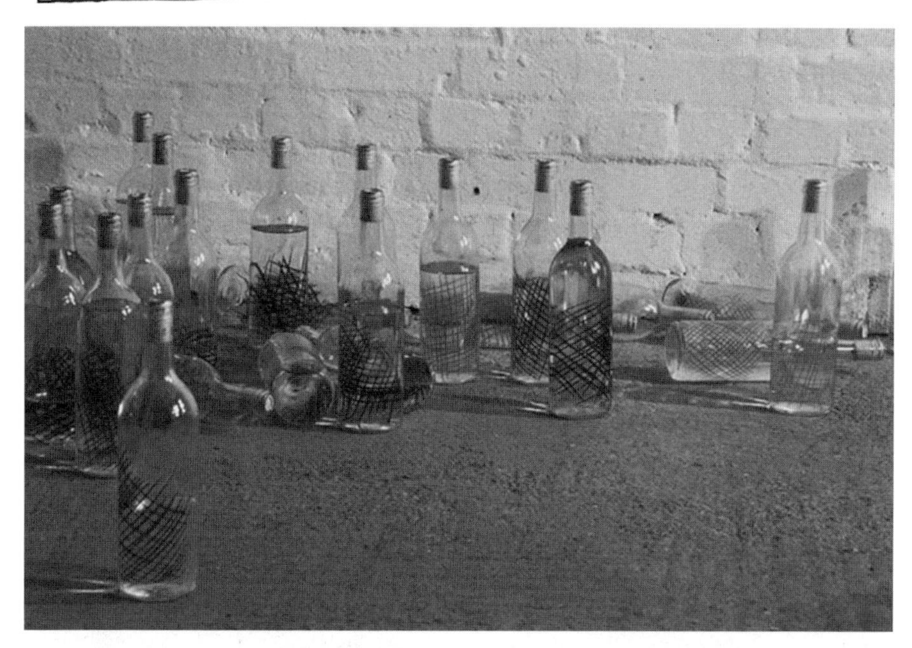

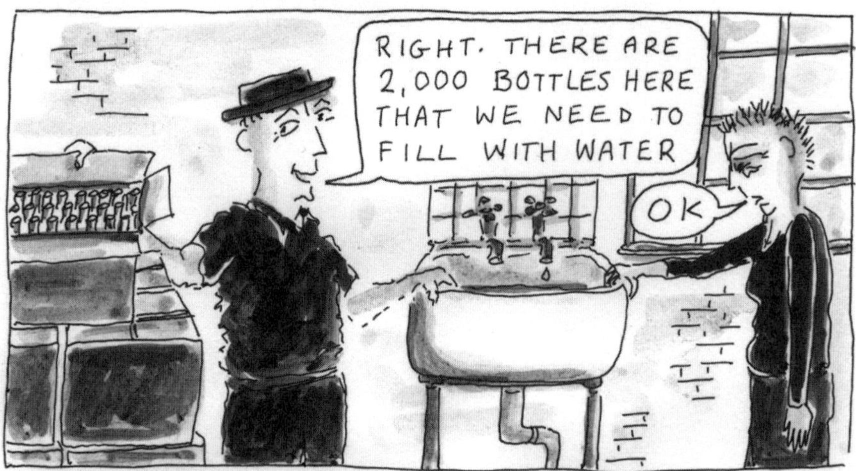
RIGHT. THERE ARE 2,000 BOTTLES HERE THAT WE NEED TO FILL WITH WATER
OK

ALTHOUGH I WAS STILL CONVINCED I HAD "DONE" MY STAGES OF GRIEF AND WAS THEREFORE "BETTER", MY DAILY CRYING CONTINUED.

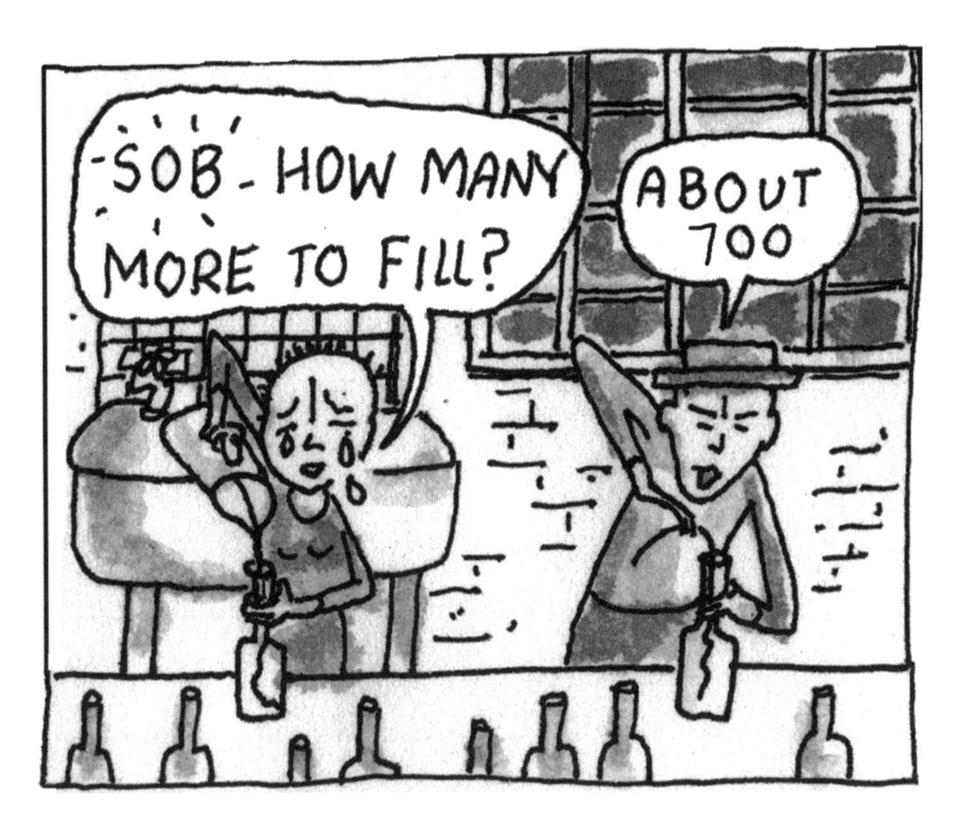
-SOB- HOW MANY MORE TO FILL?
ABOUT 700

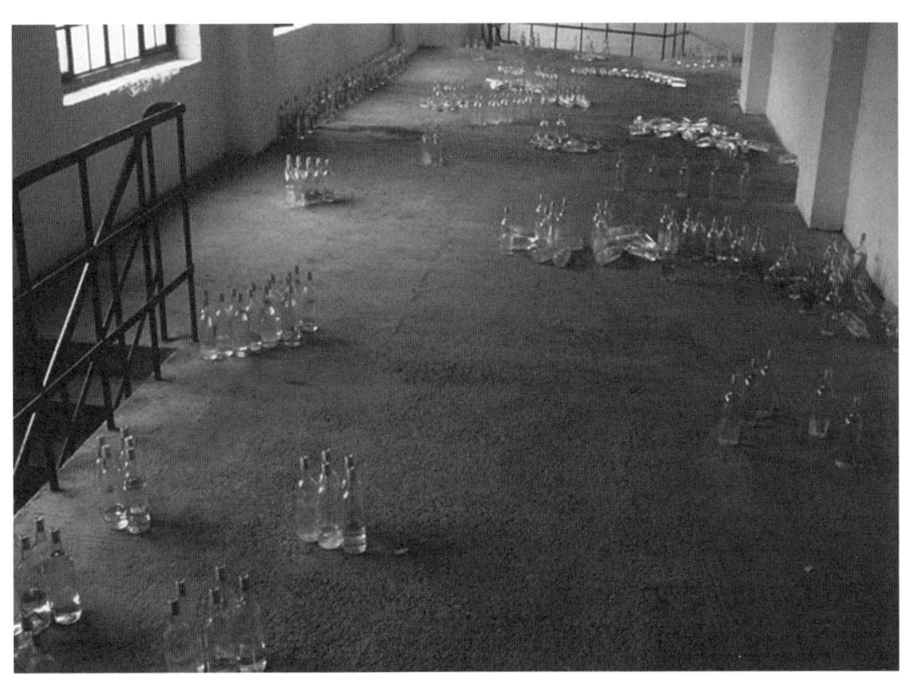

ONE MORNING MARIE DROPPED BY WITH AN IDEA.

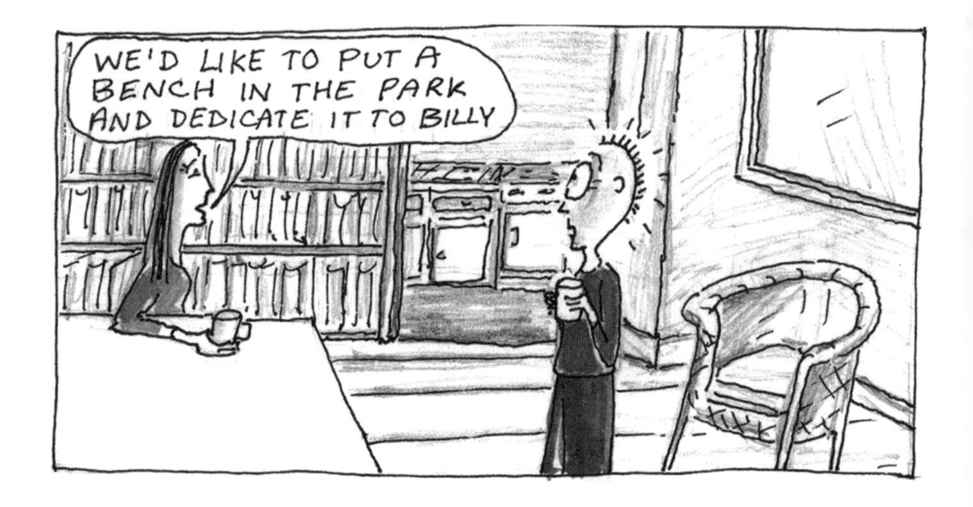
WE'D LIKE TO PUT A BENCH IN THE PARK AND DEDICATE IT TO BILLY

SUDDENLY I GOT AN "ANGER STAGE".

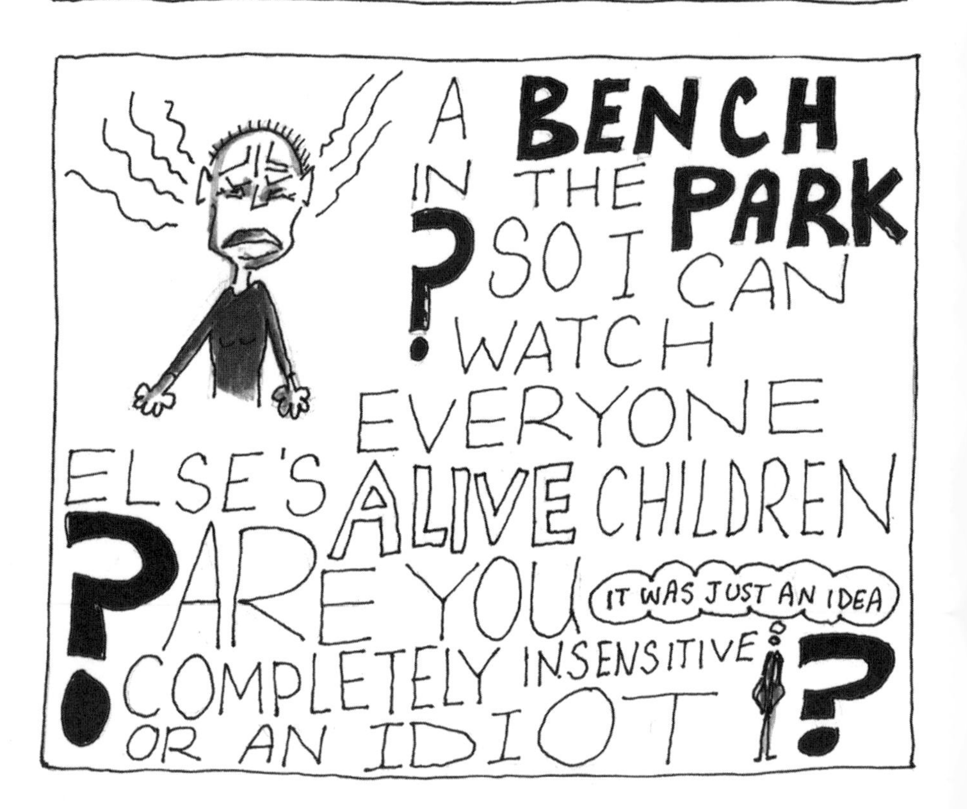
A BENCH IN THE PARK? SO I CAN WATCH EVERYONE ELSE'S ALIVE CHILDREN? ARE YOU COMPLETELY INSENSITIVE OR AN IDIOT?
IT WAS JUST AN IDEA

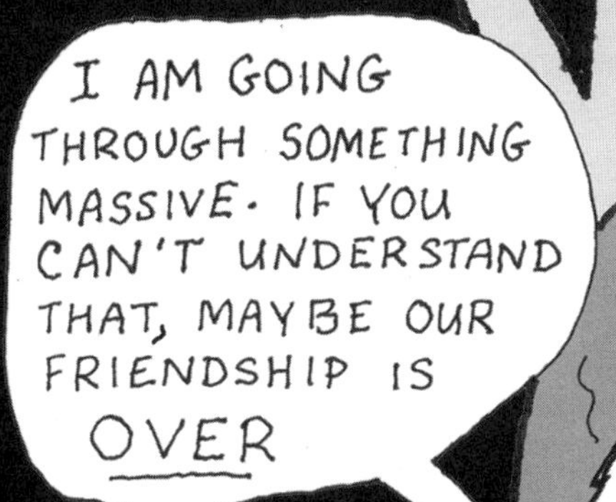
I AM GOING THROUGH SOMETHING MASSIVE. IF YOU CAN'T UNDERSTAND THAT, MAYBE OUR FRIENDSHIP IS OVER

I'VE SUPPORTED YOU AS BEST I CAN...

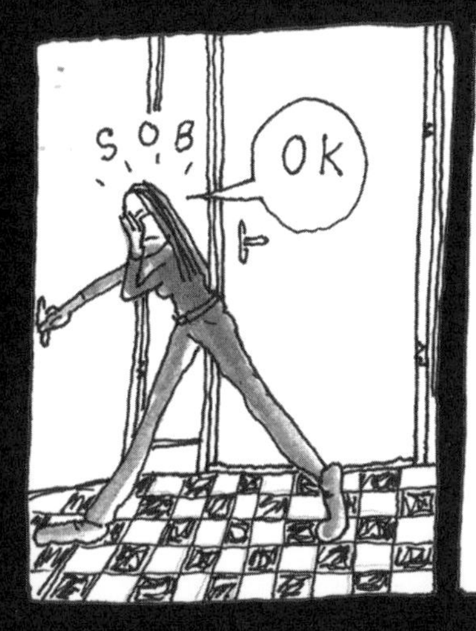
SOB
OK

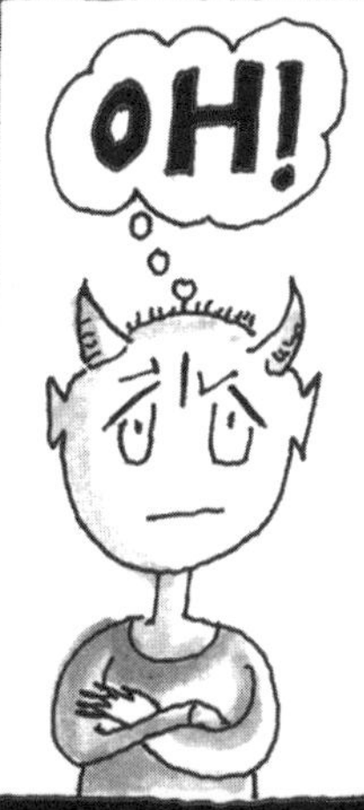
OH!

THERE! MY BEST FRIEND SINCE CHILDHOOD BRUSHED AWAY IN A MOMENTARY "ANGER STAGE" THAT I THOUGHT I'D ALREADY COMPLETED...

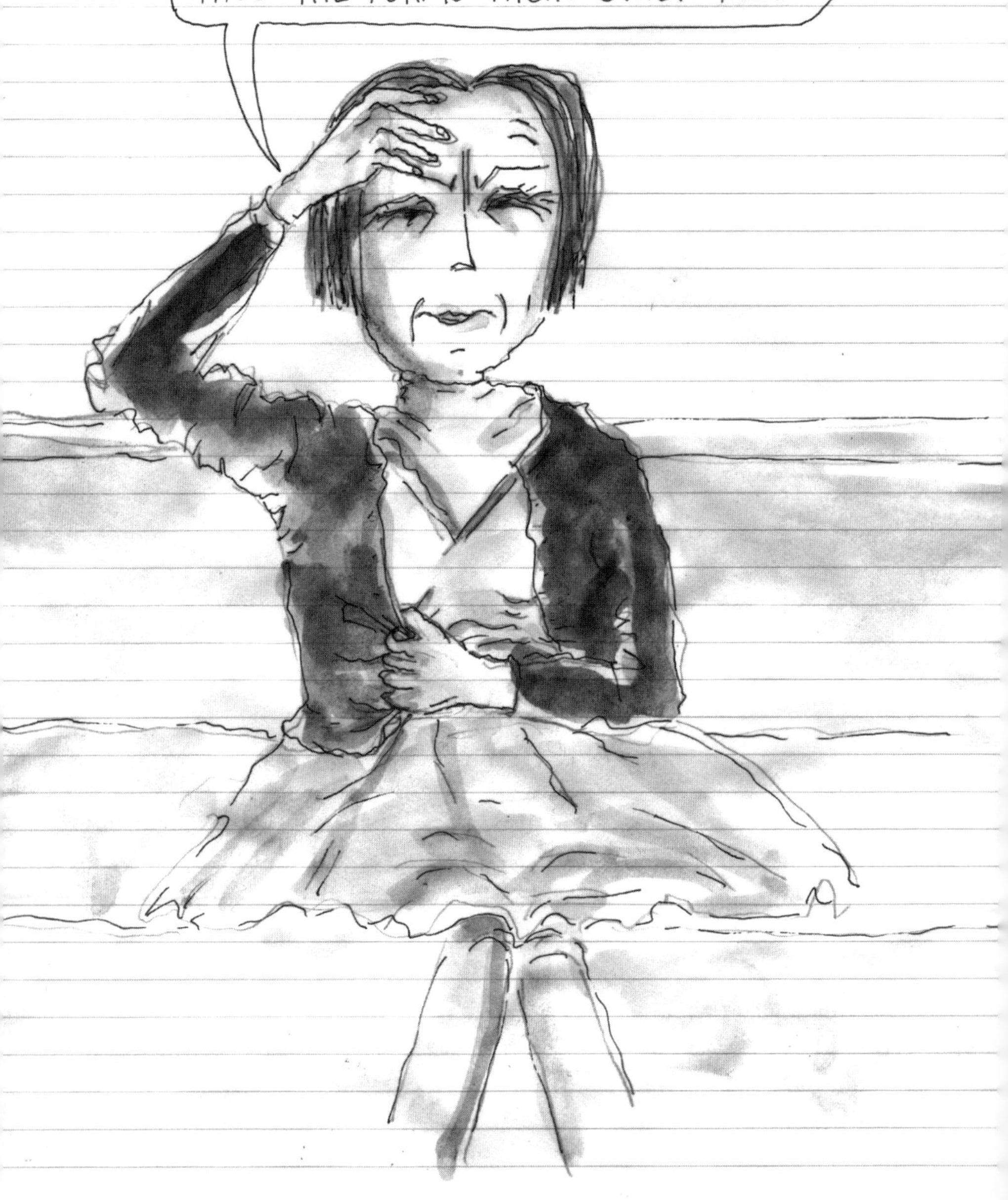
OH, THE ARROGANCE OF THE GRIEVING! I'D IMPOSED ANOTHER HIERARCHY, SANCTIONING WHO COULD GRIEVE AND THE FORMS THEIR GRIEF TOOK

Mon	Tue	Wed	Thu	Fri	Sat	Sun	Mon	Tue	Wed	Thu	Fri	Sat	Sun	Mon	Tue	Wed	Thu	Fri	Sat	Sun	Mon	Tue	Wed	Thu	Fri	Sat	Sun
1	2	3	4	5	6	7	8	9	10	11	12	13	14	15	16	17	18	19	20	21	22	23	24	25	26	27	28

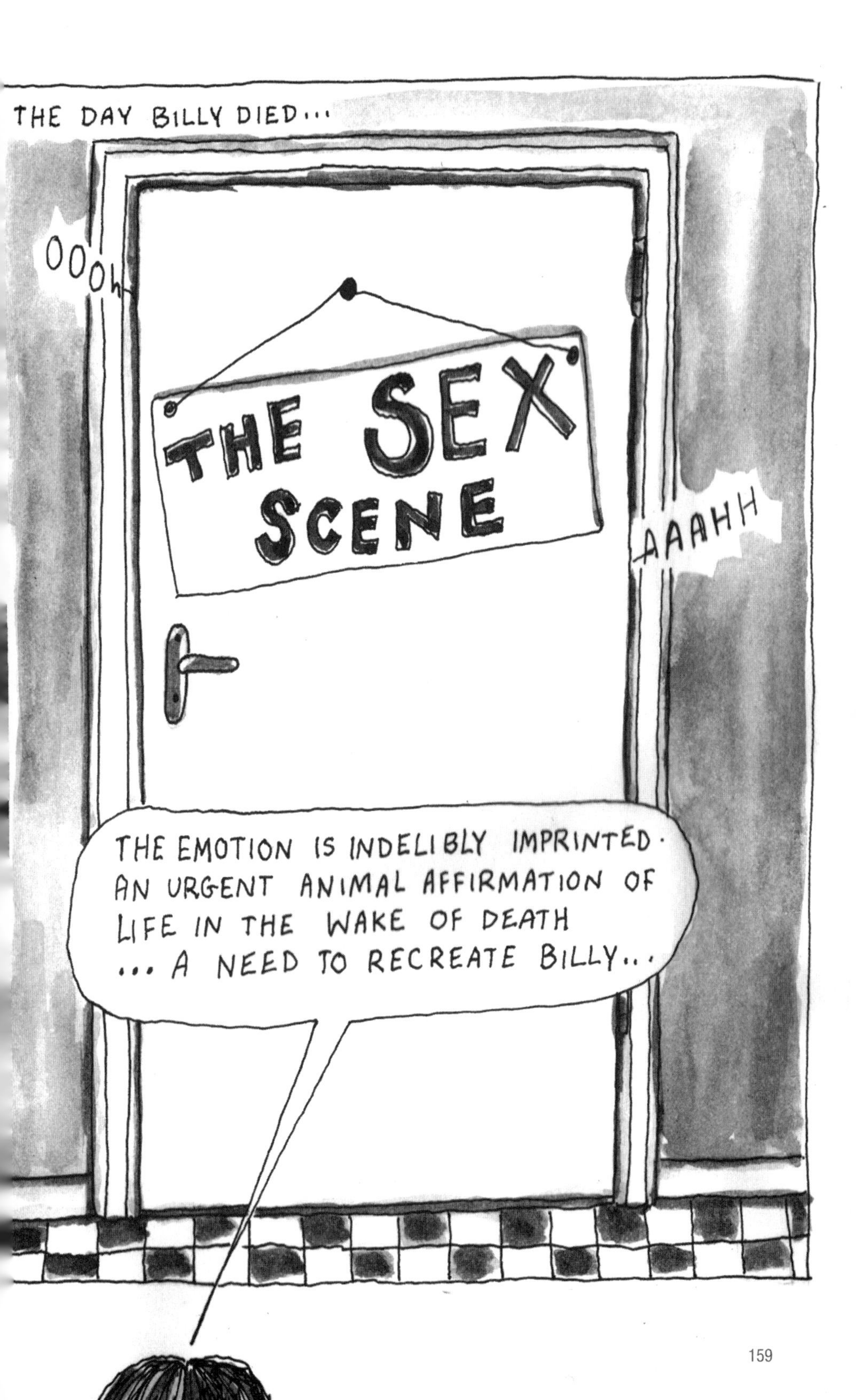
THE DAY BILLY DIED...
OOOh
THE SEX SCENE
AAAHH
THE EMOTION IS INDELIBLY IMPRINTED. AN URGENT ANIMAL AFFIRMATION OF LIFE IN THE WAKE OF DEATH ... A NEED TO RECREATE BILLY...

DESPITE THIS ACUTE NEED TO RECREATE, I KNEW JOHN AND I WEREN'T MENTALLY FIT ENOUGH TO HAVE ANOTHER BABY IMMEDIATELY

Fri	Sat	Sun	Mon	Tue	Wed	Thu	Fri	Sat	Sun	Mon	Tue	Wed	Thu	Fri	Sat	Sun	Mon	Tue	Wed	Thu	Fri	Sat	Sun	Mon	Tue	Wed	T
3	4	5	6	7	8	9	10	11	12	13	14	15	16	17	18	19	20	21	22	23	24	25	26	27	28	29	3

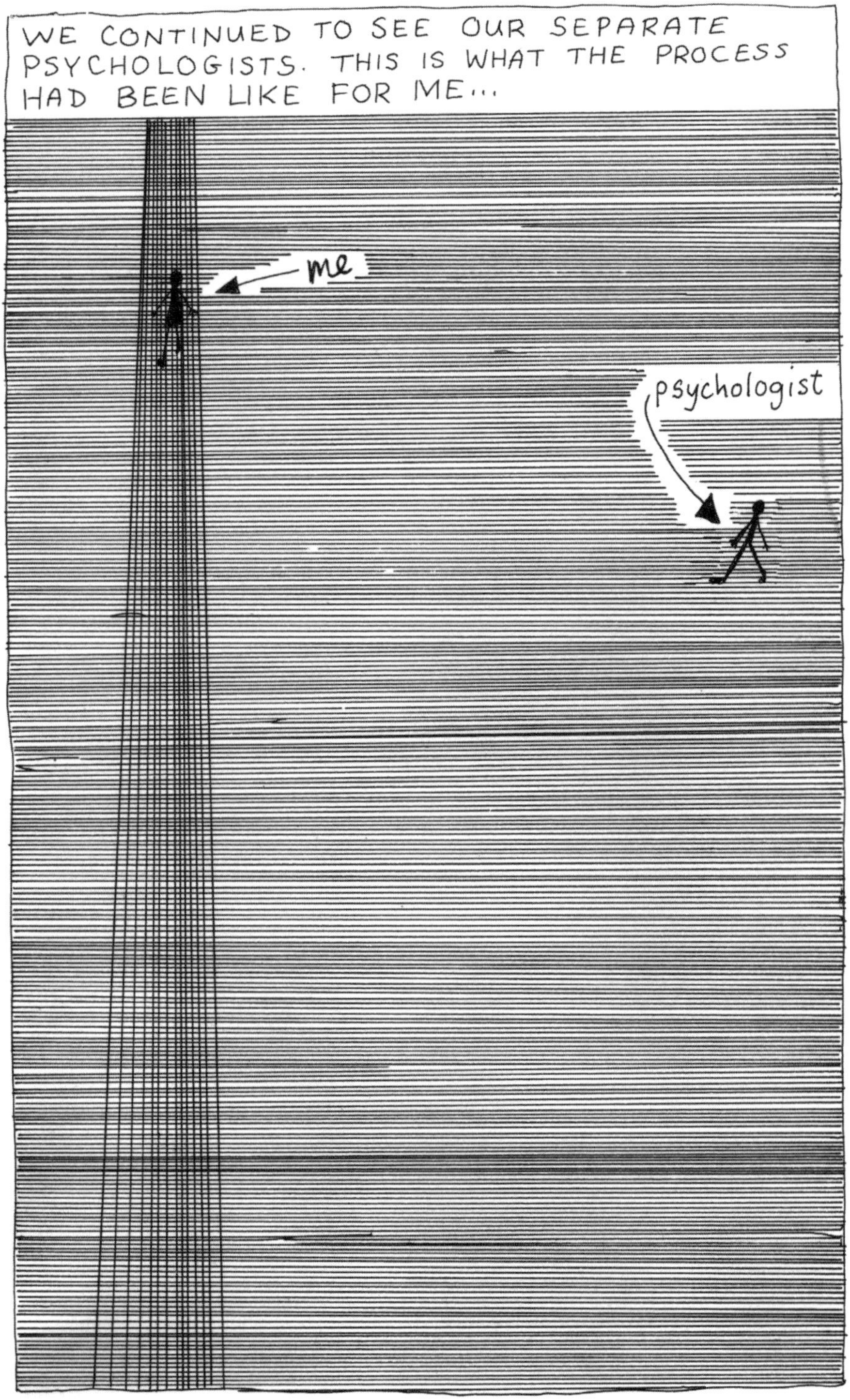

WE CONTINUED TO SEE OUR SEPARATE PSYCHOLOGISTS. THIS IS WHAT THE PROCESS HAD BEEN LIKE FOR ME...

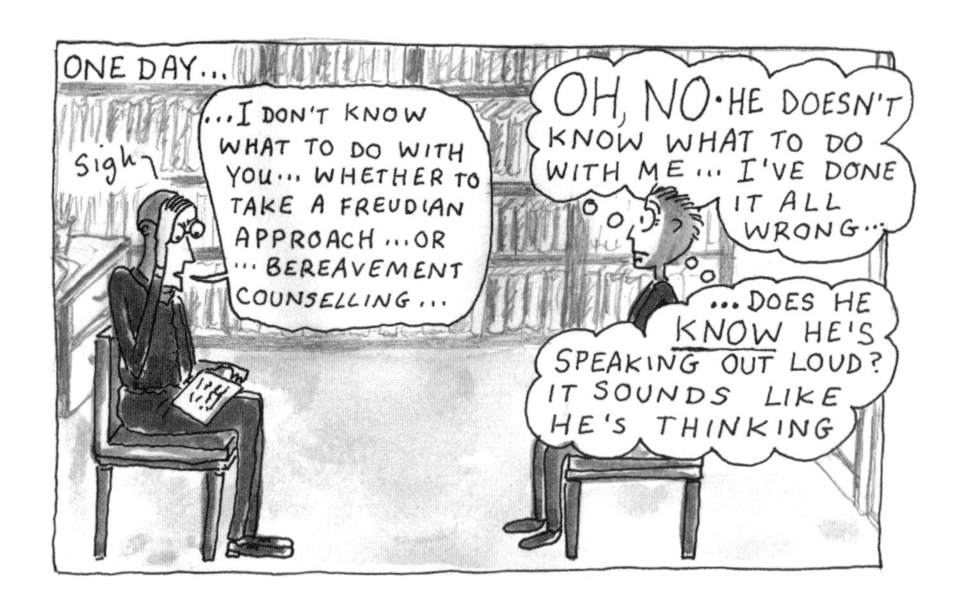
ONE DAY...
Sigh
...I DON'T KNOW WHAT TO DO WITH YOU... WHETHER TO TAKE A FREUDIAN APPROACH ...OR ... BEREAVEMENT COUNSELLING...
OH, NO. HE DOESN'T KNOW WHAT TO DO WITH ME... I'VE DONE IT ALL WRONG...
...DOES HE KNOW HE'S SPEAKING OUT LOUD? IT SOUNDS LIKE HE'S THINKING

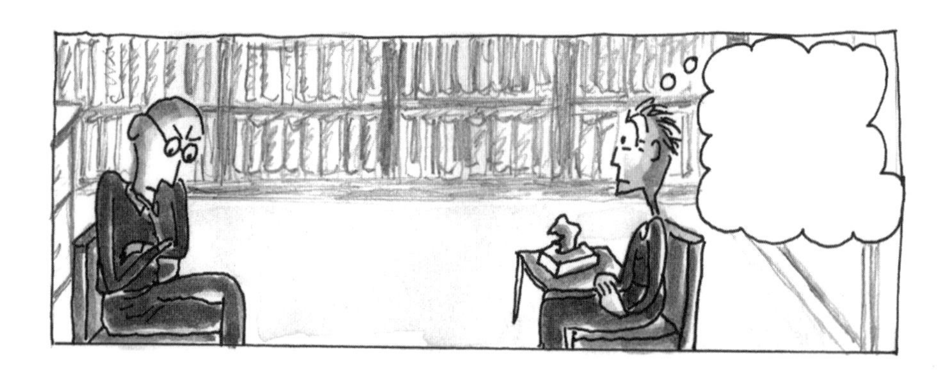

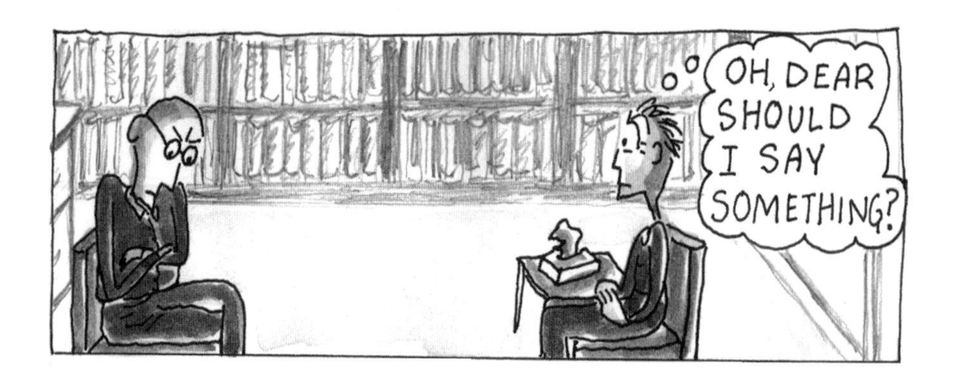
OH, DEAR SHOULD I SAY SOMETHING?

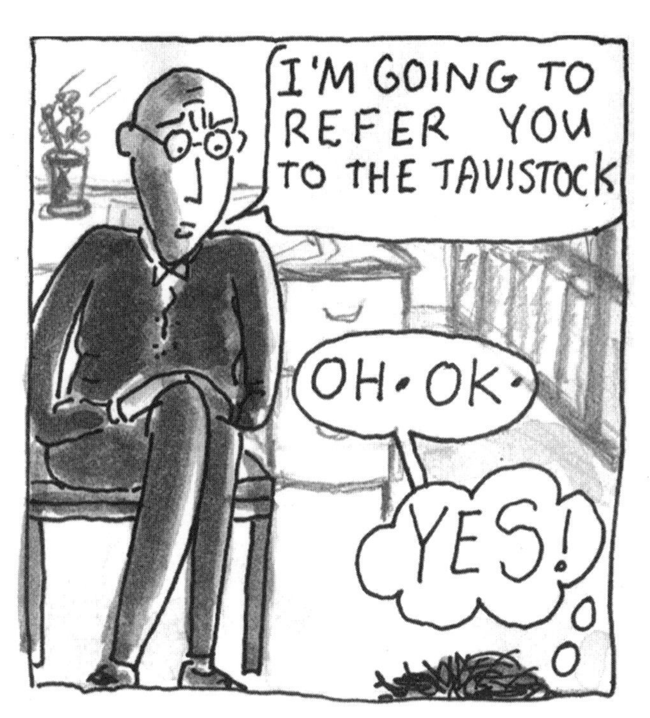
I'M GOING TO REFER YOU TO THE TAVISTOCK
OH. OK.
YES!

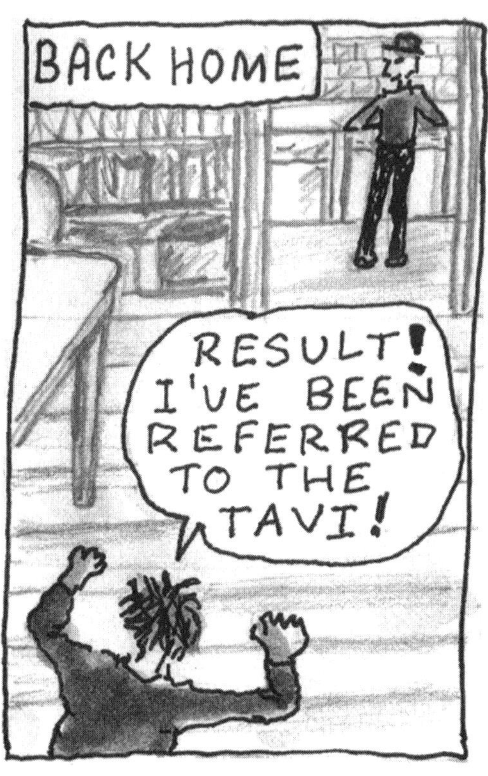
BACK HOME
RESULT! I'VE BEEN REFERRED TO THE TAVI!

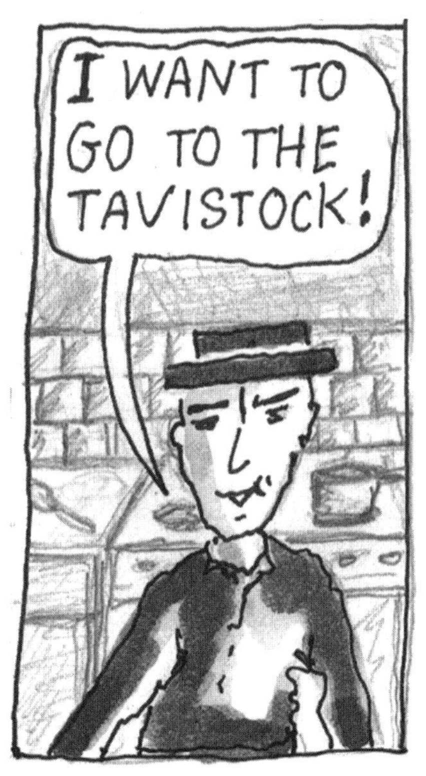
I WANT TO GO TO THE TAVISTOCK!

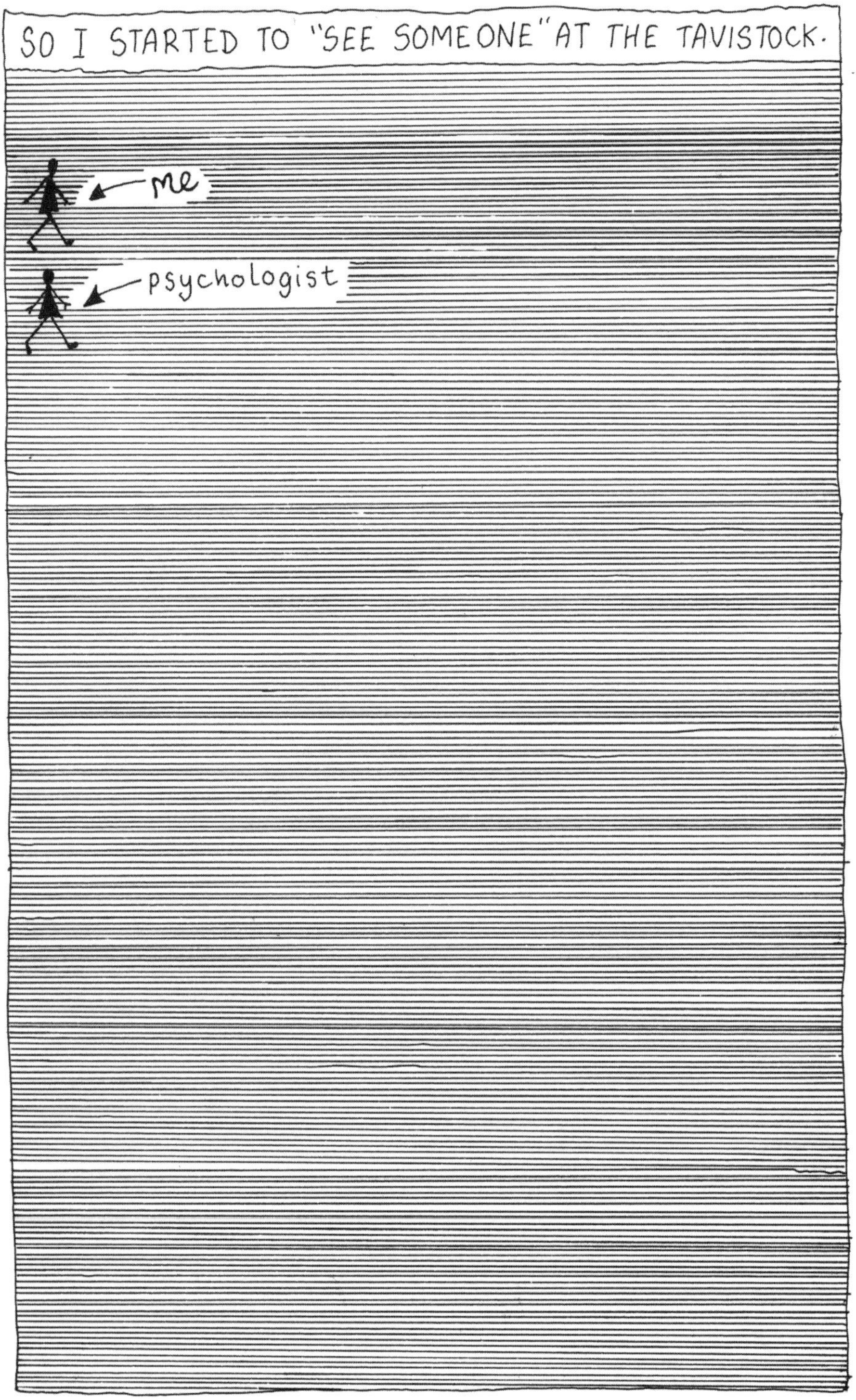

SO I STARTED TO "SEE SOMEONE" AT THE TAVISTOCK.

me

psychologist

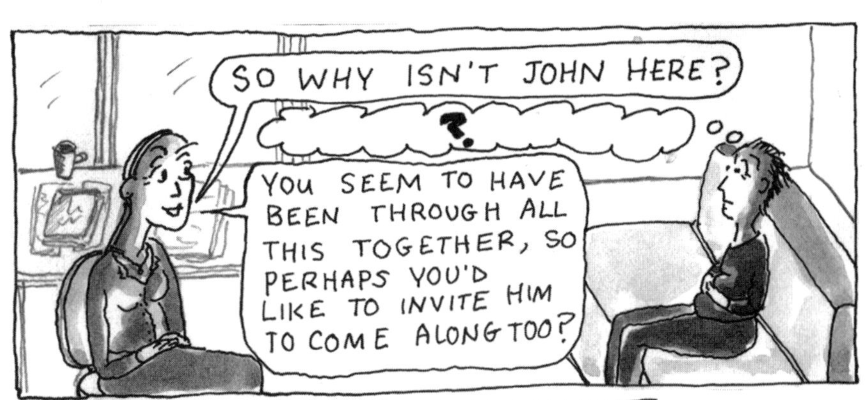
SO WHY ISN'T JOHN HERE?
?
YOU SEEM TO HAVE BEEN THROUGH ALL THIS TOGETHER, SO PERHAPS YOU'D LIKE TO INVITE HIM TO COME ALONG TOO?

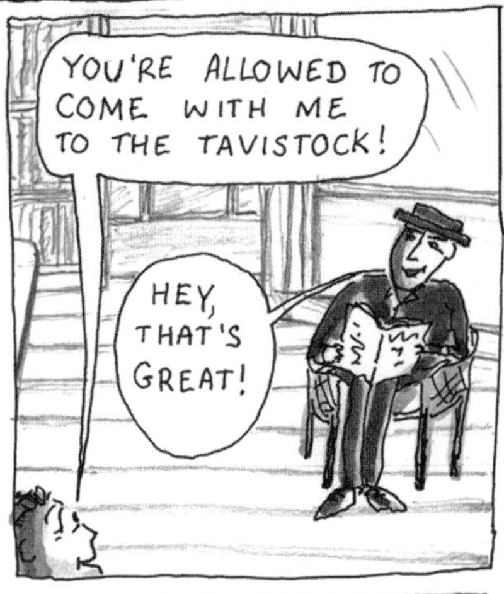
YOU'RE ALLOWED TO COME WITH ME TO THE TAVISTOCK!
HEY, THAT'S GREAT!

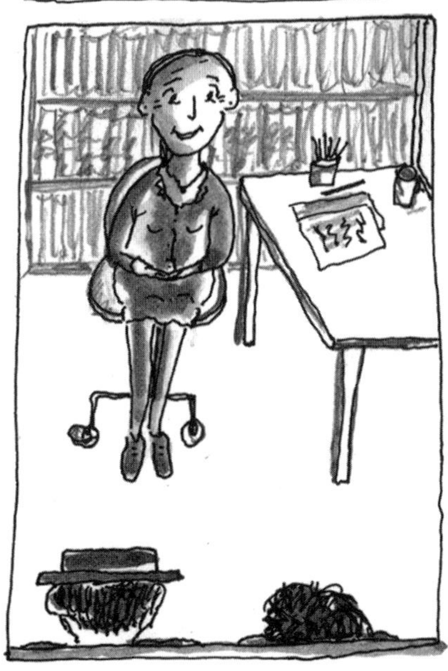

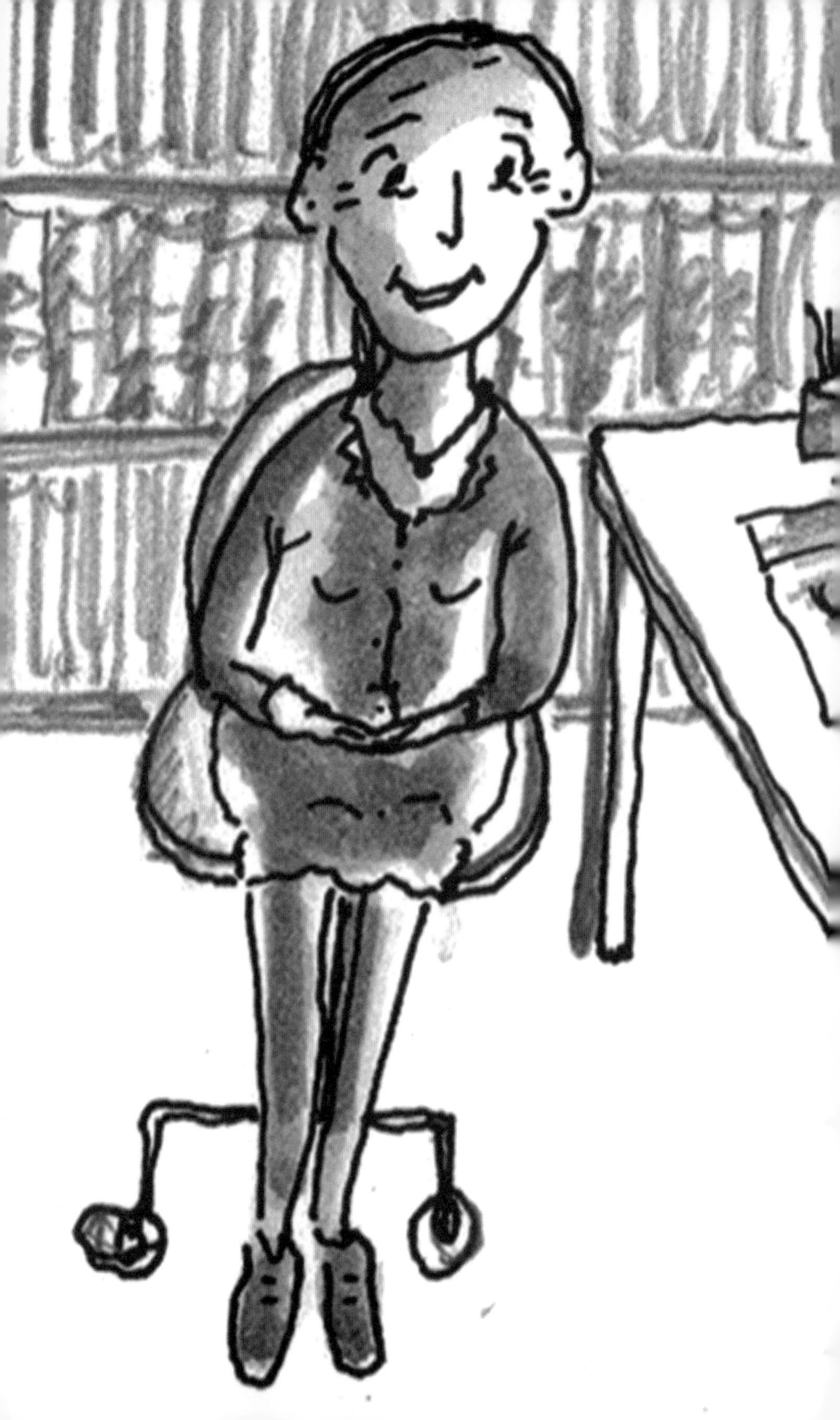

TEN MONTHS AFTER BILLY DIED I GOT PREGNANT.

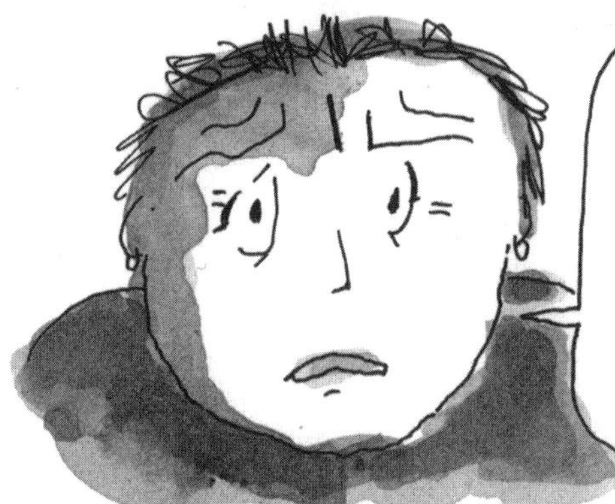

WHAT IF IT'S A GIRL? WHAT IF IT'S A BOY?

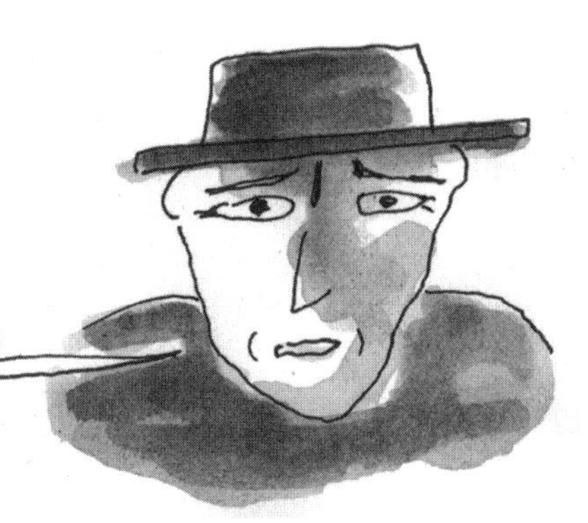

WHAT IF WE FORGET BILLY? WHAT IF THIS BABY DIES TOO?

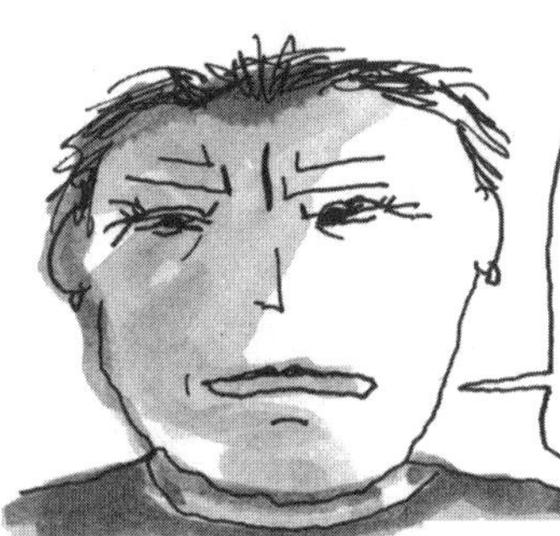

WHAT IF I LOVE IT MORE? WHAT IF I LOVE IT LESS? WHAT IF THIS BABY HAS HEART DEFECTS TOO?

ONCE OUR WORRIES WERE VOICED IN THIS SAFE ENVIRONMENT THEY BEGAN TO DISSIPATE.

I'D STARTED TEACHING AT A DIFFERENT LANGUAGE SCHOOL.

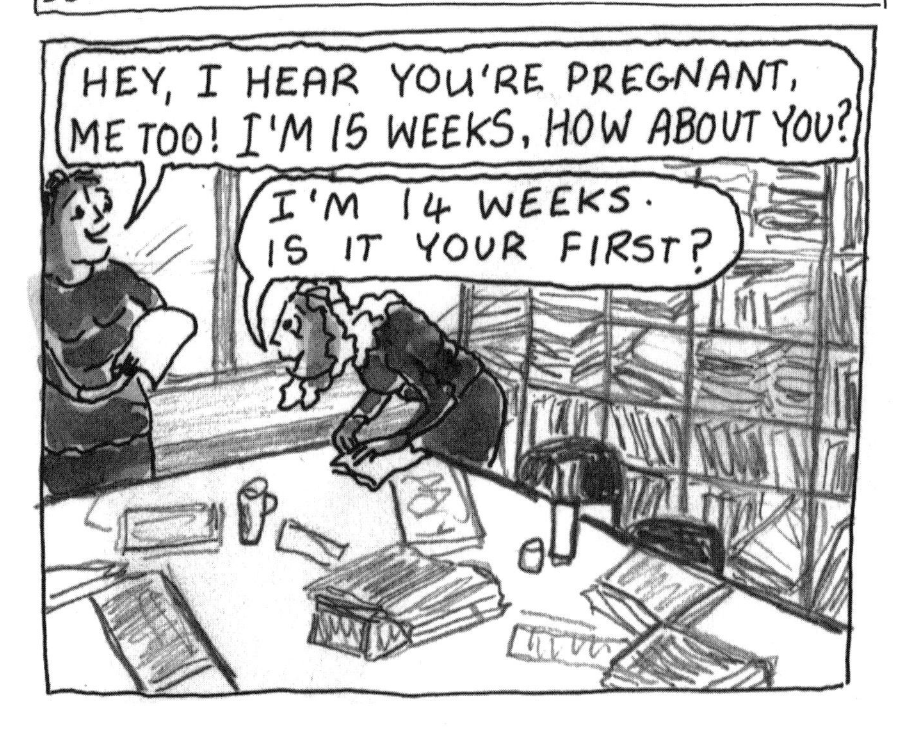
HEY, I HEAR YOU'RE PREGNANT, ME TOO! I'M 15 WEEKS, HOW ABOUT YOU?
I'M 14 WEEKS. IS IT YOUR FIRST?

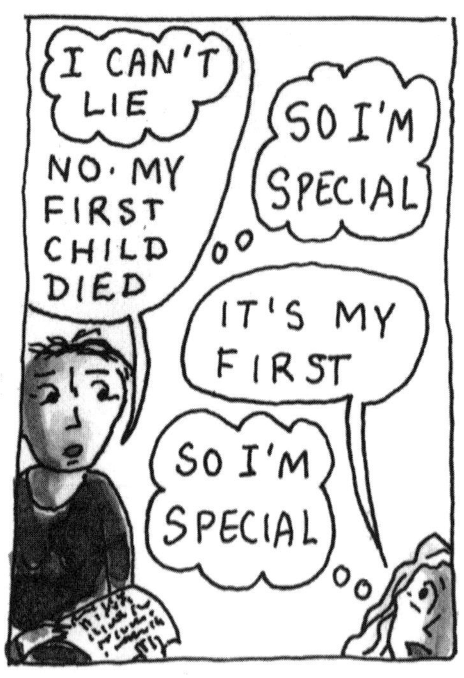
I CAN'T LIE
NO. MY FIRST CHILD DIED
SO I'M SPECIAL
IT'S MY FIRST
SO I'M SPECIAL

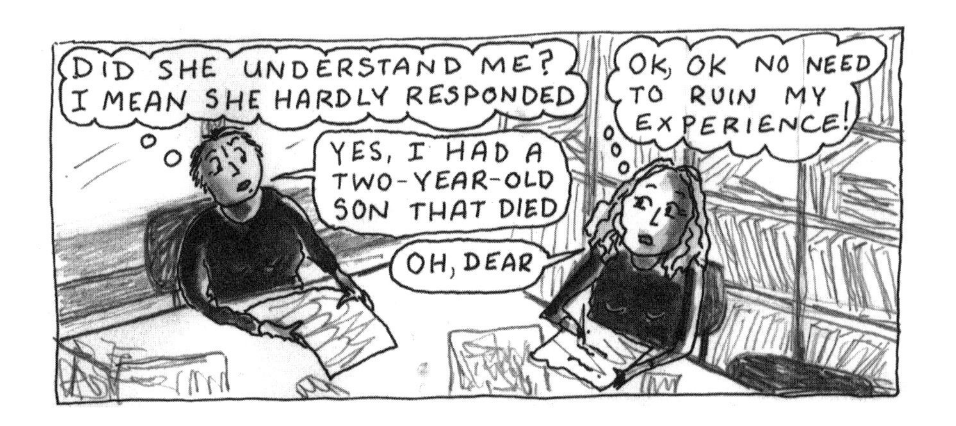
DID SHE UNDERSTAND ME? I MEAN SHE HARDLY RESPONDED
YES, I HAD A TWO-YEAR-OLD SON THAT DIED
OH, DEAR
OK, OK NO NEED TO RUIN MY EXPERIENCE!

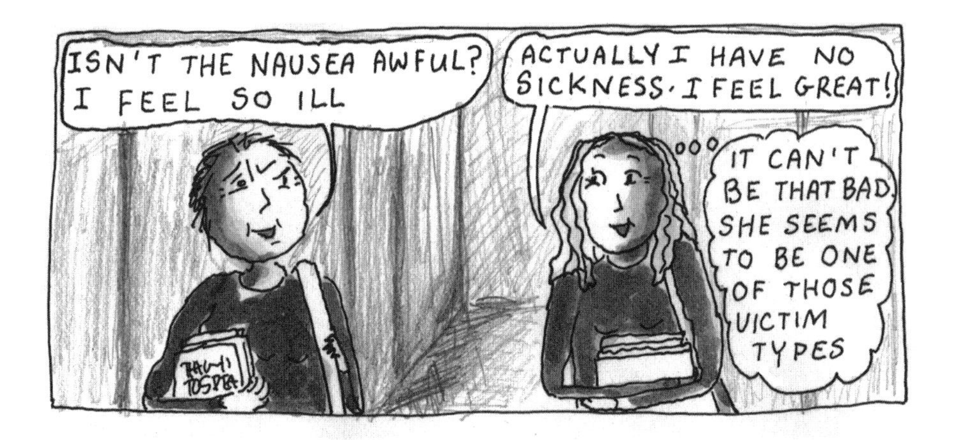
ISN'T THE NAUSEA AWFUL? I FEEL SO ILL
ACTUALLY I HAVE NO SICKNESS. I FEEL GREAT!
IT CAN'T BE THAT BAD. SHE SEEMS TO BE ONE OF THOSE VICTIM TYPES

AS WEEKS PASSED I GREW TO HATE THE TEACHING. IN THE MORNINGS JOHN WALKED WITH ME TO THE SCHOOL.

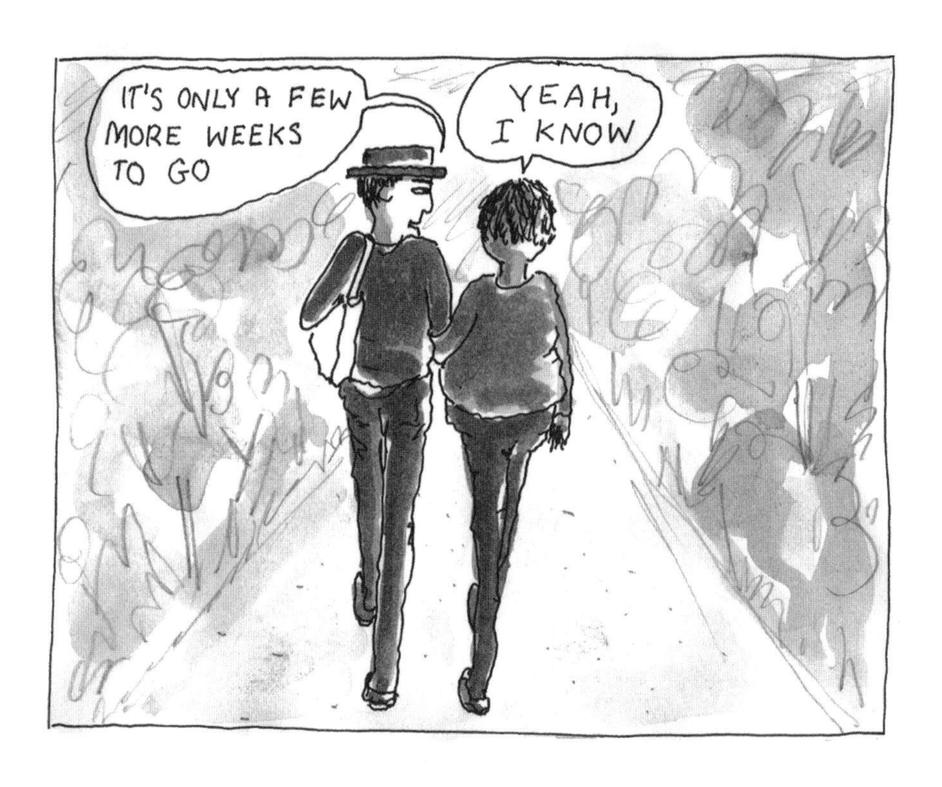
IT'S ONLY A FEW MORE WEEKS TO GO
YEAH, I KNOW

AND EVERY NIGHT I DREW.

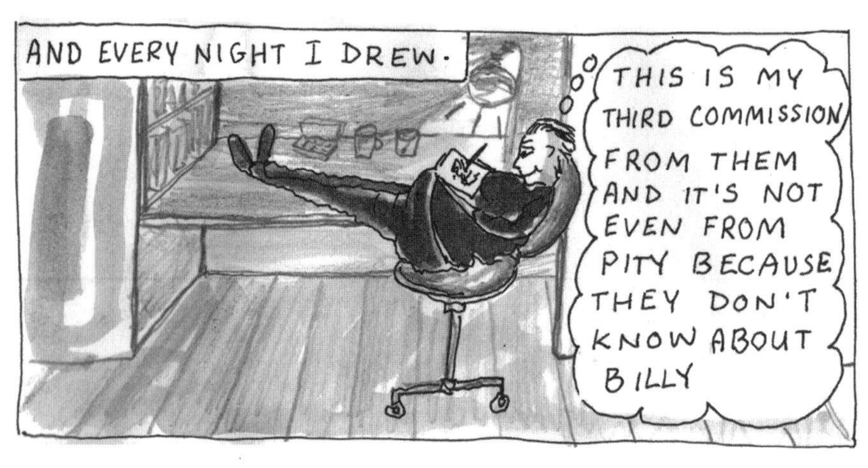
THIS IS MY THIRD COMMISSION FROM THEM AND IT'S NOT EVEN FROM PITY BECAUSE THEY DON'T KNOW ABOUT BILLY

FINALLY, TIME BROUGHT US TO THE BIRTH OF OUR SECOND CHILD, SALLY.

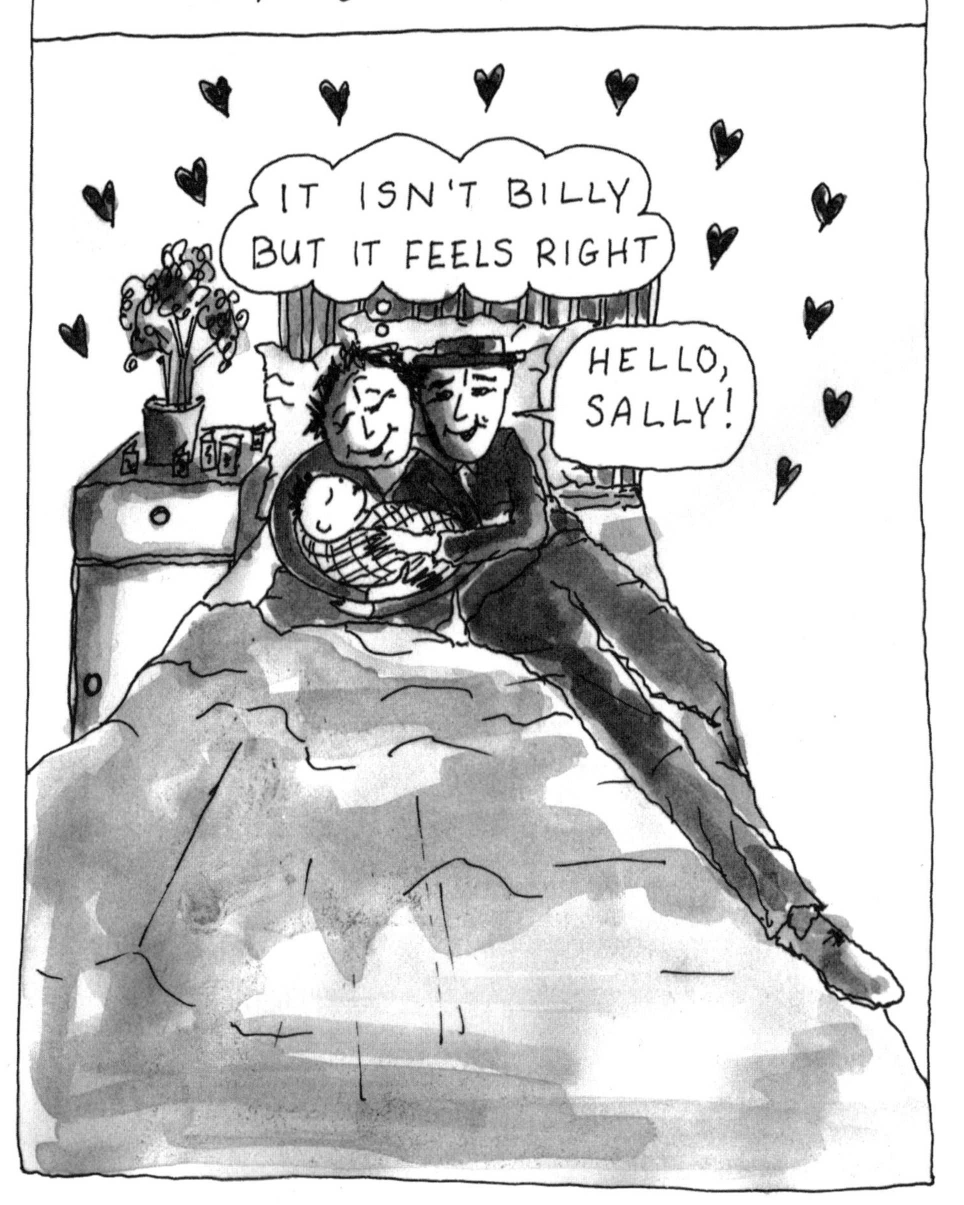

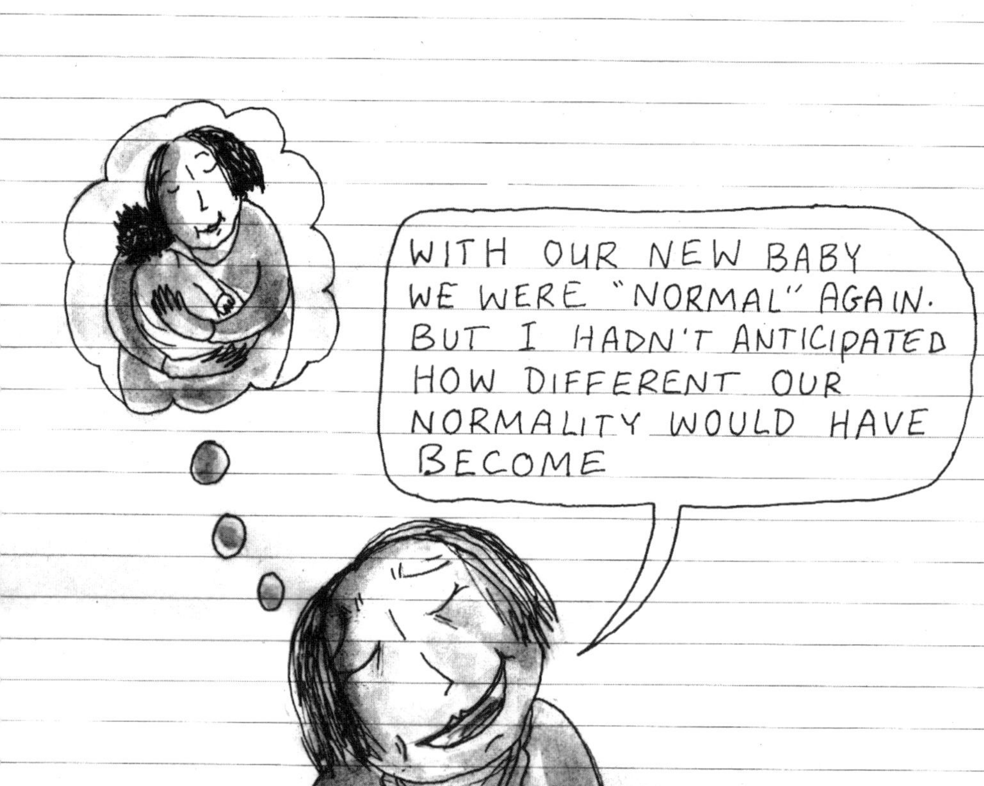
WITH OUR NEW BABY WE WERE "NORMAL" AGAIN. BUT I HADN'T ANTICIPATED HOW DIFFERENT OUR NORMALITY WOULD HAVE BECOME

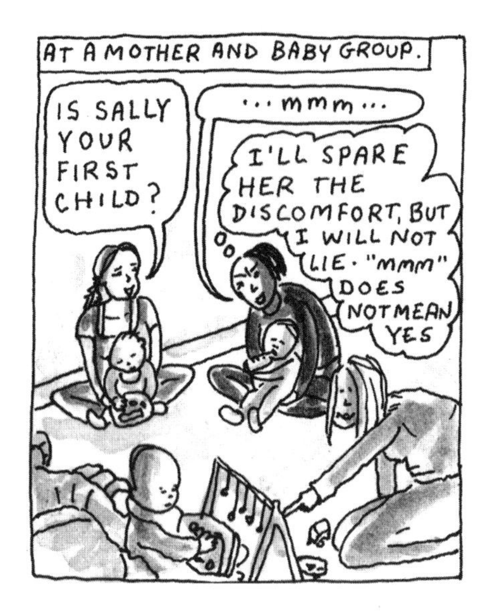
AT A MOTHER AND BABY GROUP.
IS SALLY YOUR FIRST CHILD?
...mmm...
I'LL SPARE HER THE DISCOMFORT, BUT I WILL NOT LIE. "mmm" DOES NOT MEAN YES

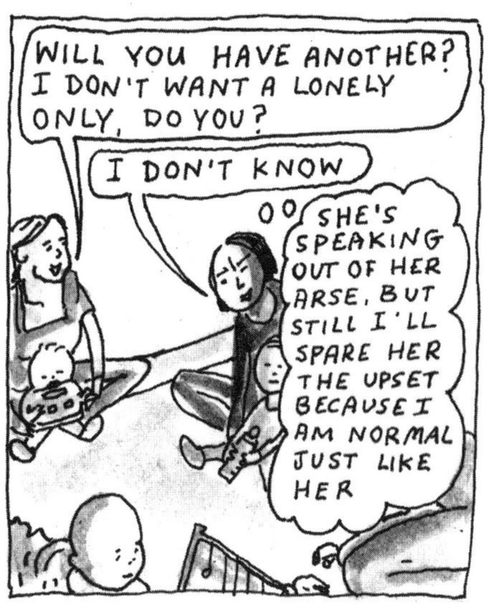
WILL YOU HAVE ANOTHER? I DON'T WANT A LONELY ONLY, DO YOU?
I DON'T KNOW
SHE'S SPEAKING OUT OF HER ARSE, BUT STILL I'LL SPARE HER THE UPSET BECAUSE I AM NORMAL JUST LIKE HER

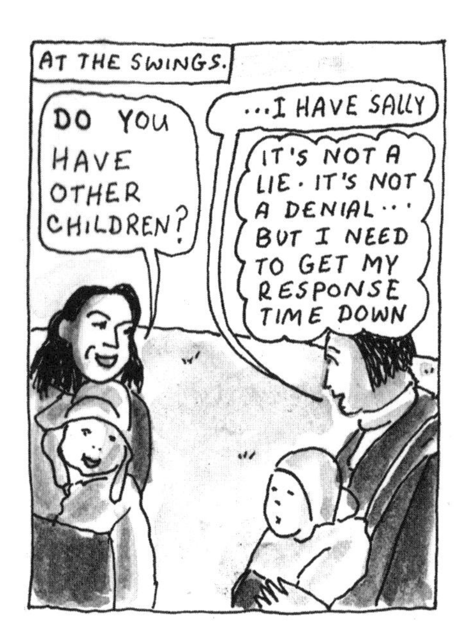
AT THE SWINGS.
DO YOU HAVE OTHER CHILDREN?
...I HAVE SALLY
IT'S NOT A LIE. IT'S NOT A DENIAL... BUT I NEED TO GET MY RESPONSE TIME DOWN

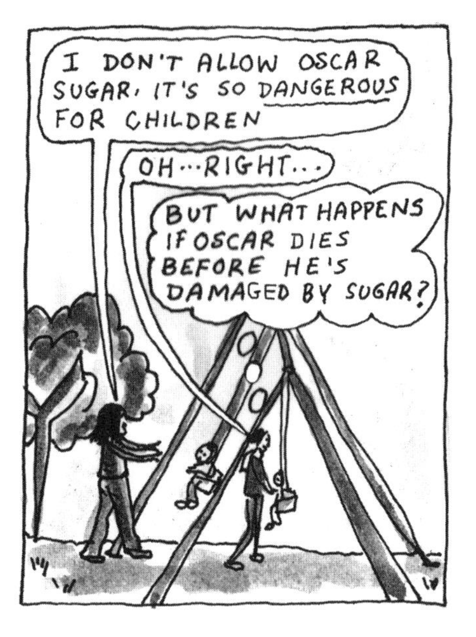
I DON'T ALLOW OSCAR SUGAR, IT'S SO DANGEROUS FOR CHILDREN
OH...RIGHT...
BUT WHAT HAPPENS IF OSCAR DIES BEFORE HE'S DAMAGED BY SUGAR?

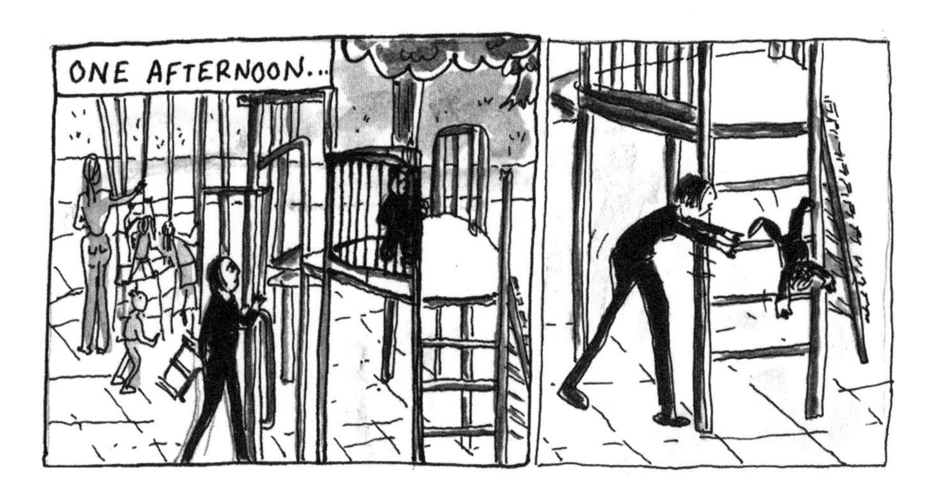
ONE AFTERNOON...

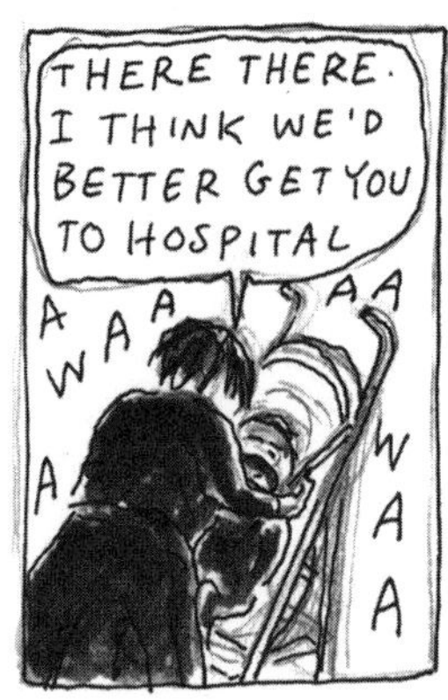
THERE THERE.
I THINK WE'D BETTER GET YOU TO HOSPITAL
AWAAA
AA
WAAA

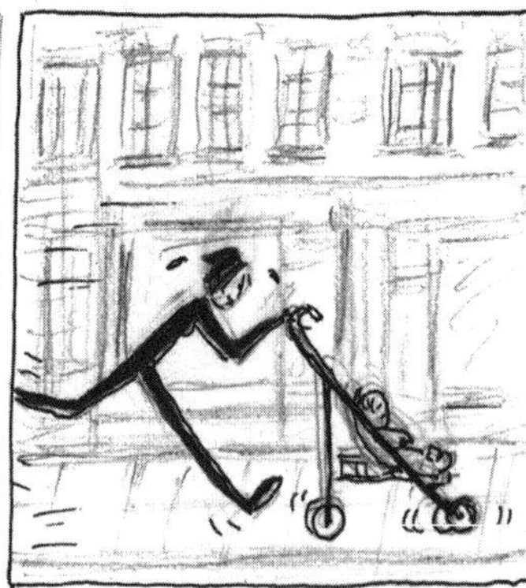

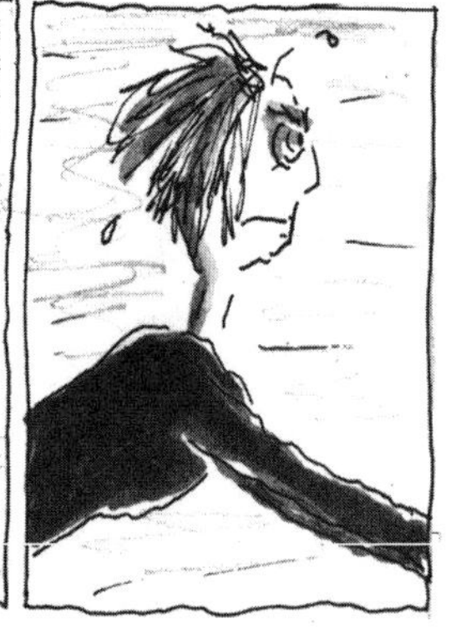

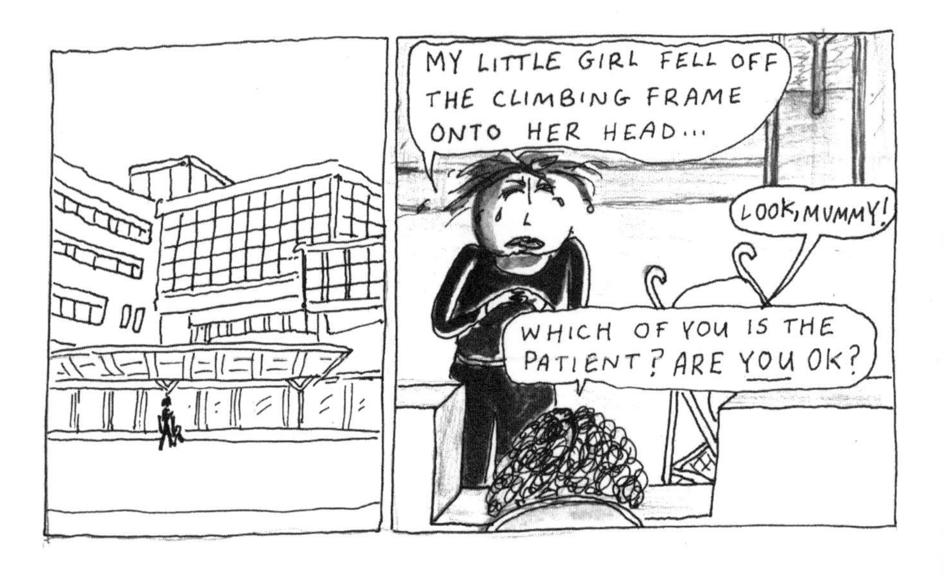
MY LITTLE GIRL FELL OFF THE CLIMBING FRAME ONTO HER HEAD...
LOOK, MUMMY!
WHICH OF YOU IS THE PATIENT? ARE YOU OK?

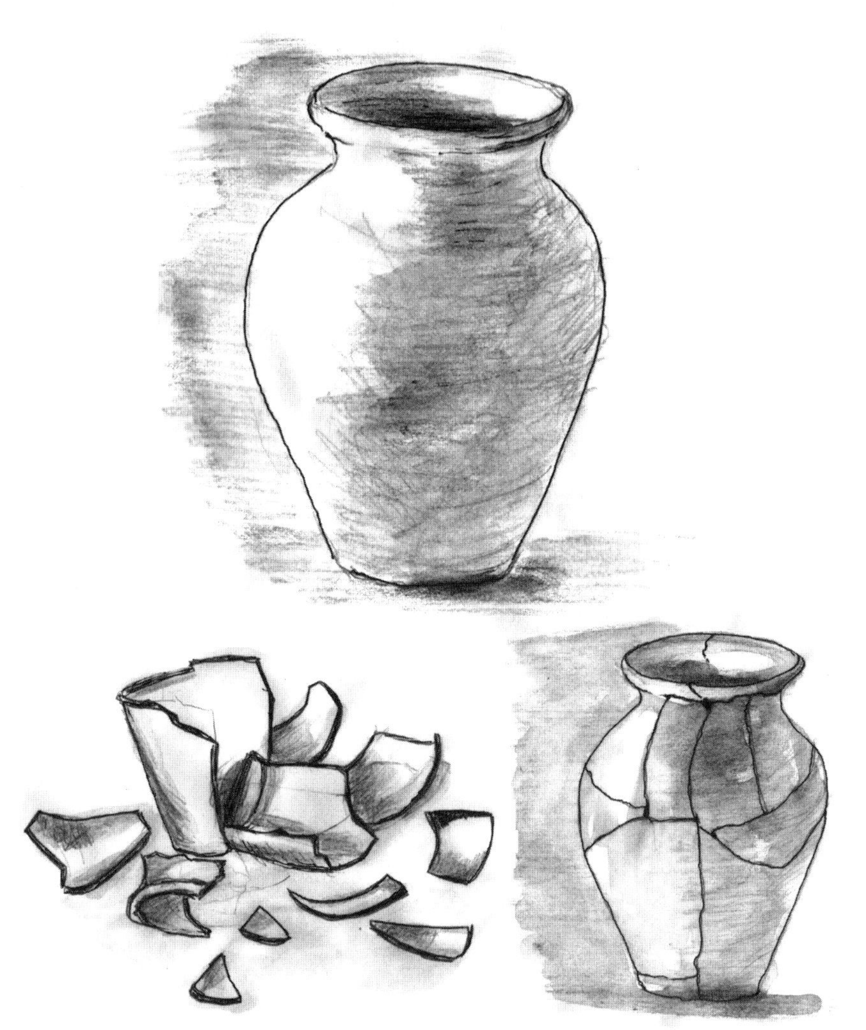

IS THIS STILL A VASE? IS THIS STILL A VASE?

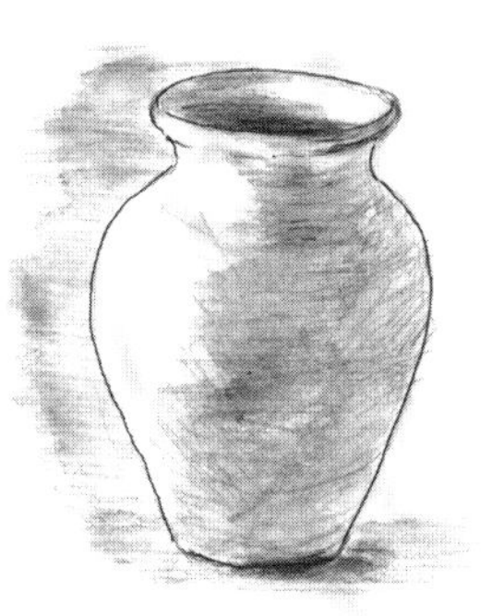

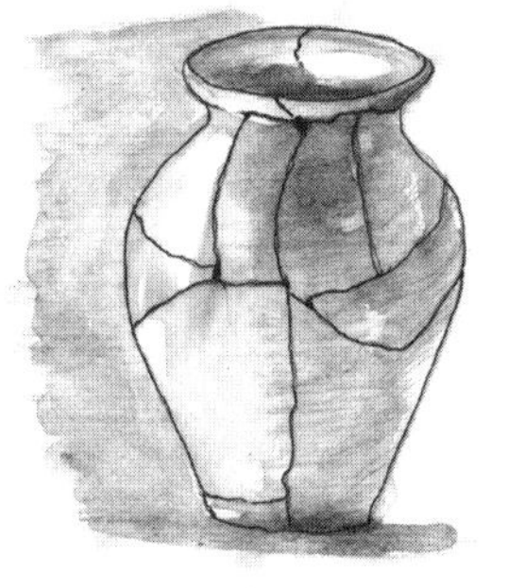

WHICH IS NORMAL?

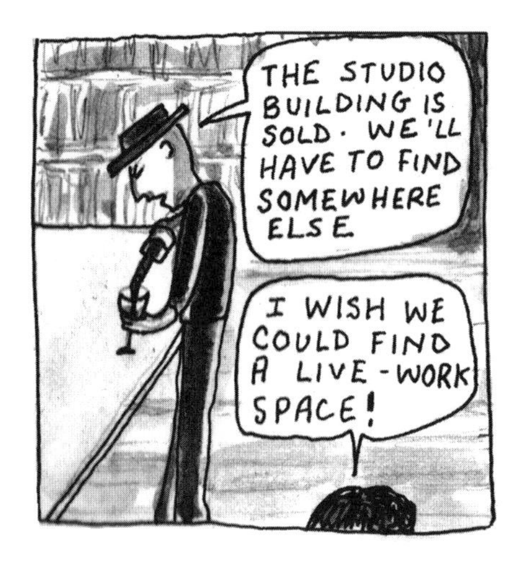
THE STUDIO BUILDING IS SOLD. WE'LL HAVE TO FIND SOMEWHERE ELSE
I WISH WE COULD FIND A LIVE-WORK SPACE!

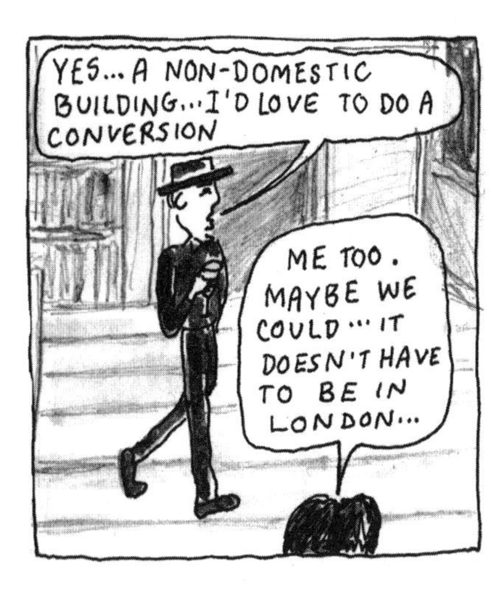
YES... A NON-DOMESTIC BUILDING... I'D LOVE TO DO A CONVERSION
ME TOO. MAYBE WE COULD... IT DOESN'T HAVE TO BE IN LONDON...

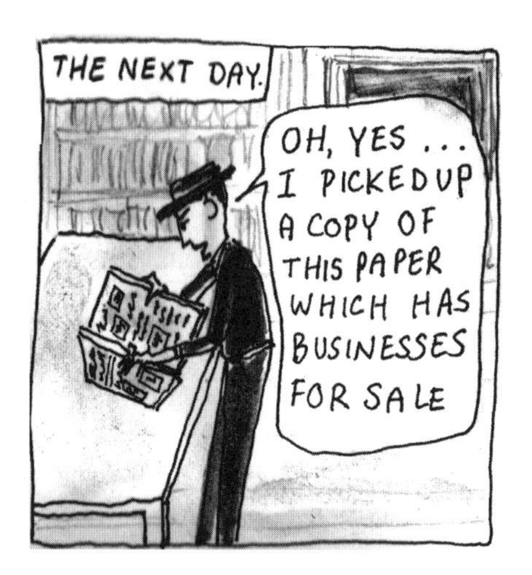
THE NEXT DAY.
OH, YES... I PICKED UP A COPY OF THIS PAPER WHICH HAS BUSINESSES FOR SALE

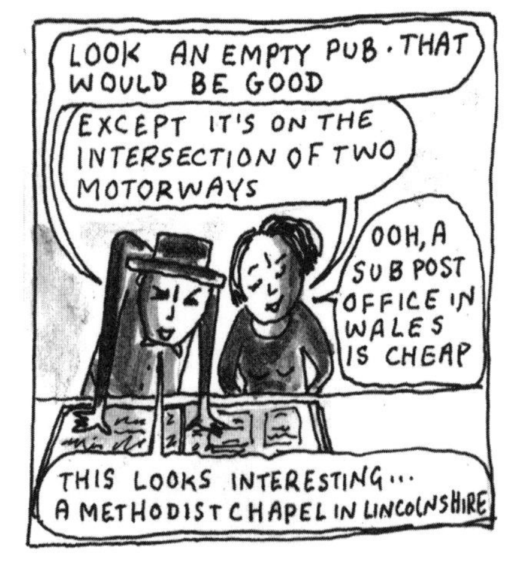
LOOK AN EMPTY PUB. THAT WOULD BE GOOD
EXCEPT IT'S ON THE INTERSECTION OF TWO MOTORWAYS
OOH, A SUB POST OFFICE IN WALES IS CHEAP
THIS LOOKS INTERESTING... A METHODIST CHAPEL IN LINCOLNSHIRE

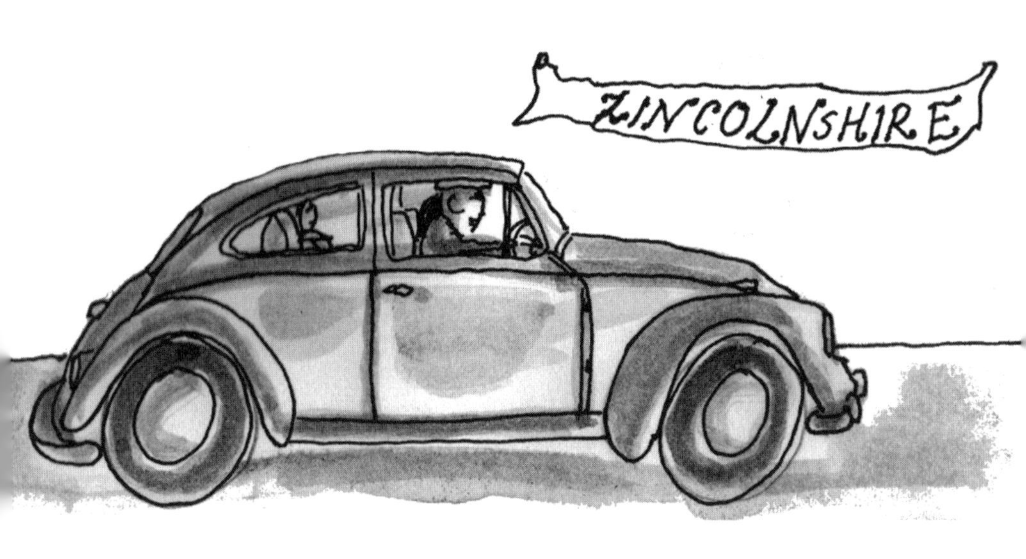
LINCOLNSHIRE

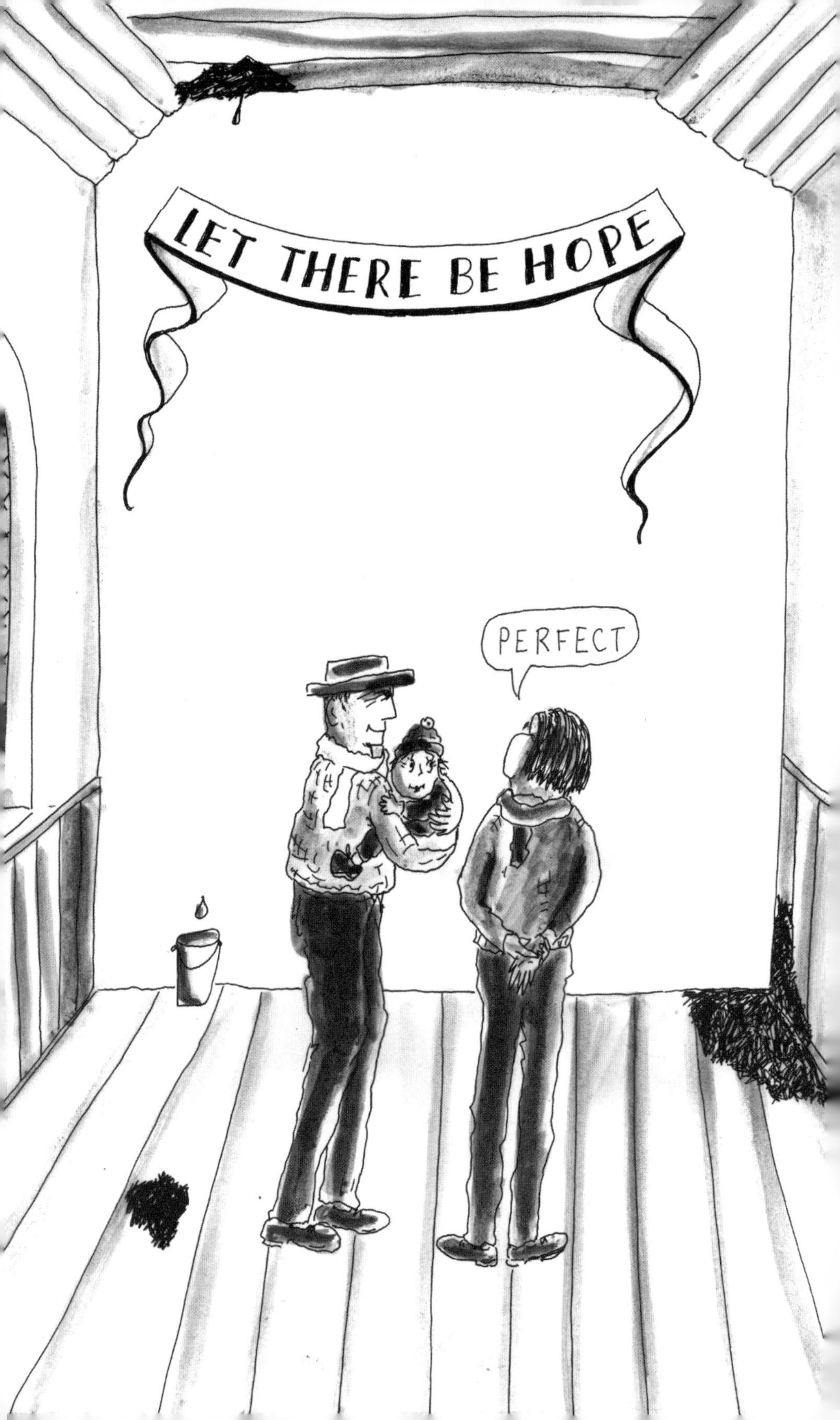
LET THERE BE HOPE
PERFECT

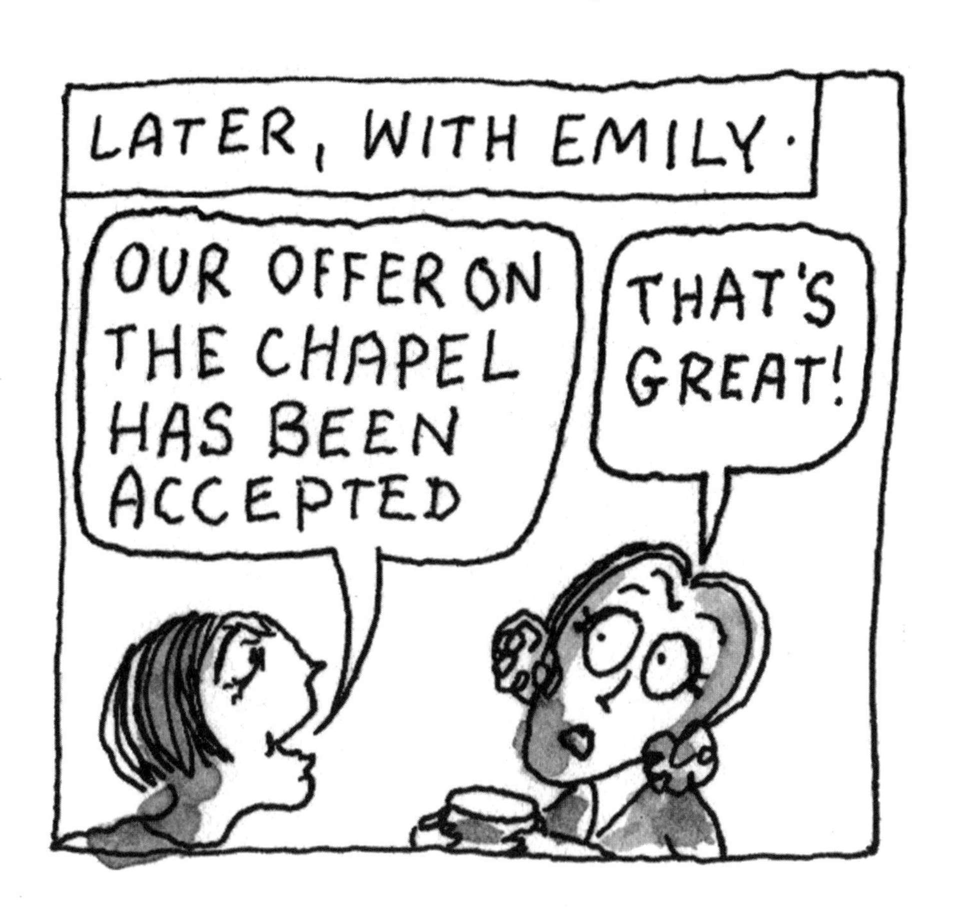
LATER, WITH EMILY.
OUR OFFER ON THE CHAPEL HAS BEEN ACCEPTED
THAT'S GREAT!

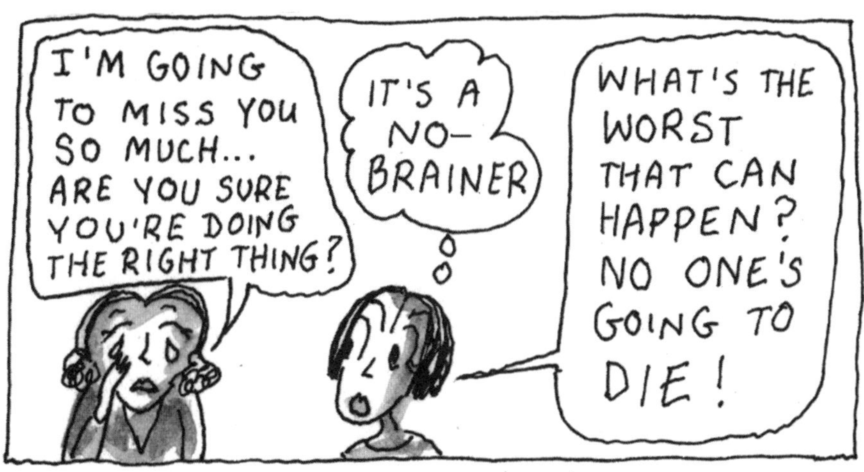
I'M GOING TO MISS YOU SO MUCH... ARE YOU SURE YOU'RE DOING THE RIGHT THING?
IT'S A NO-BRAINER
WHAT'S THE WORST THAT CAN HAPPEN? NO ONE'S GOING TO DIE!

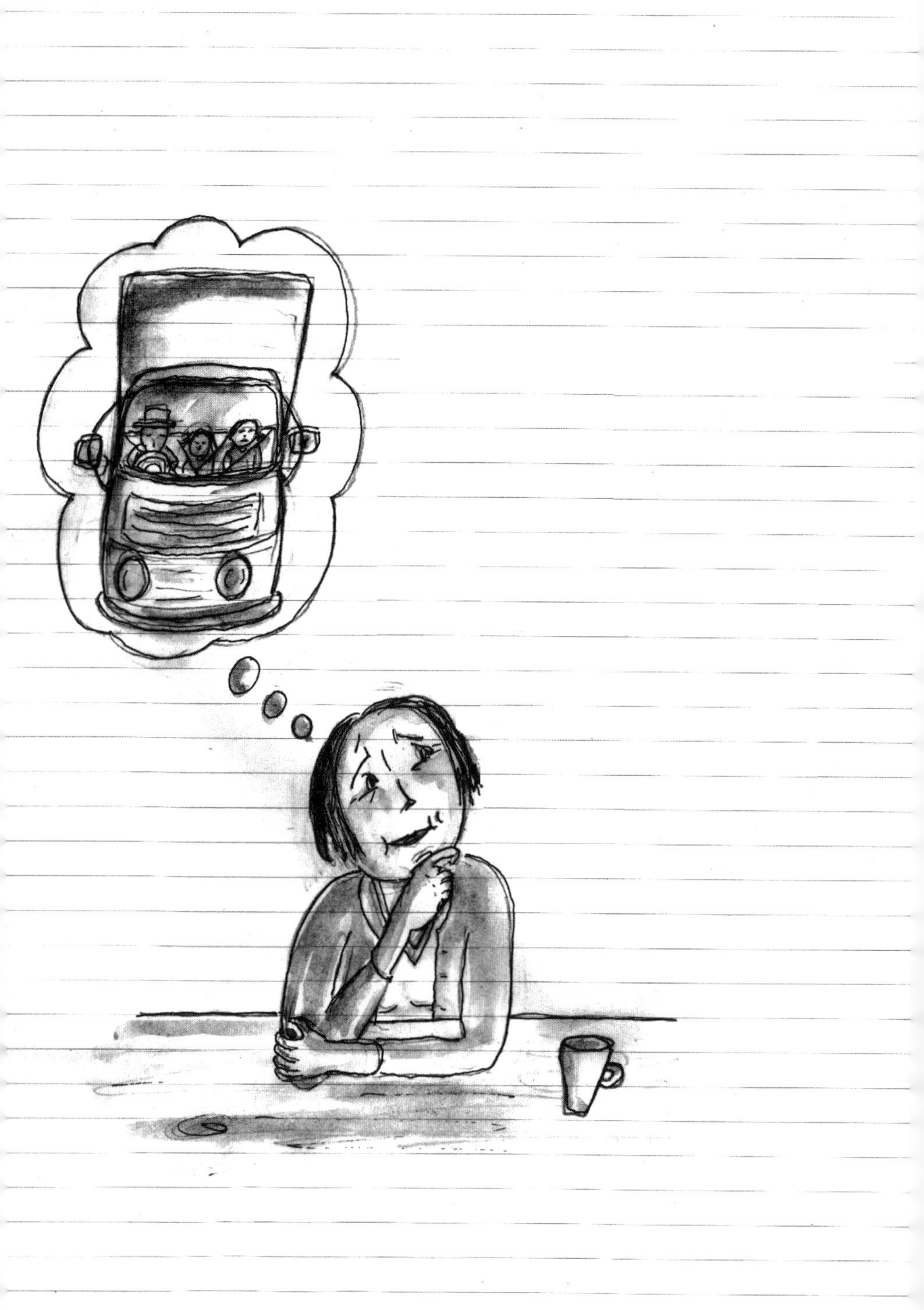

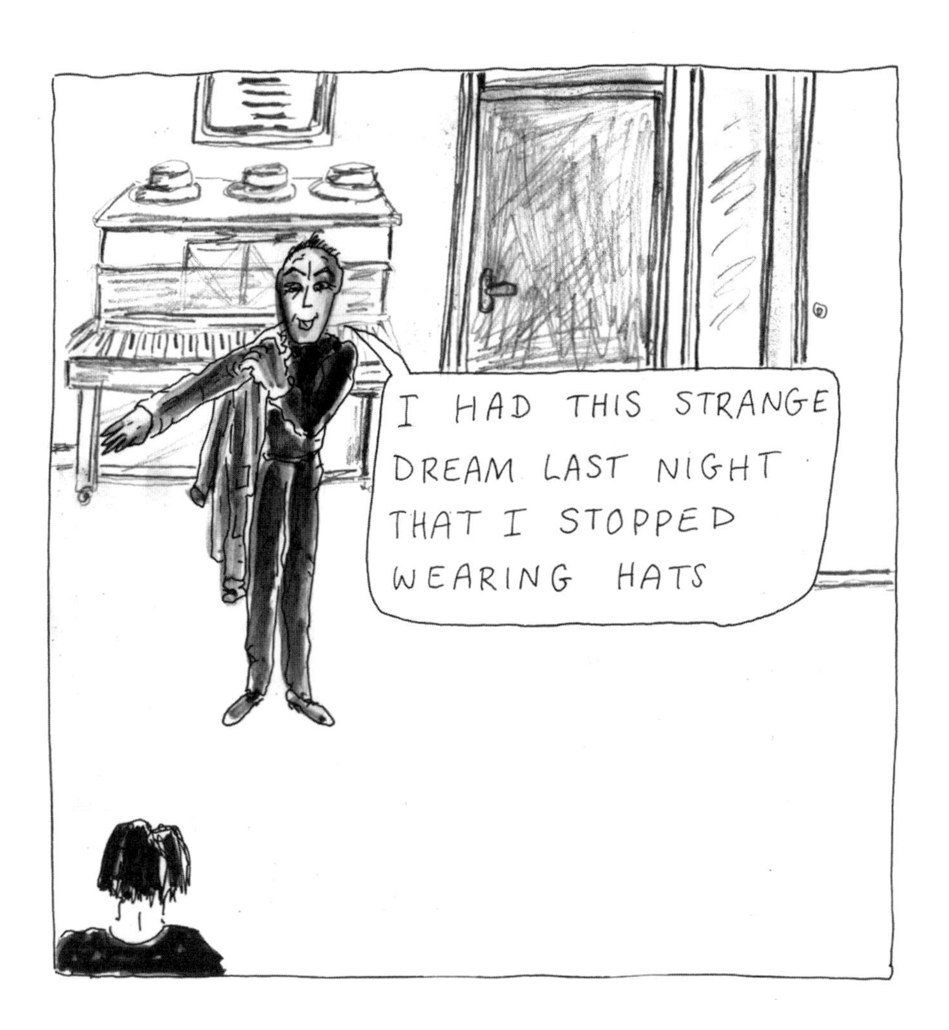
I HAD THIS STRANGE DREAM LAST NIGHT THAT I STOPPED WEARING HATS

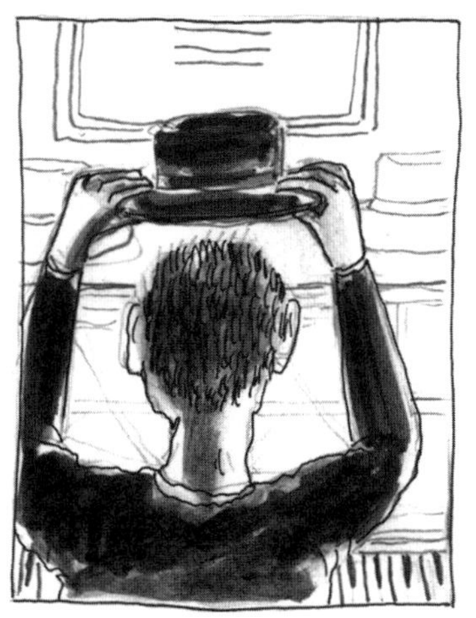

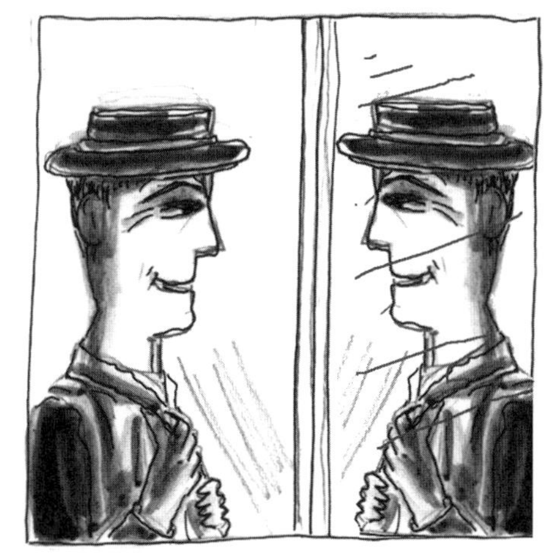

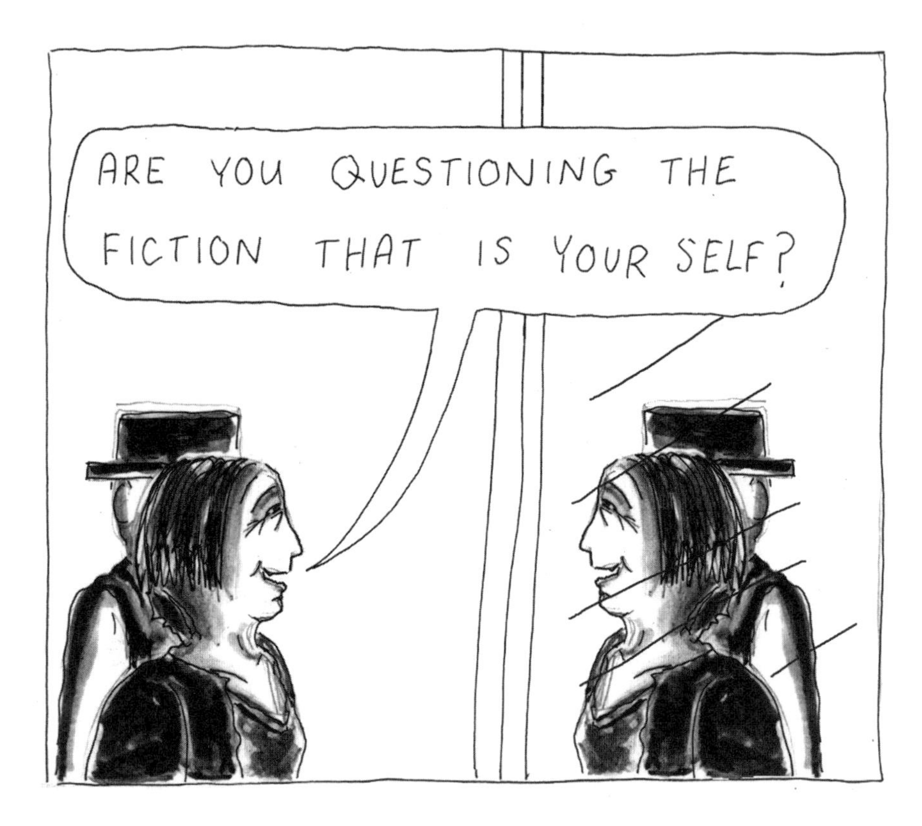
ARE YOU QUESTIONING THE FICTION THAT IS YOUR SELF?

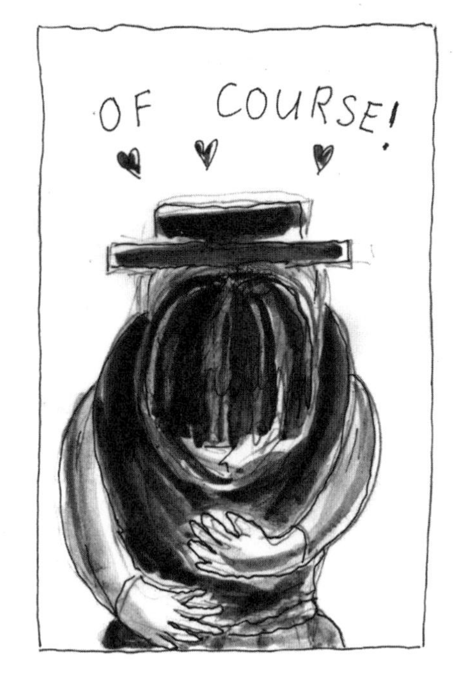
OF COURSE!

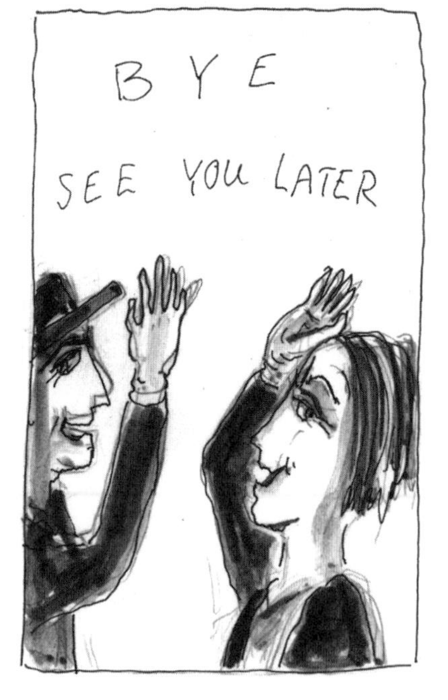
BYE
SEE YOU LATER

Sun 5
Mon 6 Tue 7 Wed 8 Thu 9 Fri 10 Sat 11 Sun 12
Mon 13 Tue 14 Wed 15 Thu 16 Fri 17 Sat 18 Sun 19
Mon 20 Tue 21 Wed 22 Thu 23 Fri 24 Sat 25 Sun 26
Mon 27 Tue 28 Wed 29 Thu 30

MEMORIES OF BILLY

Sun 5 | Mon 6 Tue 7 Wed 8 Thu 9 Fri 10 Sat 11 Sun 12 | Mon 13 Tue 14 Wed 15 Thu 16 Fri 17 Sat 18 Sun 19 | Mon 20 Tue 21 Wed 22 Thu 23 Fri 24 Sat 25 Sun 26 | Mon 27 Tue 28 Wed 29 Thu 30

In Memoriam

BILLY Edwin Plowman **STREETEN**
3 July 1993 - 19 September 1995
Billy boy, Billy boy, playing in his den,
Billy boy, Billy boy, with his band of friends,
Loved by his mum, loved by his dad,
Billy boy, Billy boy.

When Billy was alive, we made up a little song to the Robin Hood tune. At his funeral we invited everyone to sing along... Every year since, John has put an IN MEMORIAM in the newspaper. This year there was a line left out...

In Memoriam

BILLY Edwin Plowman **STREETEN**
Billy boy, Billy boy, playing in his den,
Billy boy, Billy boy, with his band of friends,
Loved by his mum, loved by his dad,
Billy boy, Billy boy.

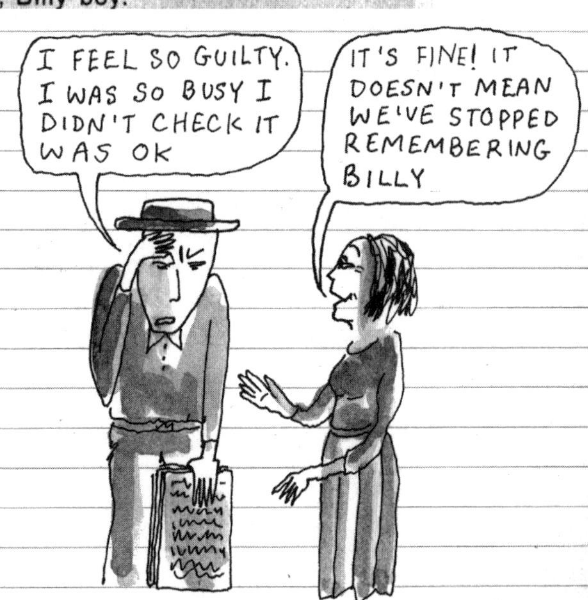

I FEEL SO GUILTY. I WAS SO BUSY I DIDN'T CHECK IT WAS OK
IT'S FINE! IT DOESN'T MEAN WE'VE STOPPED REMEMBERING BILLY

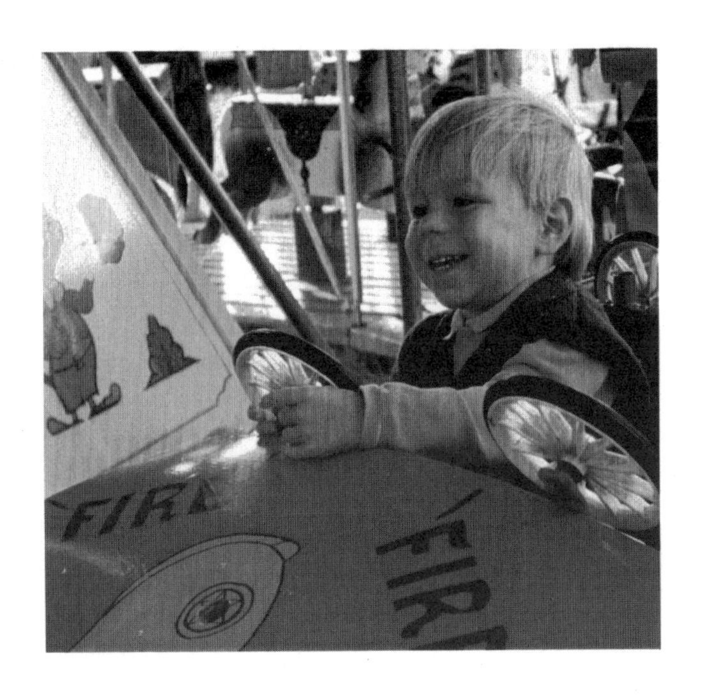

Billy Edwin Plowman Streeten

3 July 1993 — 19 September 1995

OUR MAIN MEMORIES OF BILLY ARE AROUND HIS PASSIONATE DEVOTION TO TRANSPORT. THIS FIXATION INTRODUCED A WHOLE NEW WORLD TO US.

AT THE CITY FARM, BILLY HURRIED PAST THE ANIMALS TO POSITION HIMSELF AT A PLACE WITH A GOOD VIEW OF A TRAIN TRACK.

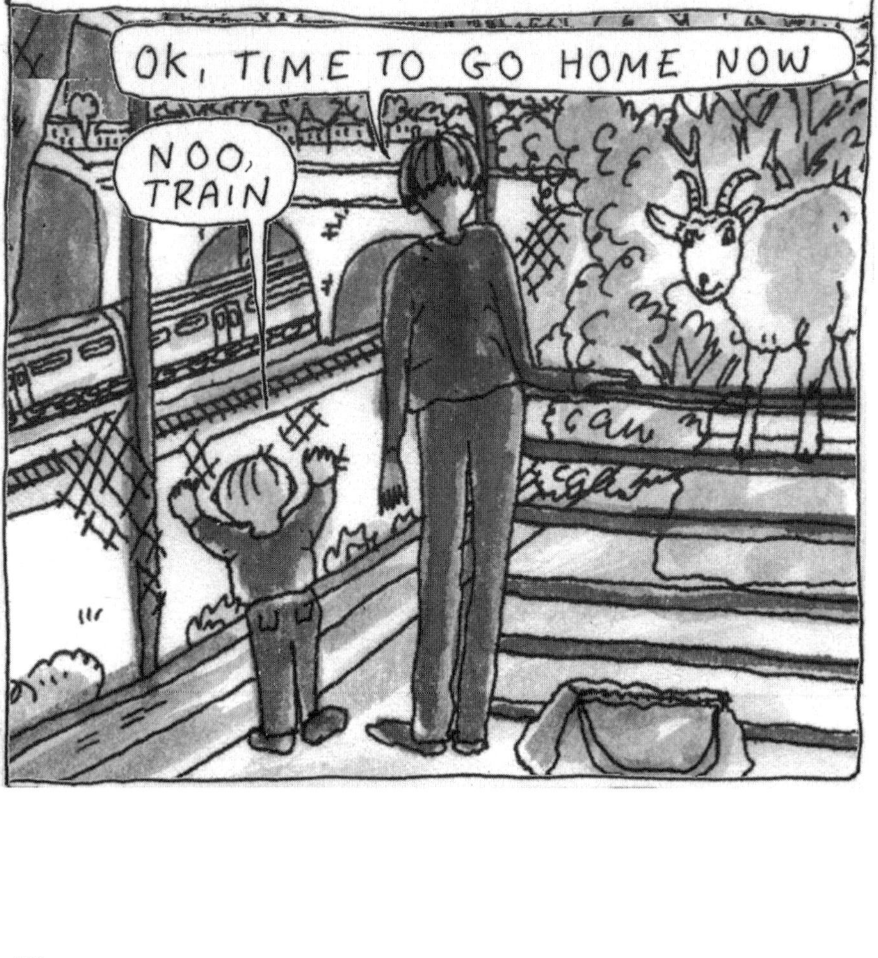

OK, TIME TO GO HOME NOW

NOO, TRAIN

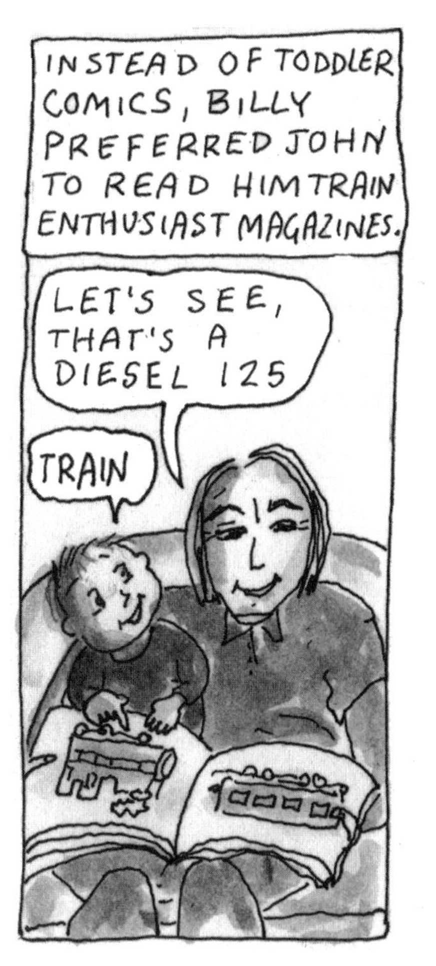
INSTEAD OF TODDLER COMICS, BILLY PREFERRED JOHN TO READ HIM TRAIN ENTHUSIAST MAGAZINES.
LET'S SEE, THAT'S A DIESEL 125
TRAIN

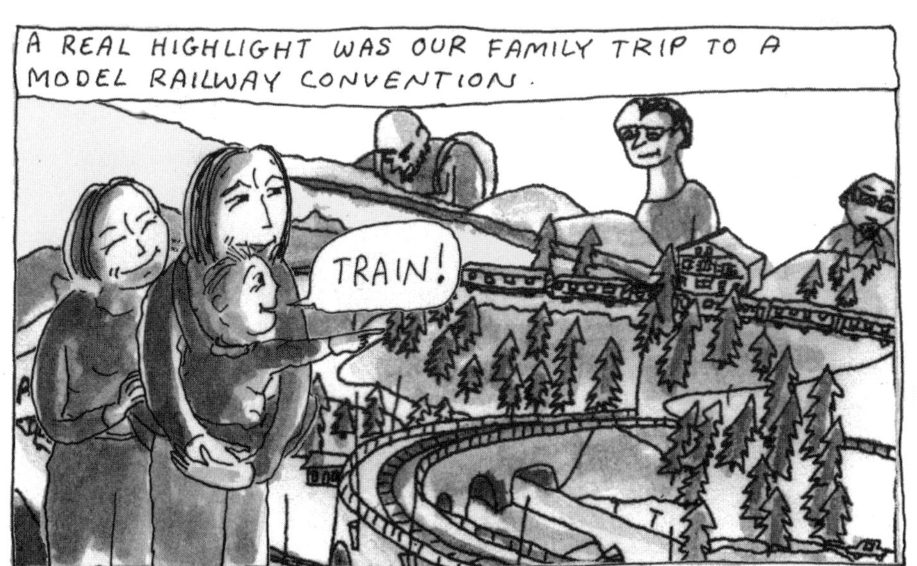
A REAL HIGHLIGHT WAS OUR FAMILY TRIP TO A MODEL RAILWAY CONVENTION.
TRAIN!

30 May 95

AND EVERY DAY HE DREW WITH INCREASING CONFIDENCE...
LITTLE REPETITIVE STUDIES OF "NEE NARS".

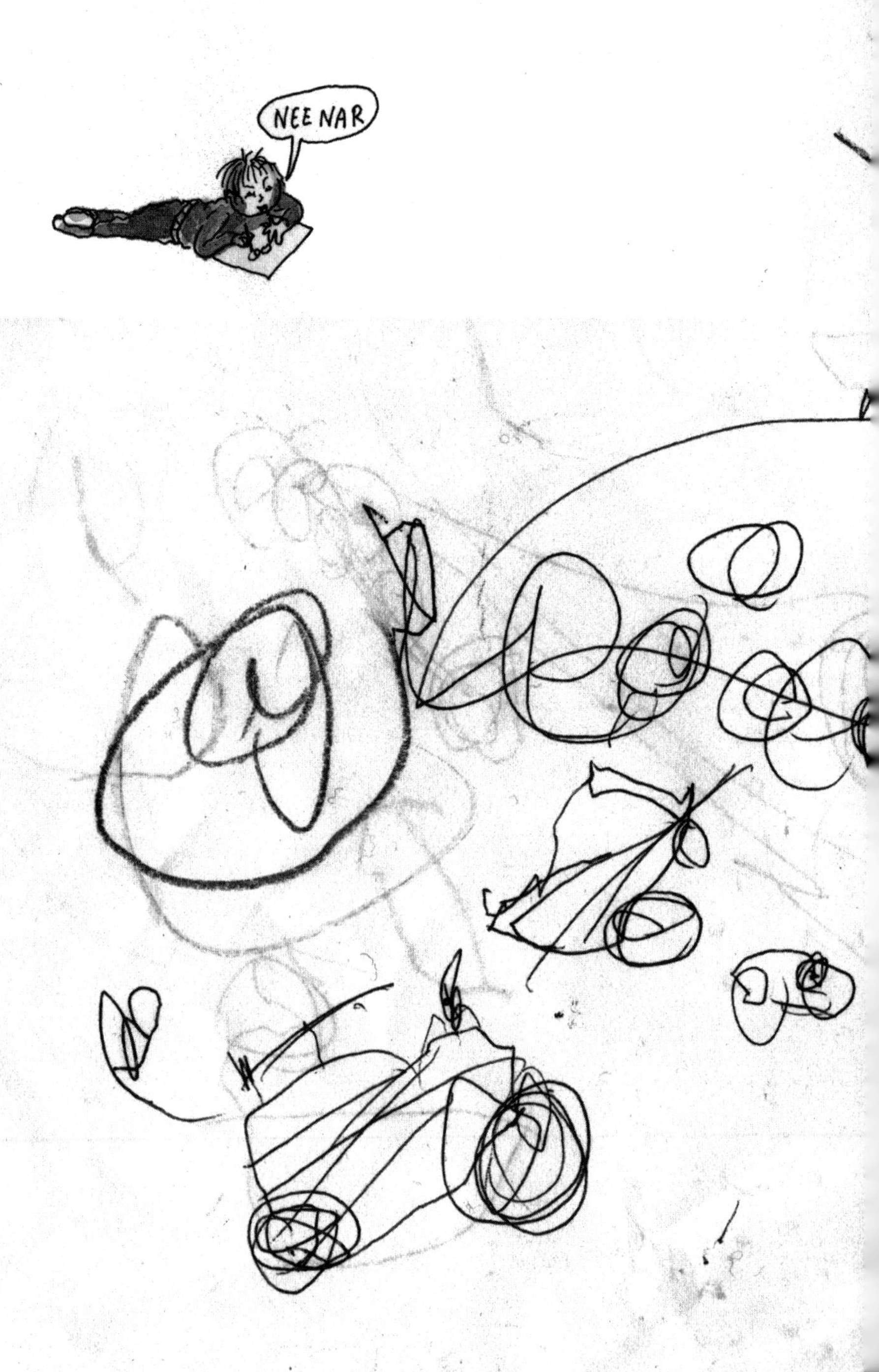

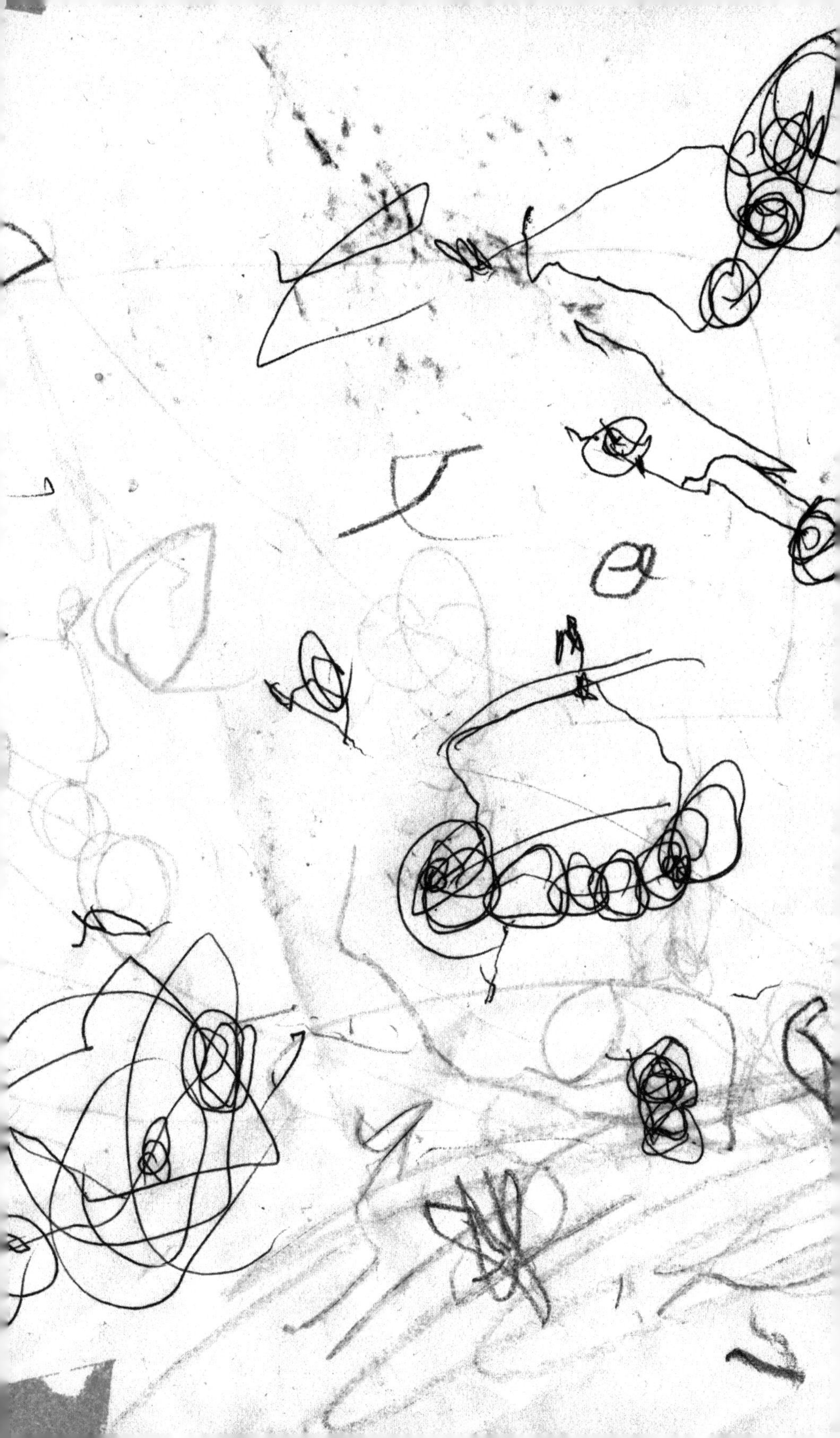

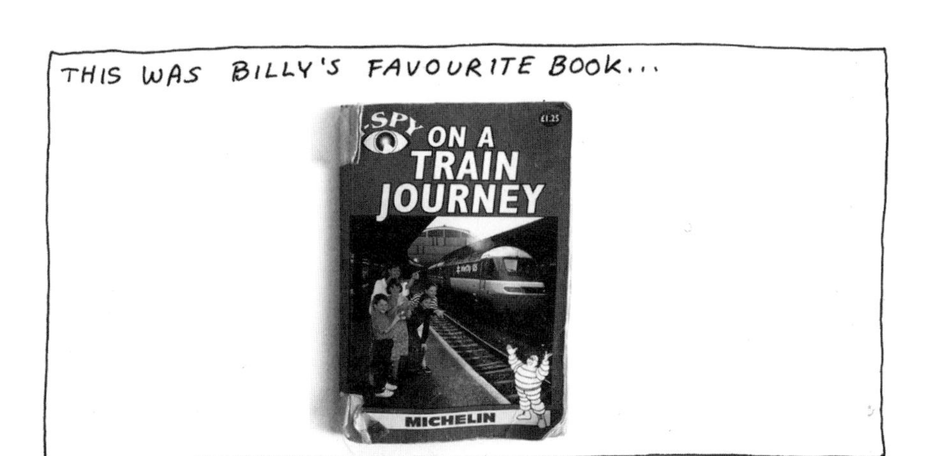
THIS WAS BILLY'S FAVOURITE BOOK...
I-SPY ON A TRAIN JOURNEY
£1.25
MICHELIN

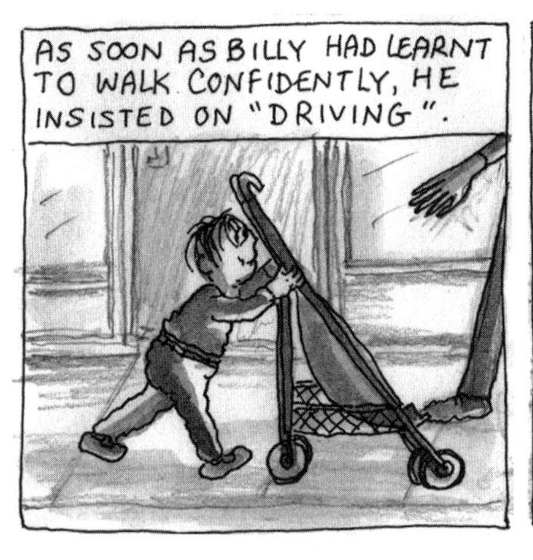
AS SOON AS BILLY HAD LEARNT TO WALK CONFIDENTLY, HE INSISTED ON "DRIVING".

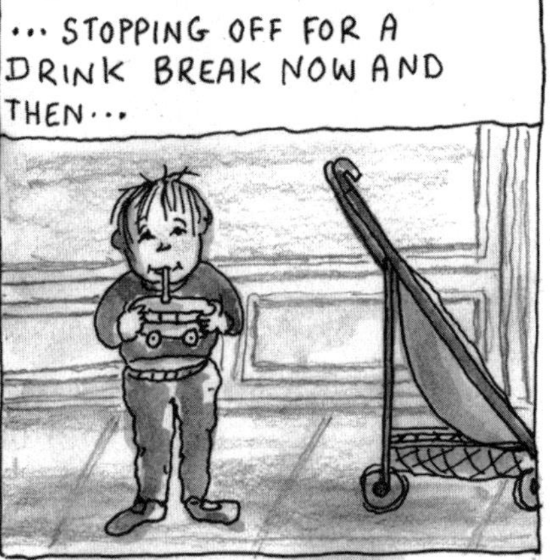
... STOPPING OFF FOR A DRINK BREAK NOW AND THEN...

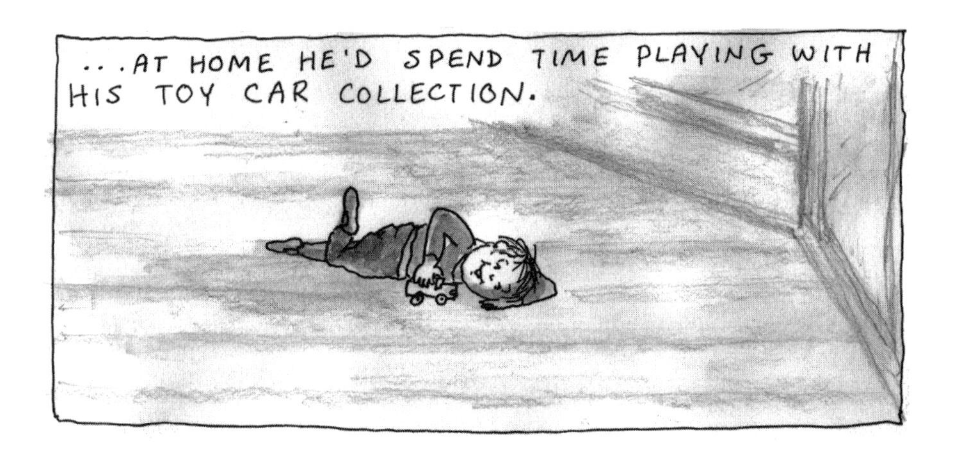
...AT HOME HE'D SPEND TIME PLAYING WITH HIS TOY CAR COLLECTION.

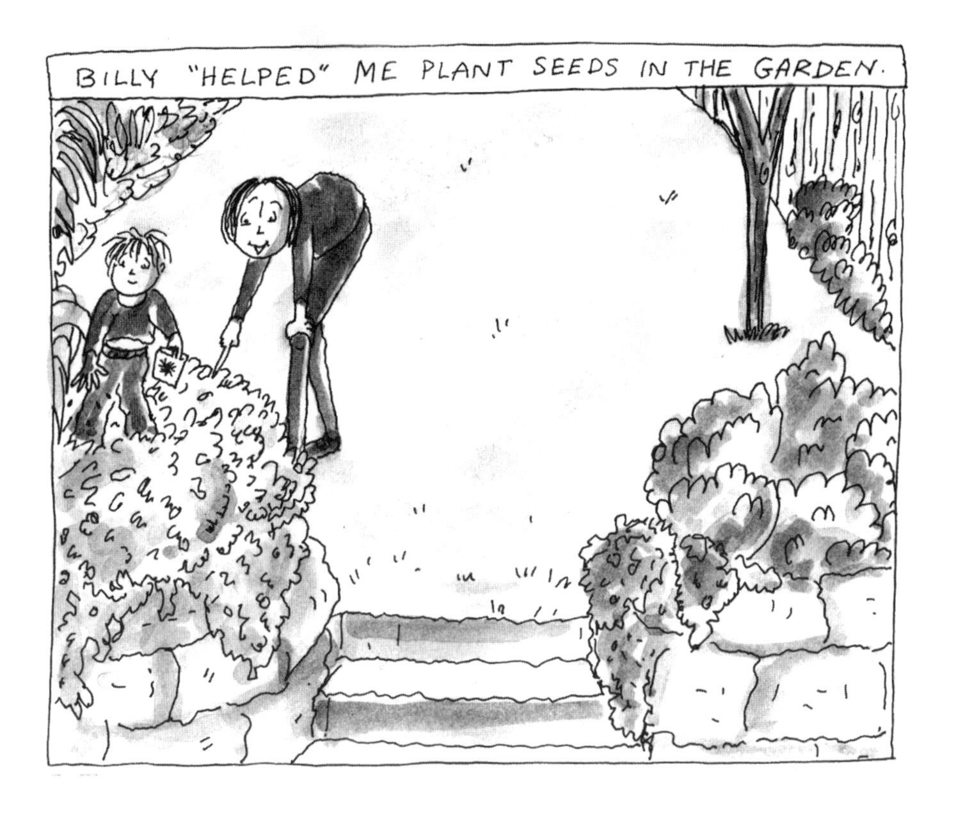

BILLY "HELPED" ME PLANT SEEDS IN THE GARDEN.

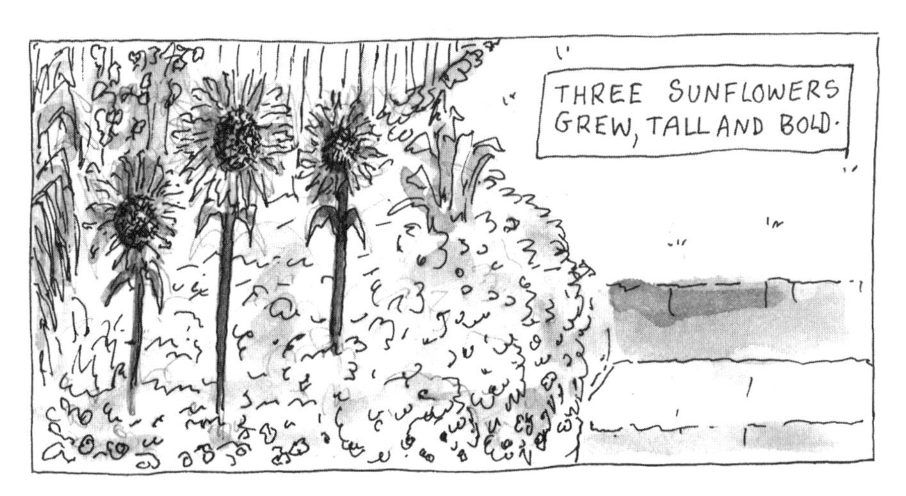

THREE SUNFLOWERS GREW, TALL AND BOLD.

THE DAY BEFORE BILLY'S OPERATION, I CUT THEM DOWN AND TOOK THEM INTO THE HOSPITAL.

The following day ...

Sat	Sun	Mon	Tue	Wed	Thu	Fri	Sat	Sun	Mon	Tue	Wed	Thu	Fri	Sat	Sun	Mon	Tue	Wed	Thu	Fri	Sat	Sun	Mon	Tue	Wed	Thu
4	5	6	7	8	9	10	11	12	13	14	15	16	17	18	19	20	21	22	23	24	25	26	27	28	29	30

AFTERWORD

I HAD SIGNED UP TO DO A MASTER'S DEGREE, FOR WHICH I WOULD EMBARK ON A GRAPHIC NOVEL. AN EARLY ASSIGNMENT WAS TO PRESENT OUR PROPOSALS TO THE CLASS.

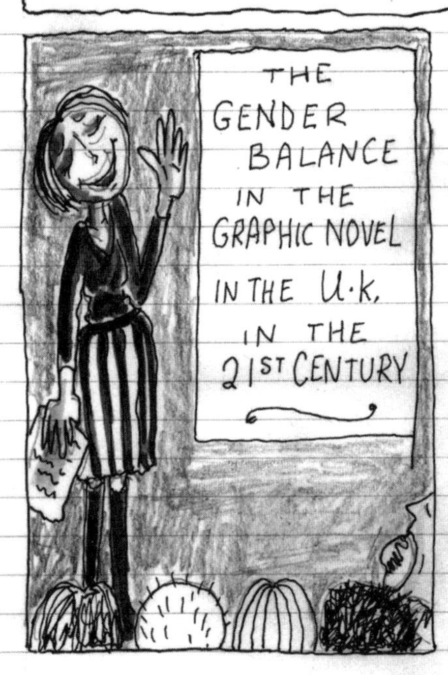
THE GENDER BALANCE IN THE GRAPHIC NOVEL IN THE U.K. IN THE 21ST CENTURY

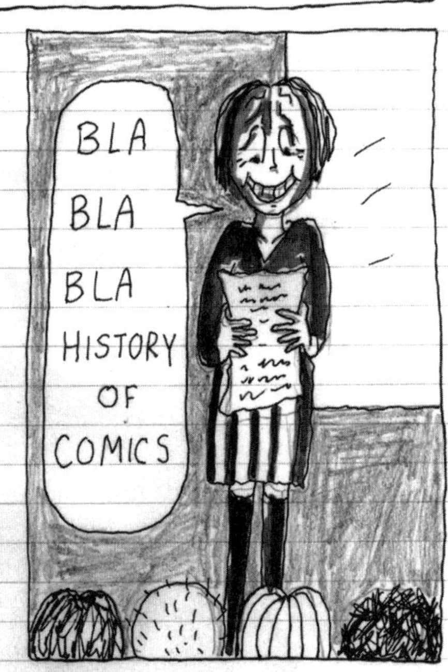
BLA BLA BLA HISTORY OF COMICS

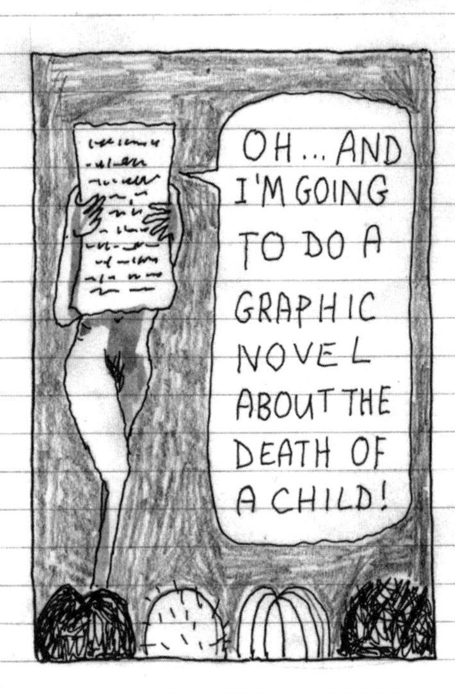
OH... AND I'M GOING TO DO A GRAPHIC NOVEL ABOUT THE DEATH OF A CHILD!

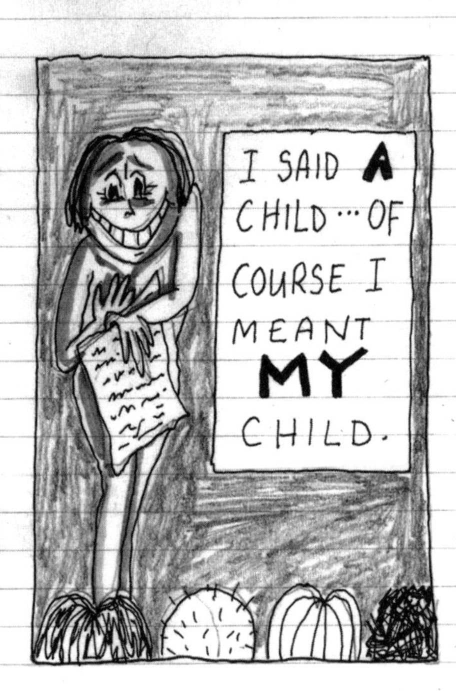
I SAID A CHILD... OF COURSE I MEANT MY CHILD.

LUCKILY THERE WAS AN OPPORTUNITY FOR CRITICAL FEEDBACK.

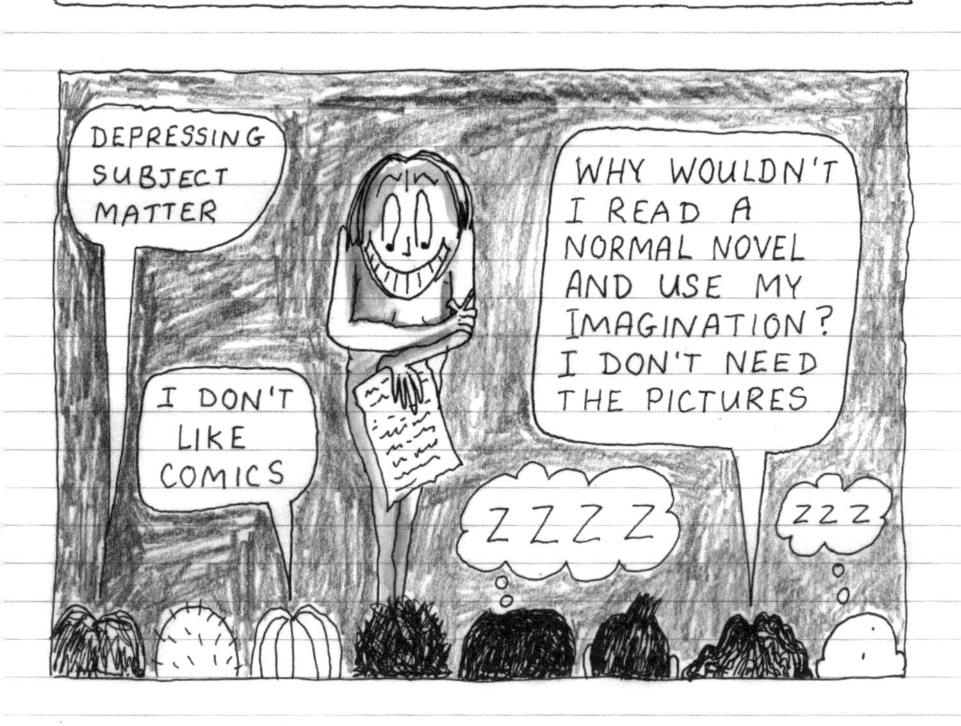
DEPRESSING SUBJECT MATTER
I DON'T LIKE COMICS
WHY WOULDN'T I READ A NORMAL NOVEL AND USE MY IMAGINATION? I DON'T NEED THE PICTURES
ZZZZ
ZZZ

I REALISED MY NARRATIVE HAD BEGUN AND THAT I HAD NO EASY TASK AHEAD.

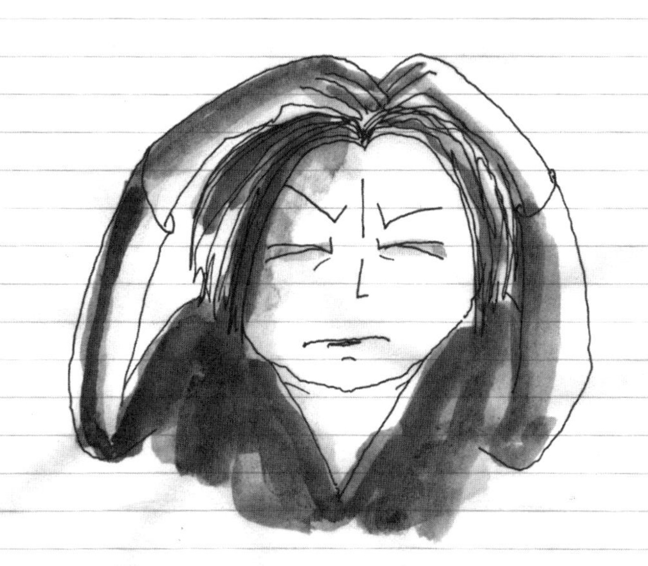

I WAS ALLOCATED A PERSONAL TUTOR.

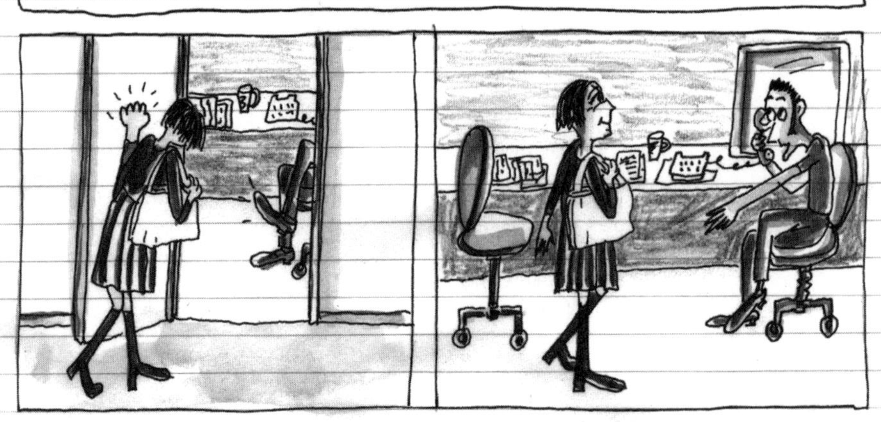

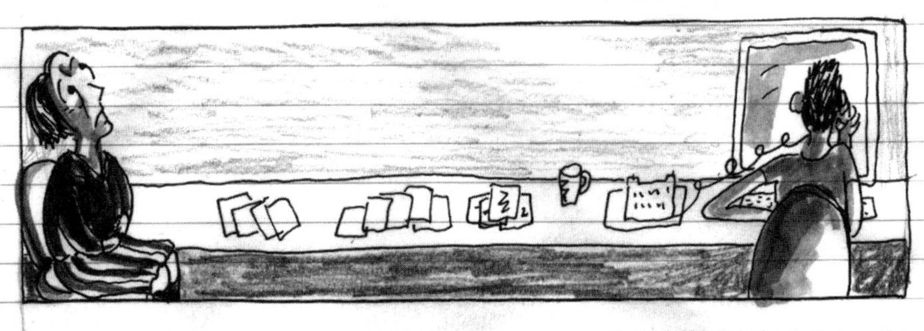

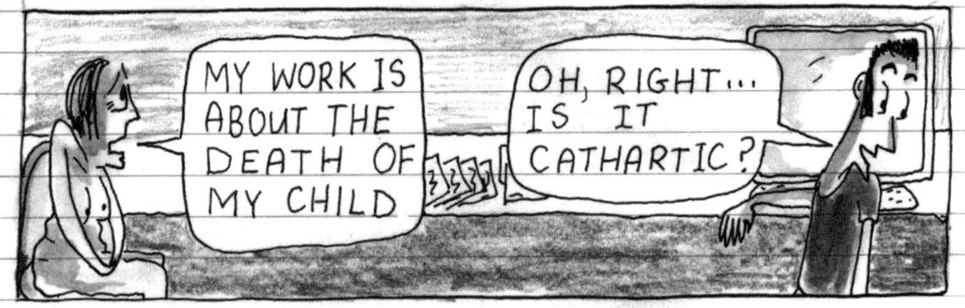

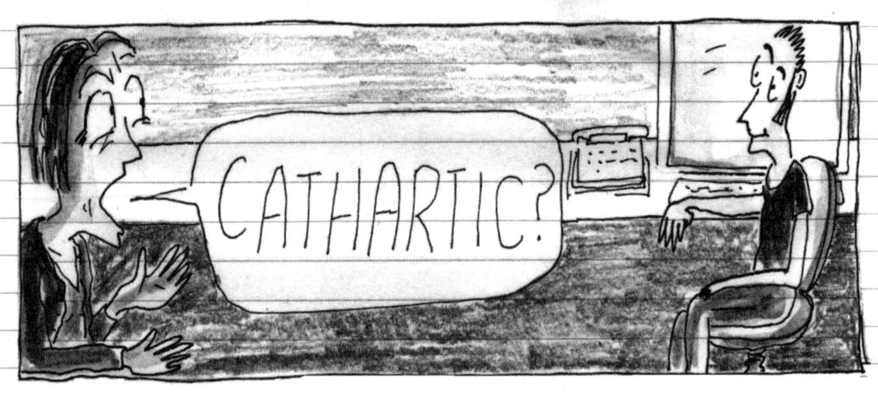

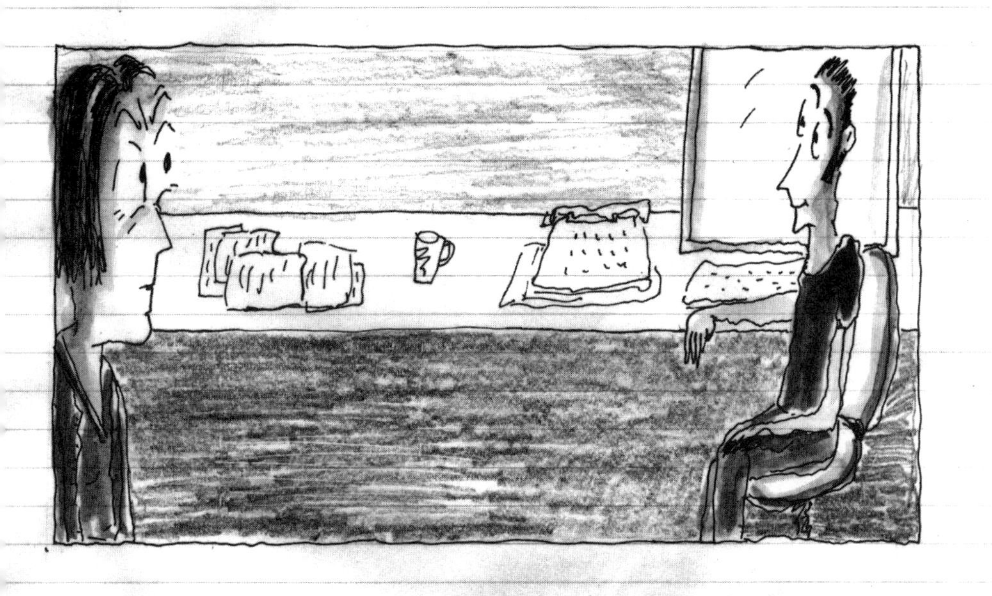

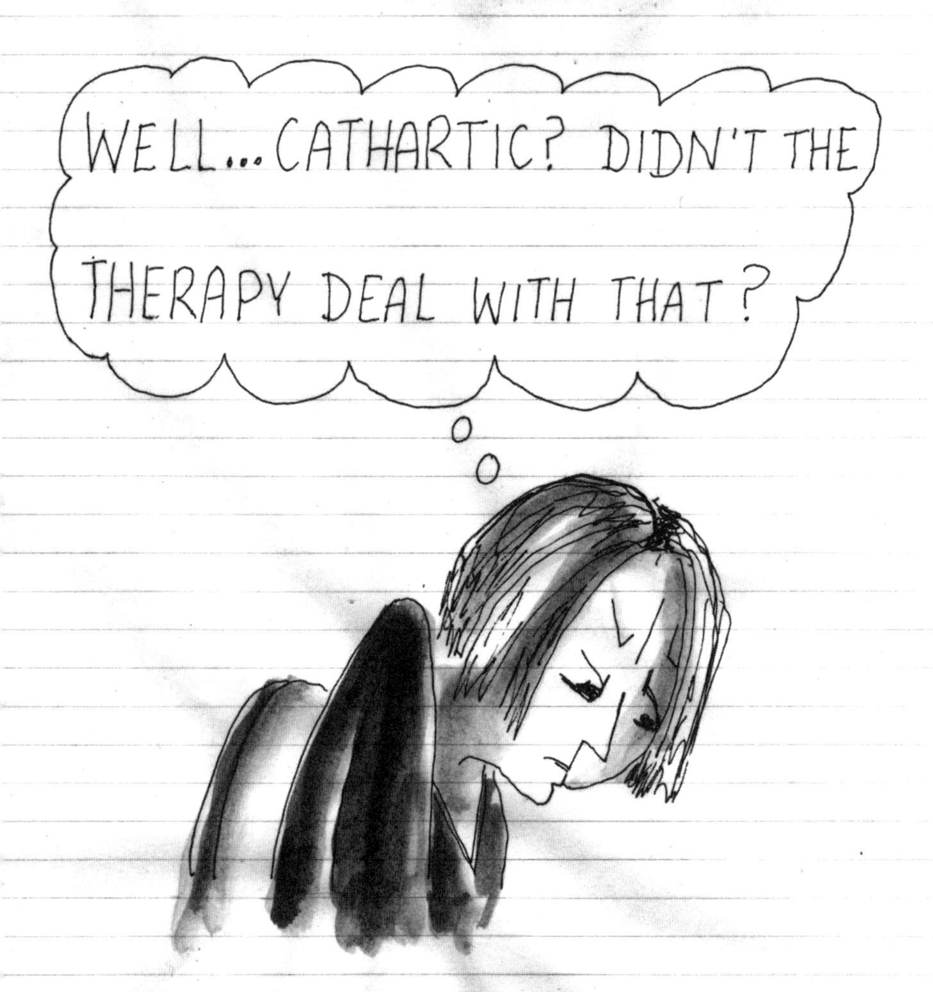
WELL... CATHARTIC? DIDN'T THE THERAPY DEAL WITH THAT?

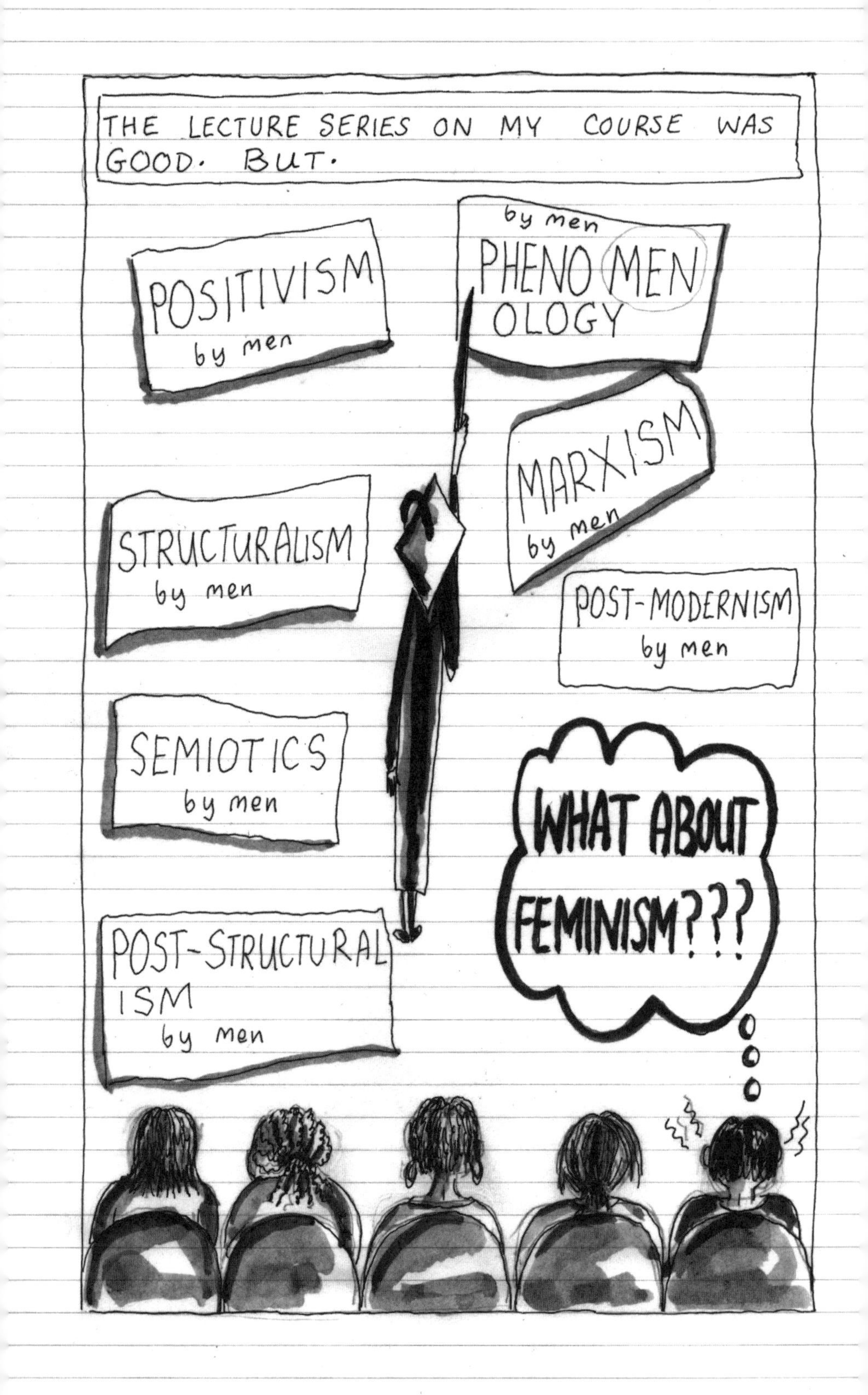

Fri 2 Sat 3 Sun 4 | Mon 5 Tue 6 Wed 7 Thu 8 Fri 9 Sat 10 Sun 11 | Mon 12 Tue 13 Wed 14 Thu 15 Fri 16 Sat 17 Sun 18 | Mon 19 Tue 20 Wed 21 Thu 22 Fri 23 Sat 24 Sun 25 | Mon 26 Tue 27 Wed 28

MEANWHILE, I ATTENDED SOME PUBLIC TALKS ABOUT "THE GRAPHIC NOVEL".

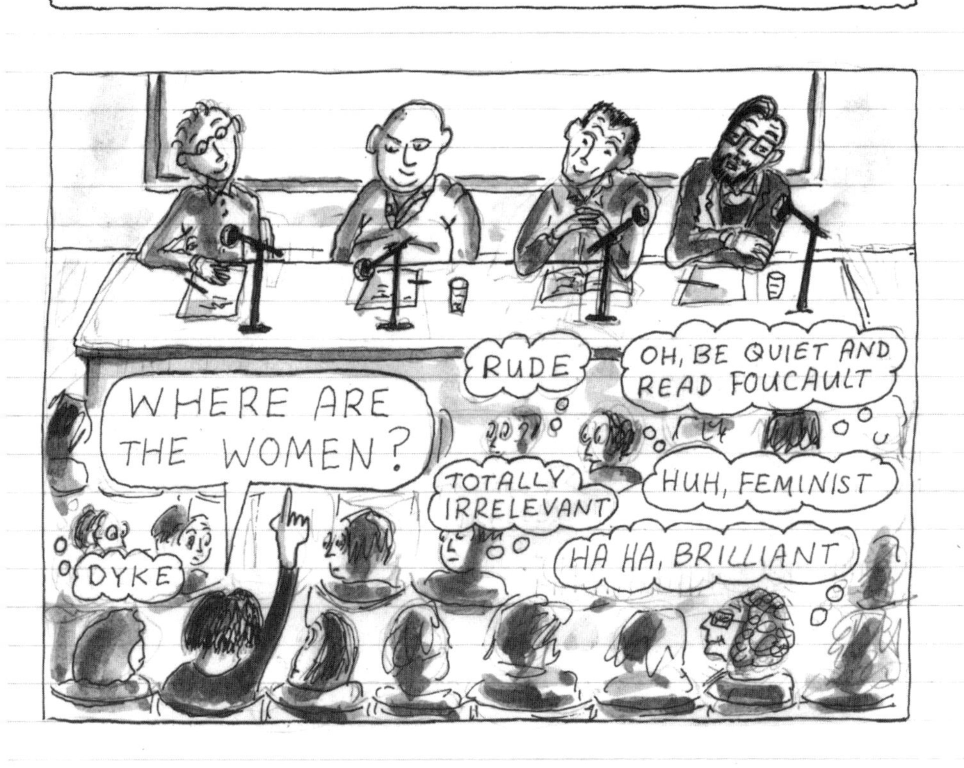
WHERE ARE THE WOMEN?
RUDE
OH, BE QUIET AND READ FOUCAULT
TOTALLY IRRELEVANT
HUH, FEMINIST
DYKE
HA HA, BRILLIANT

I GOT CHATTING TO AN ARTIST WHO'D ALSO BEEN IN THE AUDIENCE.

WOULDN'T IT BE GREAT TO HAVE A SORT OF CLUB WHERE WE COULD TALK ABOUT THE WORKS WE LIKE...

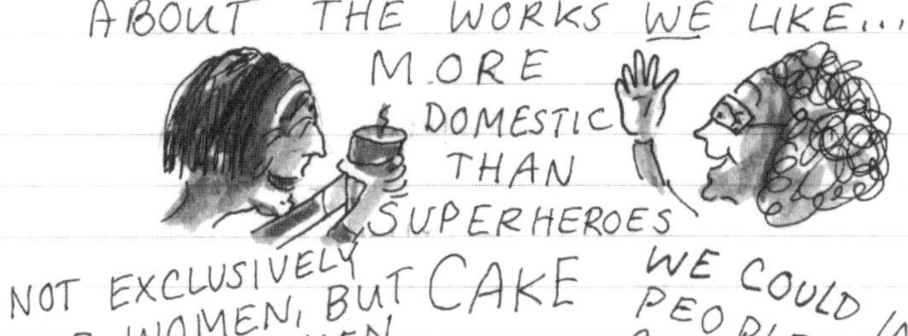
MORE DOMESTIC THAN SUPERHEROES

NOT EXCLUSIVELY FOR WOMEN, BUT WHERE WOMEN ARE COMFORTABLE

CAKE

WE COULD INVITE PEOPLE WE THINK ARE GREAT TO TALK ABOUT THEIR WORK.

LAYDEEZ DO COMICS WAS SET UP IN 2009.

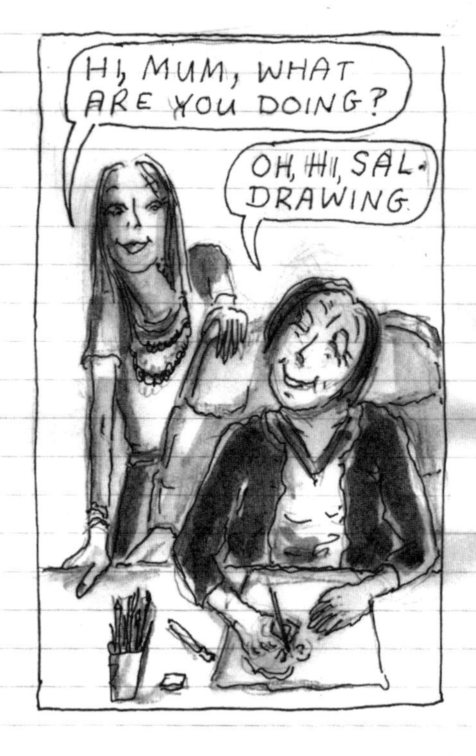
HI, MUM, WHAT ARE YOU DOING?
OH, HI, SAL. DRAWING

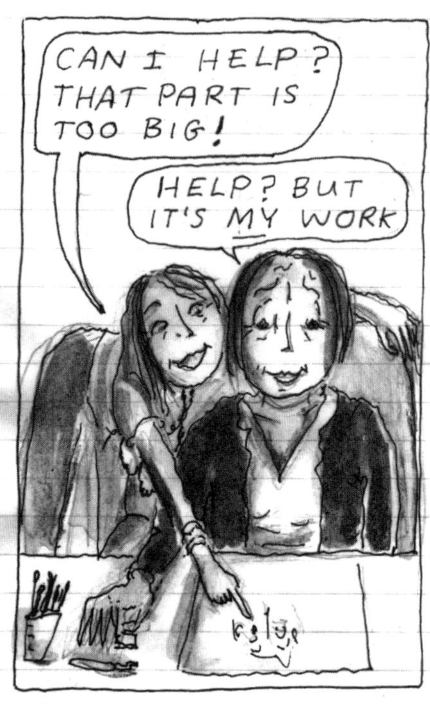
CAN I HELP? THAT PART IS TOO BIG!
HELP? BUT IT'S MY WORK

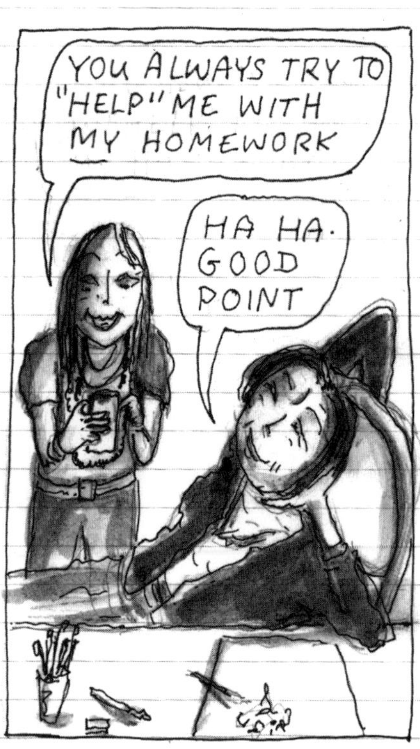
YOU ALWAYS TRY TO "HELP" ME WITH MY HOMEWORK
HA HA. GOOD POINT

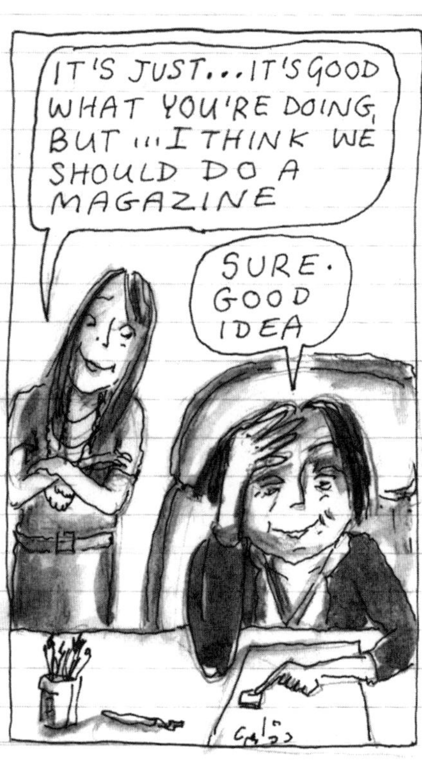
IT'S JUST... IT'S GOOD WHAT YOU'RE DOING, BUT ... I THINK WE SHOULD DO A MAGAZINE
SURE. GOOD IDEA

WE SOLD COPIES OF OUR COMIC-MAG TO FAMILY, FRIENDS AND SUBSCRIBERS.

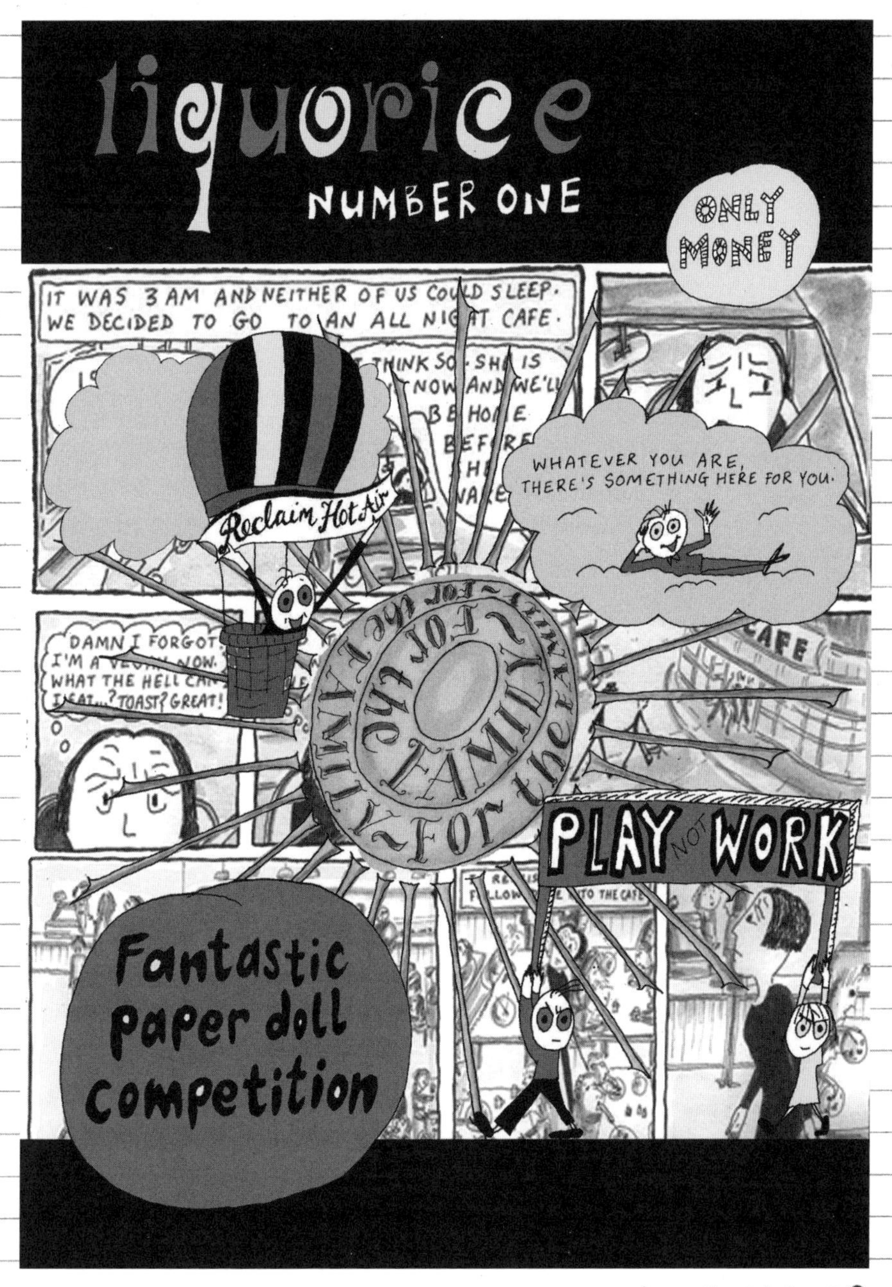

EACH ISSUE INCLUDED A CHAPTER OF "MY GRAPHIC NOVEL".

HEY! A PUBLISHER HAS SEEN LIQUORICE AND IS INTERESTED IN THE BILLY STORY...

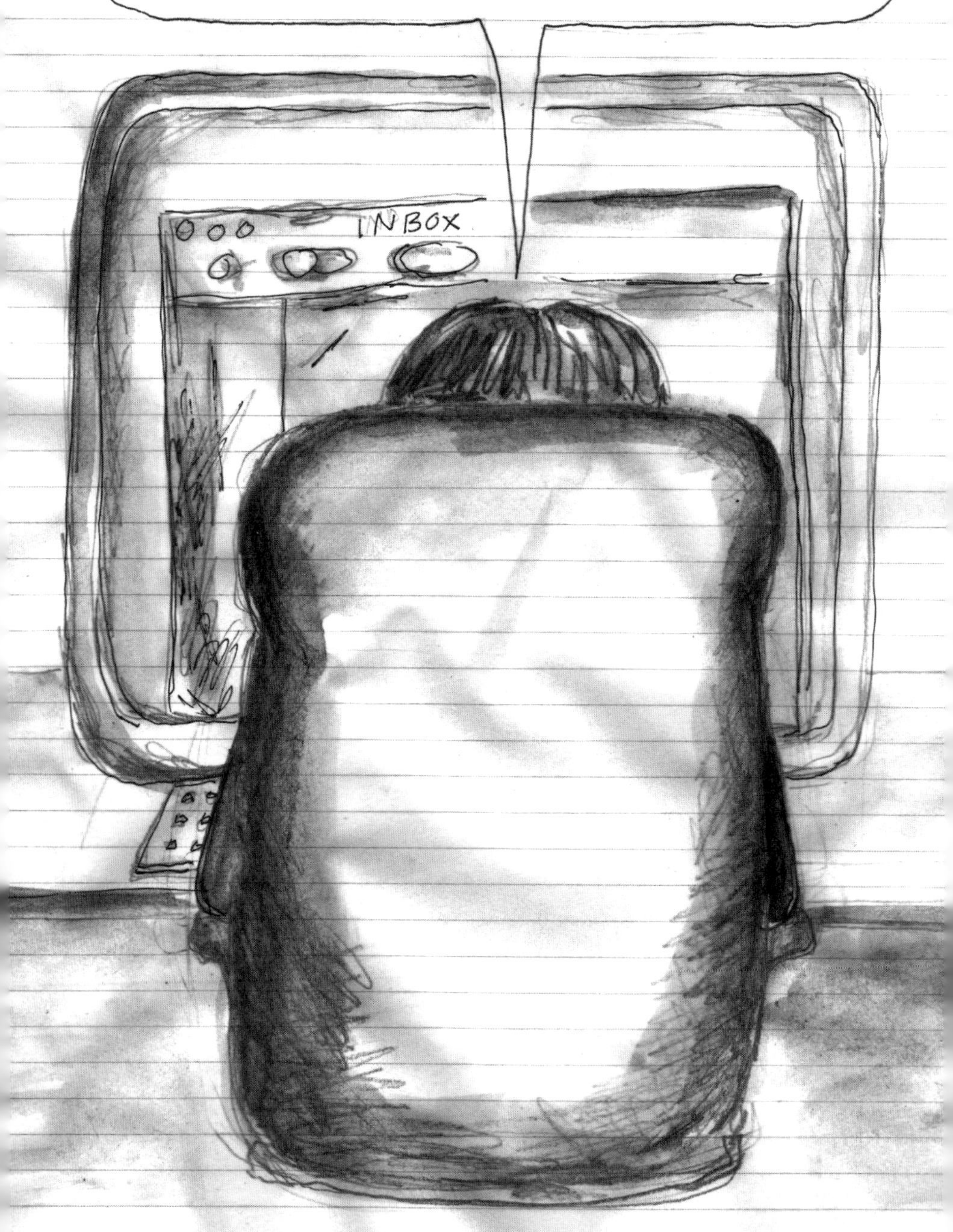

Fri	Sat	Sun	Mon	Tue	Wed	Thu	Fri	Sat	Sun	Mon	Tue	Wed	Thu	Fri	Sat	Sun	Mon	Tue	Wed	Thu	Fri	Sat	Sun	Mon	Tue	Wed	Thu
2	3	4	5	6	7	8	9	10	11	12	13	14	15	16	17	18	19	20	21	22	23	24	25	26	27	28	29

ACKNOWLEDGEMENTS

This book is about a time when I felt emotions with an extremity not experienced before or since, and here it is condensed into a story. The three-and-a-half years in the making has not been a sad experience for me, but a creatively rewarding and satisfying time. I am indebted to many people for their roles, both in the original unfolding and in the telling of it in this form. I thank them all, especially our families and friends.

Most importantly, I thank my soul mate and husband, John Plaman and our lovely daughter, Sally Plaman, who restored true happiness into our lives again. John, I thank for his collaborative approach to life with me. Sally, I thank for the idea and eagerness to start Liquorice and for the laughs we have had working on it together. A special mention to Holly, the dog, a key player in Liquorice and our lives! I thank all the essential supporters of Liquorice, who have subscribed and offered feedback. This group of people became my first readers and provided a vital testing of material.

My research into comics and the graphic novel has introduced me to a world of interesting and inspiring people. In particular, I thank Sarah Lightman, artist, curator and academic, with whom I never run out of things to talk and laugh about. This project would not have come to fruition without her friendship and the work we have done together, principally setting up Laydeez do Comics, in 2009. Thank you to all who have attended, as presenters, bloggers and audience.

Finally, I thank the team at Myriad Editions, who have been such a delight to work with. Especially Corinne Pearlman, who has given so much time and guidance to shaping the work with me from the outset.

Nicola Streeten, 2011

MORE FROM MYRIAD EDITIONS

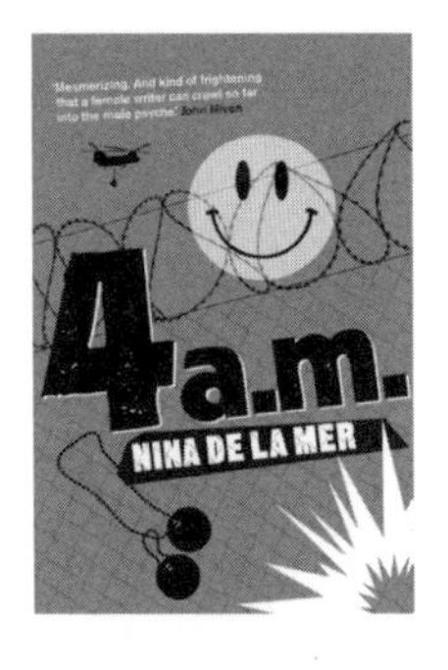

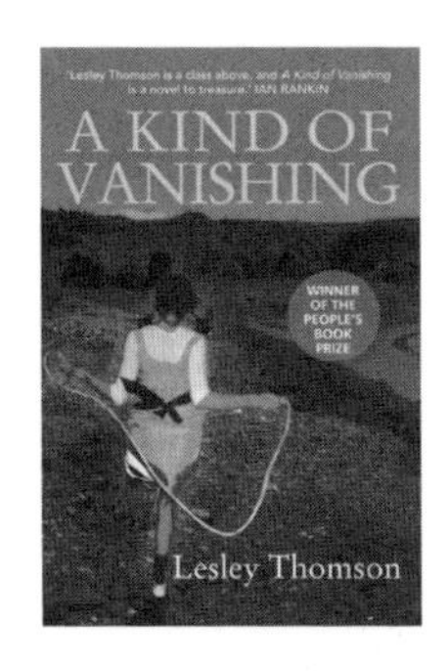

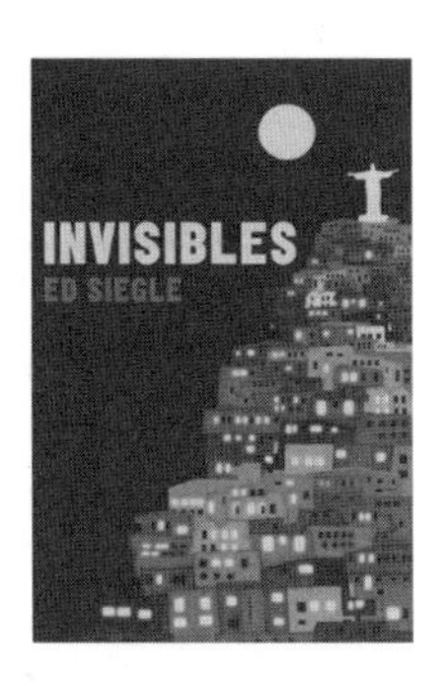

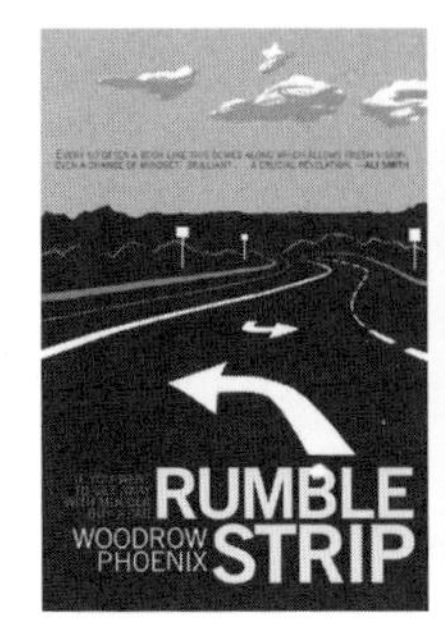

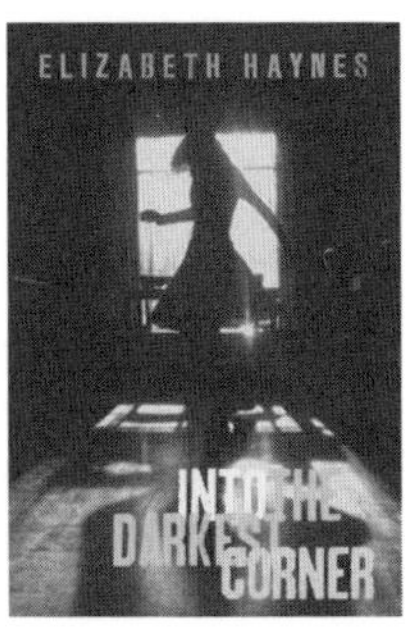

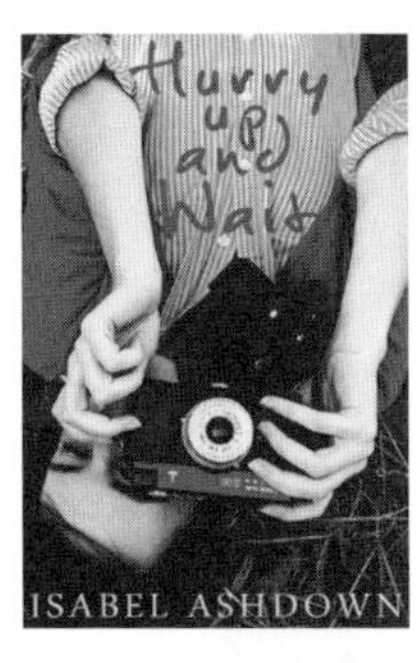

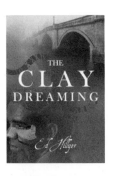

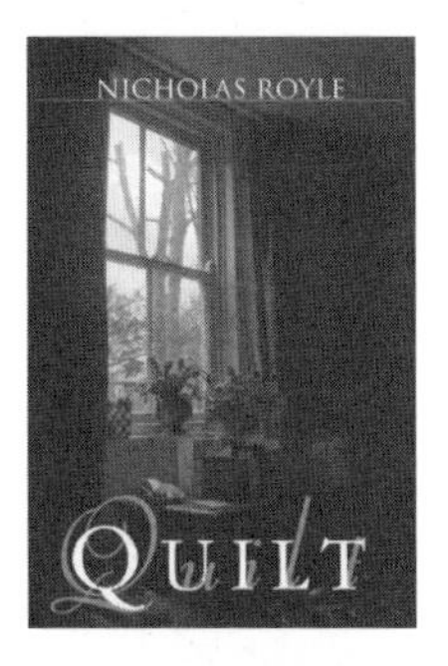

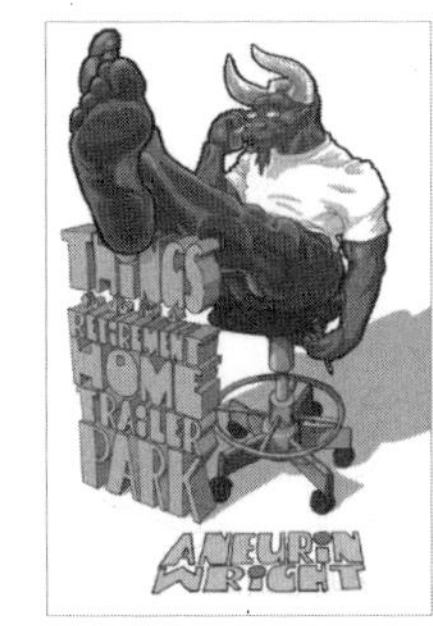

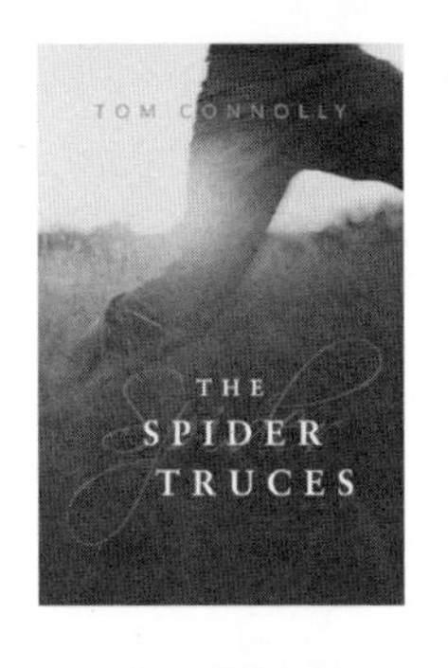

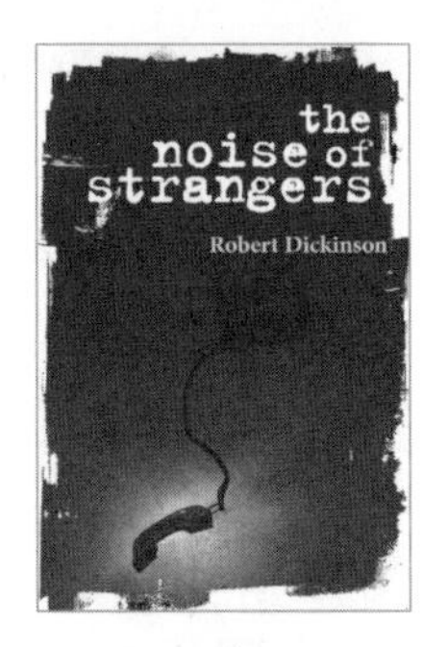

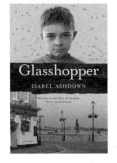

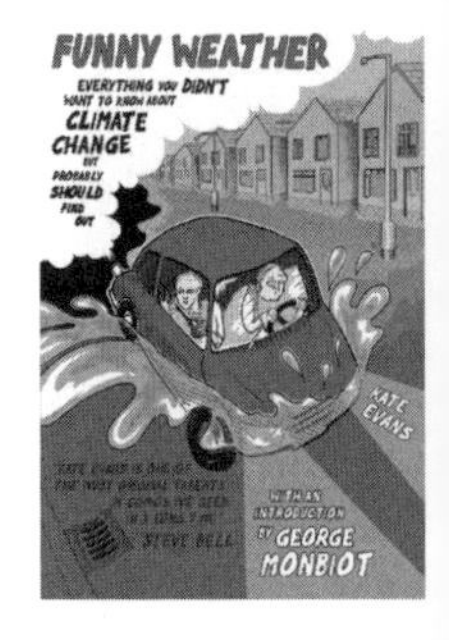

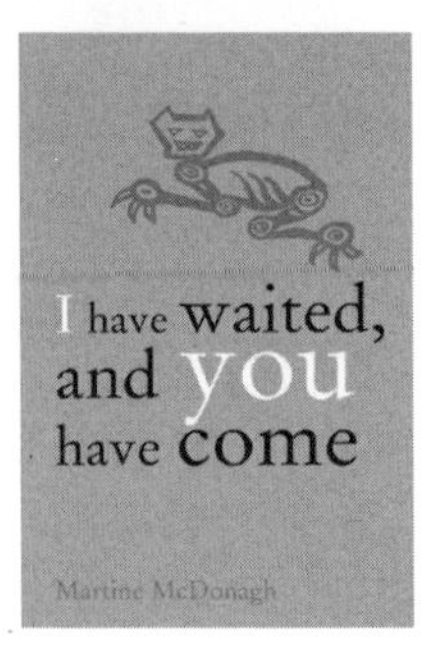

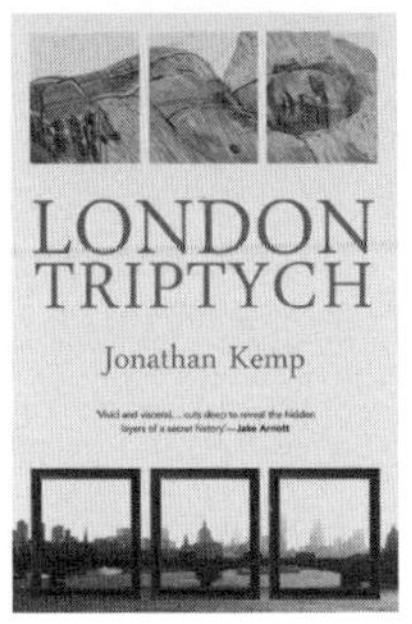

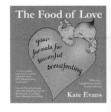